Work Practice: International Perspectives

Work Practice

International Perspectives

Edited by

Joanne Pratt
MSc, BA, DipCOT, OTR/L

Lecturer, Division of Occupational Therapy, Department of Nursing & Community Health, Glasgow Caledonian University, Glasgow, Scotland

and

Karen Jacobs
EdD, OTR/L, CPE, FAOTA

Clinical Associate Professor, Department of Occupational Therapy, Boston University, Sargent College, Boston, MA, USA

BUTTERWORTH
HEINEMANN

Butterworth-Heinemann
Linacre House, Jordan Hill, Oxford OX2 8DP
A division of Reed Educational and Professional Publishing Ltd

A member of the Reed Elsevier plc group

OXFORD BOSTON JOHANNESBURG
MELBOURNE NEW DELHI SINGAPORE

First published 1997

British Library Cataloguing in Publication Data
Work practice: international perspectives
1 Occupational therapy 2 Work
I Pratt, Joanne II Jacobs, Karen
616.8′595

ISBN 0 7506 2260 1

Library of Congress Cataloguing in Publication Data
Work practice: international perspectives/edited by Joanne Pratt and Karen Jacobs.
p. cm.
Includes bibliographical references and index.
ISBN 0 7506 2260 1
1 Occupational therapy – United States. 2 Occupational therapy – Great Britain. I Pratt, Joanne. II Jacobs, Karen, 1951– .
RM735.W577 97–5624
615.8′5′0941–dc21 CIP

Composition by Genesis Typesetting, Rochester, Kent
Printed and bound in Great Britain by The Bath Press, Somerset

Contents

Contributors

Tina Campanella MA
Director, Department for Organizational Supports
The Accreditation Council
100 West Rd, Suite 406
Towson, MD 21204, USA

Barbara Acheson Cooper Dip P&OT, BA, MHSc, PhD
Associate Professor, Associate Dean Health Sciences
Director of the School of Occupational Therapy and Physiotherapy
McMaster University, Ontario, Canada

Gary Donaldson PhD
President, Strategic Performance Solutions Corp. Organizational and Human Resource Development Consultants
9614 Sutherland Road
Silver Spring, MD, USA

Maree Dyson BAppSc(OT), GradDip(Erg), CertQA
Director, Maree Dyson Pty Ltd
PO Box 1508, Geelong
Victoria 3320, Australia

Dorothy Ferguson BA(Hons), MPH, RGN, SCM, RHV, OHNC, HVT
Lecturer, Dept of Nursing and Community Health
Glasgow Caledonian University
Cowcaddens Rd, Glasgow G4 OBA, UK

James Gardner PhD
Chief Executive Officer
The Accreditation Council
100 West Rd, Suite 406
Towson, MD 21204, USA

Rosie Hallam DipCOT, DMS
Director, RESTORE
Manzil Way, Cowley Rd,
Oxford OX4 1YH, UK

Mildrette Hill BA, MA
Student barrister, Founder and Executive Director, Black Spectrum
Chair, CHANGE
3 Dwight Court, Burlington Place, Fulham
London SW6 4NJ, UK

Ev Innes BAppSc(OT), MHPEd
Lecturer, School of Occupational Therapy
Faculty of Health Sciences
The University of Sydney, East St
PO Box 170, Lidcombe, NSW 2141
Australia

Karen Jacobs EdD, OTR/L, CPE, FAOTA
Clinical Assistant Professor
Boston University, Sargent College
Boston, MA, USA

Mary Law BSc(OT), MSc, PhD
Associate Professor, School of Occupational Therapy and Physiotherapy
and Department of Clinical Epidemiology and Biostatistics
McMaster University, Ontario, Canada

Jonathan Leach MSc, BSc(Hons)
Training and Development Worker
RESTORE, Manzil Way
Cowley Rd, Oxford OX4 1YH, UK

Margaret McKay BSc(OT), SROT
Extended Learning Support Coordinator
Glasgow College of Building and Printing
60 North Hanover Street
Glasgow, Scotland G1 2BP

Robina McDonald DipCOT, BAppScOT, MEd
Commonwealth Rehabilitation Service Greensborough
Greensborough Rehabilitation Unit, Level 1
9–13 Flintoff Street, (PO Box 369)
Greensborough 3088, Australia

Catherine Paterson TDipCOT, SROT, MEd
Director of Occupational Therapy, The Robert Gordon University
Department of Occupational Therapy
Woolmanhill, Aberdeen
Scotland AB9 1GS

Jeraldine Perron MS, OTR/L, FAOTA
Director of the Occupational Therapy Assistant Program
Mount Ida College
Newton, MA, USA

Joanne Pratt DipCOT, OTR/L, BA, MSc
Lecturer, Division of Occupational Therapy
Department of Nursing and Community Health
Glasgow Caledonian University, Glasgow
Scotland

Debra Stewart BSc(OT)
Occupational Therapist at Erinoak, Mississauga, Ontario and Professional Associate, School of Occupational Therapy and Physiotherapy, McMaster University, Ontario, Canada

Susan Strong BSc(OT)
Occupational Therapist, Program Evaluation/Quality Assurance
Hamilton Psychiatric Hospital and Professional Associate, School of Occupational Therapy and Physiotherapy, McMaster University
Ontario, Canada

Rwth Stuckey BAppSci(OT), Grad Dip Ergonomics, MESA, Cert Erg
7 Glenthorn Avenue, North Balwyn, 3104, Melbourne
Australia

Acknowledgements

A number of colleagues assisted in the process of compilation of this book. Their help is acknowledged with gratitude. They include:

All the primary and contributing authors;
Practitioners who shared their thoughts and experiences with the authors;
Joe Chambers, Rwth Stuckey and Employment Service Scotland for photographic support;
The models and their employers who agreed to have themselves photographed at their work;
Ainsley Asprey for computing support;
And finally, to patient families and understanding friends.

Preface

Engagement in productive or work activities, including paid employment, is fundamental to human endeavour. Much effort in the practice of occupational therapy is directed towards goals which will enable clients to develop and maintain their ability both to participate and to direct their involvement in activities which are meaningful to them. What is meaningful to the individual is, of course, embedded in their personal perceptions of their needs, desires and abilities. The environment with its physical, social, cultural, economic and political elements often provides diverse contexts for these perceptions. *Work Practice: International Perspectives* began as an attempt by the editors to compare and contrast work practice (defined here as those therapeutic interventions and programmes in occupational therapy which aim to enable clients to undertake and maintain participation in productive activities) in two countries in order to find shared meanings and to evaluate the reasons for differences in professional practice. The resulting text has emerged from invitations to authors in five countries to share in these discussions.

The text, which is based on a person–environment framework, provides evidence that occupational therapy has broad and unique capabilities related to improving individuals' work performance. This book, with its three sections and twelve chapters, first offers an introduction to the diversity of work patterns given cultural, gender and historical factors. Catherine Paterson next reminds us of our own historical legacy of work programmes in occupational therapy, while Jerrie Perron and Margaret McKay document present-day programme models in the US and the UK. Section II attempts to provide a framework for the utilization of occupational therapy concepts in response to the breadth of environmental demands. Barbara Cooper leads a team of authors from McMaster University in Canada to present a well-informed chapter which will help to deepen readers' understanding of the broad concept of 'environment'. Chapter 5 is a practical overview of the legislation which drives the statutory provisions in three countries. Mildrette Hill's contribution to the chapter is particularly interesting and provocative as it considers UK legislation from the perspective of both a service consumer and a disability advocate. The text then moves on to the range of activities that can be undertaken by the practitioner when addressing clients' needs. These chapters, in Section III, focus on specific areas – neuromotor, psychosocial, cognitive – of functional performance to highlight the ways in which programmes can be structured to direct effort towards the achievement of specific, client-driven goals. The need for client-driven goals is reinforced by Gardner and Campanella in their chapter on outcome measures in work practice. The text concludes with a forum for a discussion of the challenges and issues likely to be faced by those employed in this area of practice in three countries as the new century opens. It is intended that this book will provide a broad and sound understanding of the field for students as well as act as a useful resource for clinicians and managers. More importantly, it is hoped that it will foster discussion within and across professions such that we continue to develop our practice in response to the goals towards which our clients strive.

Joanne Pratt
Karen Jacobs

Section I

Overview

1

The Nature of Work and Work Patterns

Rwth Stuckey

Learning objectives

Upon completion of this chapter the reader should be able to:

1 Define the occupational performance area called work.
2 Describe historical patterns of work organization.
3 Describe factors relating to the work of women, children and migrants.
4 Understand the issues which impact on humans in industrialized work.

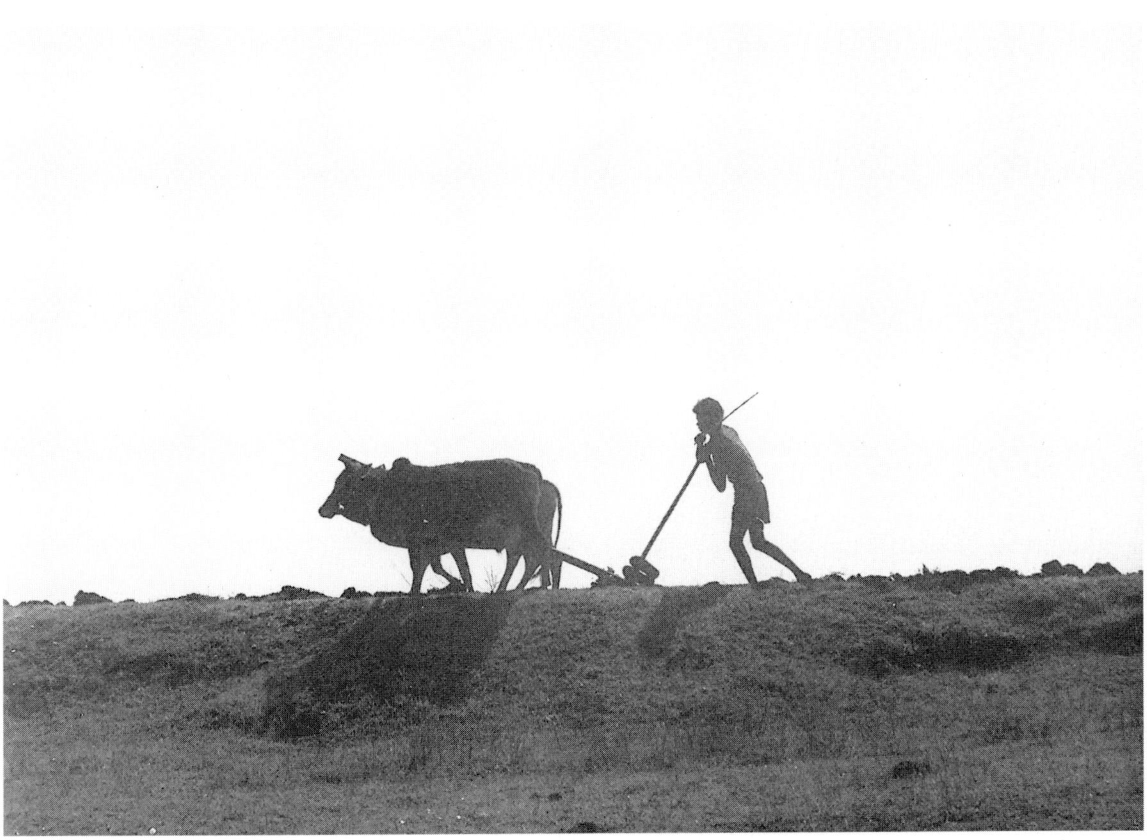

Defining work

There are many ways to define work: work is activity; productive activity; paid labour; employment; synonymous with toil; often conceived as unwanted and painful; something avoided if possible; a burdensome necessity; engaged in because we have to, are obliged to, or because we want to; work is productive, creative activity; a moral ideal; an expression of what people do to be truly human; work is an expression of human purpose.

Humans have an inherent or innate urge to explore and control their environment, fulfil their basic needs and find efficacy and competence. Through work we can exercise our powers to shape and form the objective world and appropriate it to our needs.

Work is commonly the basis of social life, confers a sense of identity and status, and provides a source of self-respect and meaning. Through work people offer a product or service which is necessary or helpful to their social environment and so gives the individual the opportunity to contribute to the community. Work adds value to the human condition, needs are met, a new commodity is created; new ideas or feelings are evoked; and in this process work itself becomes a highly valued commodity. Work is a necessity for earning a living, whether undertaken by the individual or by others, through payment, force or persuasion.

Most people want to work and feel the need for work even when they find the task itself unsatisfying, dull or meaningless. Herzberg saw humans as innately active and productive beings for whom the idea of activity and work is attractive and involving as a form of individual expression (Herzberg, 1966). Herzberg's model of work motivation describes humans as working for intrinsic and extrinsic 'motivators'. Intrinsic motivators include personal achievement, recognition, responsibility and advancement of status: factors relating to the individual and the job itself. Extrinsic motivators, or hygiene factors, include pay increases, competent supervision, improved working conditions or job security; factors which stem from and relate to the organizational context of work, and are therefore divorced from the direct influence of the individual.

In socialist writings productive labour is seen as the individual's essential activity and potentially the main avenue to human self-development and fulfilment. Marx says 'the object of work is . . . the objectification of man's species life,' in which he can 'contemplate himself in a world that has to be created.' (Marx, 1961: 114).

An historical association of work and labour with misery and anguish is evident in the early roots for the words from the Latin (*labor*) and English (labour), which are analogous with extreme physical effort and suffering. The same word is used for work and for birthing pain in English, German, French and Greek. The etymological root of labour is the same as that of labara, to stumble under a burden. The root of the French, word for work is derived from '*tripalium*', a form of torture. In Greek and German, the word for work is related to that for poverty. More contemporary language denotes work with a sense of dignity, and acknowledges its contribution to the transformation of nature and human beings (Arendt, 1958).

Generally the more interesting, creative and varied the work, the higher the reward; while the more mundane, repetitive and routine the task, the poorer the reward. Employment is simply one form of work.

Modern work

Work is perceived differently in different circumstances. Western employers managing industry in undeveloped countries often complain that the local people, by Western standards, are poor workers, unreliable and lazy. In contrast, people from resource-rich subsistence cultures find the work discipline of Western industrialization alien and unnecessary.

The industrial revolution saw the development of the idea that one should work to gain money, then spend to buy one's material wants as a consumer; the basis of capitalist production. In previous times, the generation of income was not seen as the essential basis for livelihood. The concepts of employment did not include regular and full-time employment in a single occupation.

Typically, modern work is restrained by imposed scheduling and discipline, workers have little autonomy and the product is made for the benefit of someone else.

Employment is affected by interacting factors relating to regulations, legislation, economic, political and social demands and increasingly sophisticated technology, at a local, national and global level. Marx described industrialized work as:

> 'often routine, oppressive, stultifying, alienating of the body and the soul. Industrial forms of work mutilate the labourer into a fragment of the man, degrade him to the level of an appendage to the machine, destroy every tenant of charm in his work and turn it into hated toil . . . work not only demands activity in the form of a job it imposes a time structure on the waking day.' (Marx, 1961: 645)

Within the 'global economy' there is an increase in multinational power and the concentration of ownership; a decrease in the number of companies competing in markets; and an inequitable distribution of industrial work, particularly hazardous and arduous work, to undeveloped regions. Unfortunately, the continuing move from agriculture to industrialization is impacting on the global environment with the abuse and overuse of natural resources and ever increasing pollution from emissions.

Factors which impact on modern work include the increase of automation; de-skilling, with the use of sophisticated technology; and an exponential increase in output and decrease investment in people power and capital. The availability of instant worldwide communication, the development of international division of labour and the decreasing relevance of local or regional market forces in determining patterns of employment, are moving basic trade from a local to an international process. The vast increase in the volume of available information is contrasted with an increasing specialization and fragmentation of knowledge and a redistribution of wealth to knowledge-based occupations. Structural unemployment reflects a decreasing demand for unskilled and semi-skilled workers; and a widening gap between the information rich and information poor. Ever higher educational qualifications operate as rationing devices for entry into secure employment.

The economic role of work

> *'The first thing that matters about work is to have it.'*
>
> (The Fabian Society, 1884)

The fundamental motive for work in modern society is economic. Without money, survival is difficult. The cultural norms of society dictate the methods and motives for activity and work. Subsistence workers respond to the economy of scarcity, most Westernized societies respond to a capitalist and consumer economy.

All living species undertake activities related to survival, and these are reflected in work behaviour, the division of labour, the organization of social groups and the use of communication. The gradual accumulation of new patterns of behaviour introduces and underpins cultural development and innovations, and is diffused into social groups and taught to children. Forms of social organization – rules, laws, ideas and beliefs, morals and religion – reflect and fashion behaviours and motivations, and encourage specific work ethics. Children are socialized into culture by parents and teachers and social expectations are inculcated, including preparation for work. The currency of contemporary society is money, and the fundamental motivation for activity, production and work is economic. Without the legal tender of the society survival as an accepted member of that society is practically impossible, and the basic tool for achieving the currency is paid work.

The development of work and work ethic

> *'work is of two kinds, first altering the position of matter at or near the earth's surface relative to other such matter; second, telling other people to do so. The first kind is unpleasant and ill paid; the second is pleasant and highly paid.'*
>
> (Bertrand Russell, 1872–1970)

Primitive work patterns

In primitive societies, people worked to satisfy most of their own needs, producing their own commodities, and exchanging any excess for other goods they wished to consume.

Hunting and gathering was the work pattern from the Stone Age to about 8000 BC. The people were nomadic, following the seasons and vulnerable to the environment and the availability of food, fruits and herds of wild animals. They hunted, fished and gathered fruits and vegetables, carrying out no cultivation of their own. They had simple weapons and tools for hunting and cooking and made their clothing from skins and foliage. They functioned as small family groups of twenty or thirty people, their motivation for work being fundamental: food, shelter, clothing and protection. They had some gender-based work division: men hunted, women gathered. The work was constant, but the hours of work varied with the availability of food. If the group had sufficient to eat for the day, work could cease. Hunting and gathering is still undertaken by some Pygmy groups in the Congo, Kalahari Bushmen, tribes in New Guinea and Amazon Indians.

Herding provided a more reliable and secure source of food and therefore more control of the family group's destiny. Herders were often nomadic, moving to find feed for their animals, but with domestication of cattle and sheep they were able to satisfy most of their needs from their own resources. Their motivation was still one of subsistence and their need to work related to the availability of supply. Some herders began to cultivate cereal crops, creating new tools and using animals for power. Contemporary herders are found in some areas of Tibet and among Bedouin and Masai groups.

As agriculture and horticulture continued to develop, the numbers and species of animals used for food and power and the reliability of food supplies increased. Communities were established around the farming families and grew to villages over time. Work tasks included: crafts and services such as weaving, building and pottery for the community. As surpluses of goods developed, links were created with other villages and exchange and marketing began. This created social bonds and led to further job division and specialization.

Early villages had a work leadership structure, and as hierarchical structures became more sophisticated subordinates were paid. Early trading and payment involved barter and, later, currencies developed using shells, then money. As villages continued to grow and towns began to develop, job division became clearer – farmers and herders looked after the animals, craftworkers and tradeworkers supplied most services, and priests, magicians and chiefs did no manual work. Work continued to be fundamental to the way of family life, but as these communities developed it was also seen as a way to material prosperity for the family.

Ancient Greece and the Roman Empire

The Ancient Greeks and the Romans regarded work as activity only fit for slaves. Slaves made up a large portion of the population and were regarded as a form of capital which returned a modest yield for minimal expense. They could be sold or bartered for goods. Work was highly organized, with an authoritarian military rule, a subservient slave class and large export markets. Slaves were prisoners of war from various battles and were held on estates or in households. Their treatment and work varied according to their owner; they were compelled to work by law and punished if they refused. They earned no pay and often worked alongside paid free men doing identical work. Some were skilled in trades or teaching, others were craftsmen or women.

Aristotle considered that the householder should only provide for the immediate needs of the group, and that any surplus consumption was improper. It was considered noble only to think or administer. Citizens (not slaves) undertook learning, the arts and politics, and held skilled craftsmen in high regard. Working for wages was not considered becoming, and as slaves were available to do the work this did not cause problems.

Large groups of slaves worked in mines, workshops or on farms. The motivation for work was one of fear of punishment. Division of labour, based on skill, was present in the metal, pottery and other craft industries. Women worked only in the household, doing craft-based work.

For the Ancient Greeks and Romans the motivation to work was not simply for survival. It was to expand empires, win wars, build huge buildings, and be generally associated with greatness. The whole system was underpinned by the availability of cheap slave labour. It deteriorated with a decrease in the number of prisoners of war, an increase in costs of their upkeep and the growing ethos of Christianity.

The feudal system

At its height in the Middle Ages the feudal system was based on economic and social stratification. All land was owned by the king. It was held by barons and knights living in manors in exchange for military service. The land was then allocated by strips to serfs, who received protection and provided work, military service and a proportion of their produce to the manor.

This paternalistic and dependent structure relied heavily on an acceptance of authority. There was little division of labour on farms, but some specialization of different crafts within the manorial system. The manorial village was the basic social and economic unit; specializing in different kinds of manufacture and produce, which was then sold to other villages and towns.

The manorial owners regarded work as inferior to mind activities or idleness. However, during this time, monastic orders were developing and influencing village life. They condemned idleness as sinful, and taught that manual work disciplined the soul, was ennobling and a way of serving God. Supporting the attitudes within the power base of the feudal structure, they also taught that intellectual work was superior to manual work.

During this period independent craftworkers developed their own workshops and began to sell goods direct to the public. Organized labour guilds attempting to improve rights and conditions were formed. The products from agriculture and handicrafts were the necessities of life.

The motivation to work was a need for provision for the family; and a sworn obligation to the manorial head. The only direct economic reward for this loyalty was the permission to farm a small area of land and keep a portion of its produce. Work was also seen as a moral and religious duty, an act necessary for salvation, and enforced by law.

Early industrialization

The feudal system collapsed in part as a result of the Black Plague, and because of changes in the economic and social structures. Villages and towns continued to grow and service industries developed. The serfs began to revolt against their privations and some ran away to better jobs. Most of the population still lived in the country but, as landlords found it was more profitable to pay wages and charge rent for the land, tenure was withdrawn and small craftworkers driven out of business. Although technically without continuing obligation to the landlords, their pay levels and working conditions were still controlled by the ruling class. Many preferred poverty at home to work in the developing industries.

The end of the feudal system saw an increase in the size of farms and a revolution in farming methods. Improved machinery, cropping methods, breeding strains, fertilization and drainage increased productivity, and farms began to supply towns with food. Product specialization developed within farms and regions. With the development of industries there was increased use of machinery and increased division of tasks between machines and humans. This new division of labour gradually forced the elimination of many ancient trades and saw a decline in the use of animals as energy sources. The introduction of unskilled factory work saw women and children removed from the home and farm duties to machine minding.

Having rebelled against the feudal system and its poor working conditions, the free men were now earning a wage. However the earnings were fixed by the local Justice of the Peace, who was often also the employer. Home-based businesses were virtually eliminated and people went out to work, often having to live away from home. Although the new industries offered better wages than traditional work, the new work conditions were considered so arduous that people preferred not to work at all.

The Industrial Revolution

The Industrial Revolution saw the development of large-scale, intensive use of machinery, and employment in industry and commerce. Major technological changes took place including Arkwright's spinning-Jenny (1769) in the textile industry, Watt's first steam engine and the smelting of iron and coal. Josiah Wedgwood started mass production in the pottery industry. Railways and steamboats were built for industrial transport, telephones and telegraphs made widespread communication and travel possible nationally and internationally. There was a vast increase in the industrial use of natural resources including iron, coal, oil and rubber; and a decrease in the use of traditional resources such as wood and animal substances. The supply of raw materials became central to the development of foreign and colonial policy and control.

Small-scale subsistence farming virtually disappeared, and the majority of workers ceased to be employed in agriculture. However, despite decreased numbers of workers, agricultural production levels were maintained through improved work practices on large-scale, high-volume farms.

Employment increased in other industries servicing manufacturing, such as transport, mining, commerce and administration. Towns and cities grew rapidly as industry centralized and a new concept of 'going to work' developed. Work and home became two separate spheres of life. Individual self-sufficiency decreased and job specialization increased.

The changing work ethic

A work ethic is a system of values and expectations that emphasizes the moral and psychological importance of work and other productive activities within a particular culture and society. Work ethic and work discipline are interrelated, and are dependent on the motives of all parties involved in the labour equation. A work ethic is fundamentally a product and a reflection of a social and economic environment.

An industrialized work ethic demands continuity and constancy of attendance, precision, team work, and uniform regularity of work times and speeds. As the usual source of labour in the industrialization process is people who have been accustomed to agricultural and subsistence work patterns, this work discipline has to be imposed.

The work ethic and discipline imposed during the Industrial Revolution is known as the Protestant work ethic. This developed during the spread of the Protestant religion and contains some premises of related practices. It was considered at the time to be a progressive and radical reform helping to change attitudes for the good of the workers. It promoted concepts such as dignity and self-discipline as fundamental to self-fulfillment, and suffering in the cause of work as a worthy and honourable pursuit. The creation of work discipline was necessary for the success of industrial reform and the development of modern capitalism. Workers who were unwilling to comply with the expected work behaviours were sometimes forced into virtual slavery, placed in closed communities or compounds and isolated from their social networks and communities. In 1700, a law book was developed at the Crowley Iron Works which was an entire civil and penal code spelling out the details of the required work ethic and discipline for the 'refractory' workforce. The practices which were imposed included the use of timesheets, time keepers, informers and fines. Josiah Wedgwood, in his attempts to discipline his workforce, introduced the first recorded system of clocking into work. Around the mid-18th century 'time thrift' and the importance of frugality, order and regularity were taught in schools and preached about in churches. Children from the age of 4 went to workhouses where they were employed for at least twelve hours a day in manufacturing work, with two hours of schooling to habituate them to constant employment, labour and fatigue.

As the workforce became adapted to the new work ethics incentives had to be introduced to keep them involved. With improvements in working conditions and the changes in the nature of industry and employment the emphasis has moved from the rights of the employer to a consideration of all the parties involved. Traditionally industrial welfarism or any concern about the health of the worker was a result only of the fact that a healthy worker was thought to be more productive.

Most employers saw the exploitation of workers as a right of the fit, the strong, and the powerful. The work ethic of welfare capitalism assumes that the provision of basic comforts to workers will return loyalty and a sustained working effort to their benefactor. Modern occupational welfare programmes are based on the premise that a happy healthy worker will be more productive. Modern industrial training is commenced in the discipline of education systems and continued in well-regulated workplaces. Much of the early Protestant work ethic remains in contemporary work practices and wider social and cultural standards. The inherent emphasis on the importance of employment as a means of fulfilment within Westernized societies is becoming a major concern with the development of mass long-term unemployment.

The development of mass production

The Industrial Revolution saw a new class, 'the industrial proletariat', established along with the development of industrial discipline, and the evolution of trade unions. Industries were established by entrepreneurs. The entrepreneurs were mostly middle-class merchants and some ex-craftsmen who were not well educated but successful in their own trades, and who had the required capital and a faith in the ideas of progress and new technology. Under the developing ethos of the Protestant work ethic they lived simply, not spending their new wealth but reinvesting in their industries. Some were idealists who had visions of building a total new work system, such as Robert Owen (1771–1858), who attempted to create a model community around the mill he managed by improving housing and working conditions and providing schools. Others were unscrupulous, authoritarian, exploiters of available labour. Their motivation was to make money for themselves (Argyle, 1989).

A new class of managers developed who managed the production processes and controlled and disciplined the workforce. The new elite were the engineers, technical staff and company managers who designed, engineered and controlled the use of the industrial equipment. Machinery and processes were designed with humans as the basic model. Technology could do faster and more accurately what people did with their hands and brain. Workers programmed, monitored and corrected deviations. The work was machine paced, with the workers responding as another cog in the machine.

In 1776, Adam Smith, a Scottish economist, wrote a book, *The Wealth of Nations*, advocating the advantages of the division of labour. His proposed system was reliant on interdependence and cooperation between workers, who all worked at the same speed and with the same efficiency. He hypothesized that this process would move to an international interdependence with countries specializing in the production of specialized commodities. This formal and planned process of work specialization within industries involved workers concentrating on different aspects of manufacture and eventually combining the subassembled components for the finished item. It was very successfully integrated into mass production. In 1911, Henry Ford of the Ford Motor Car Company took this idea of process specialization and combined it with the development of the assembly line, a conveyor on which the various parts are progressively assembled and gradually build up to the final product. In this process each operator has a single task to perform as the partly completed article passes by. Ford established these lines on the principles that the work should both come to the operator and be at waist height so energy was not wasted through stooping.

Assembly lines were introduced to many industries along with interchangeable parts. The basic principles of mass production were overcoming the traditional costs of the inefficiencies of human labour in the industrialized process, time, efficiency and employment costs.

It was argued that mass production increased work specialization. It therefore provided more task variety to which individuals could be better matched according to their skills and abilities, and that particular jobs such as those of trades people could become more skilled and satisfying.

On the contrary, the move to assembly operations from Smith's concepts of division of labour was a move from worker interdependence and cooperation to cooperation without any personal contact. The greater variety of work with more narrow areas of task specialization led to reduced worker training and knowledge, decreased technical control and challenge and increased repetition. In successive-stage manufacture, the worker has no contact with the product as a whole, or its purpose, which leads to decreased identification with the process, and the loss of a sense of workmanship or pride in the final output. Jobs were simpler and could be learnt faster and done with increased skill and speed. However, mass production often lead to boredom and increased inefficiency of the worker. Industry size and workforces continued to increase and the depersonalizing process continued. In this process, the worker was exchanging labour and skills for wages and using the wages to buy commodities.

Coordination, synchronization in response to mechanical precision; rapidity, repetitiveness and time restraints, were the marks of the new industrial regime and its related infrastructures.

Large towns developed an urbanized working class, largely powerless, alienated from their social supports, and discontented with factory work. Trade unions grew up among skilled craftworkers and took over from guilds, and the Marxist ideology was developed. The Protestant work ethic espoused hard work as the condition for salvation of the soul, while workers were motivated by hunger and the need of a wage to buy food.

As sufficient skilled workers adjusted to the new working conditions, innovators and entrepreneurs continued to develop the industrial processes. The development of new financial, materialist and competitive values had a major impact on social structures and related economic, political, cultural, scientific, philosophical and religious practices.

Work had moved from primary industry to a secondary and tertiary industry. Industry was urban-based and work groups cooperating in production could be based at entirely different locations. The development of occupations was based on knowledge only, not skills. For the first time work related to 'knowing what', not 'knowing how'.

Contrary to previous production units created for the purpose of the social groups such as the family, the industrial structure was based on social units created specifically for the purpose of production. At a local and national level wherever industrialization developed there was a need for supportive administration and organization such as regulations and laws. Work was done at fixed hours according to production demands and unrelated to the natural order and influences of seasons and day and night.

The management and regulation of time was essential to the process of industrialization. Early work patterns were based on natural work rhythms such as birds and animals waking or cows being ready for milking, fires needing stoking or crops harvested. Time was task oriented, many jobs had to be finished once they were started or done at a particular point of the day or night. There was little differentiation between work and life and the time in the working day was largely dependent on weather, daylight and the tasks to be done. Within the industrialized system the acceptance of time was as a commodity to be spent, lost, wasted or saved. In employment there was now a distinction between the employer's time and the worker's own time; the employer was obliged to use and not waste the employees time. Time had become money (Thompson, 1967).

The Industrial Revolution was most important as it established the basis for work practices found in industrialized countries today.

Post-industrial and modern work

> *'Machines are worshipped because they are beautiful and valued because they confer power; they are hated because they are hideous and loathed because they impose slavery'.*
>
> (Bertrand Russell, 1872–1970).

The Industrial Revolution was underpinned by the development of steam as a power source. Other technological developments which have since led to periods of work change have related to railways, electricity, chemicals, internal combustion and plastics, nuclear power and the many recent developments in automation. People are increasingly interacting primarily with machines.

Technology frequently dictates modern work environments and work behaviours. To a great extent, the machinery often exceeds the workers in their ability to programme, feedback and monitor, unless problems occur.

The majority of people are employed in labour-intensive service industries – selling, teaching, management and administration, transport, the media, health care and tourism. There is a decrease in capital-intensive employment. There is a drive for maximum outputs with the smallest possible investment in labour. Economies are increasingly based on information, and the number of people employed collecting, processing, storing and retrieving data is rapidly increasing over the numbers in agriculture and manufacturing.

The dominant Western model of economy which developed during the Industrial Revolution in the United Kingdom and spread to Europe and North America has become the 'preferred' model for development at an international level.

The principles of mass production, division of labour and job specialization continue to be promulgated. Time and motion studies and Taylorism (Taylor, 1964) from the turn of the nineteenth century made it possible to standardize every job in order that a simple set of movements could be used, and piece rates and payments could be established. Every worker could carry out a very simple task in which they could become an expert and for which they could be paid according to the volume they produced (Barnes, 1963). Efficient production comes at the cost of worker stress and boredom.

There is a growing disparity between management and workers as educational and knowledge-based demands increase and skill-based task requirements decrease. There is decreased job loyalty and increased mobility in less skilled jobs, many workers change employers and occupations, moving according to personal needs.

Early expressions of frustration with industrialized work systems were countered by laws introduced to protect the employers and prevent unionism as we know it today. Conditions in many countries have improved considerably with the rising influence of trade unions and occupational health and safety regulations (see Chapter 5, Legislation). However many blue-collar workers continue to be alienated and discontented with their ever diminishing role. Workers are generally assumed to be inherently lazy, incapable of self-discipline and driven solely by economic needs. Much of the frustration with modern work stems from the fact that while work is an economic necessity, the work content provides little stimulation or satisfaction (Jones, 1982). For many workers this has meant work is no longer a central life interest and is simply the method by which a living can be made to buy needs. Work is undertaken to sustain consumption.

As work becomes increasingly automated it is decreasingly dependent on the participation of individual producers, already in some production the process of industrialization is no longer dependent on human input. In many work environments the design and layout of machinery dictates work posture, reaches, mobility and dexterity and makes no allowances for individual human variations.

In the late 1930s, ergonomics, or 'human factors engineering', was developed and recognized as a profession. Ergonomics is the science of optimizing the functioning of systems by adapting them to match human capacity and needs. The inclusion of ergonomic principles and practices into workplace design and work activities attempts to overcome the mismatches which have developed in the industrialization process, recognizing the positive links between productivity and human comfort. The implementation of ergonomic principles considers the human within the total work environment, including the physiological, psychological, social, systems and environmental factors. Ergonomics practitioners attempt to balance all these presenting variables to the best possible benefit of both the worker and the production process (Grandjean, 1988).

Working hours

Working hours have been regulated since working guilds or statutes in the Middle Ages in Europe. Work was commonly done between sunrise and sunset with a break for food at noon and perhaps one other break. If shorter days were worked in winter or for lack of light, pay was reduced. Workers averaged 10½ hours work per day, six or seven days per week. With the removal of holidays and saints days this averaged around a 54-hour week over a year.

During the reformation, there were more people competing for jobs, saints days were reduced and work hours extended. As late as the eighteenth century in Britain and the United States and the late nineteenth century in Germany and Japan, 12–14 hour work days were common, six days a week, often using child labour. A gradual decrease in the number of holidays and the difference in summer and winter hours, and an increased number of people seeking work because of the need for wages led to increased sickness and absenteeism. Since the 1830s hours have been reduced progressively, a limit of 8 normal daily hours set, and in 1919 an International Labour Organization (ILO) international agreement was reached reducing work days to five-and-a-half then five days per week. Paid holidays and sick leave allowances were also introduced, under pressure from organized labour movements.

Unemployment

'to be idle is no longer considered rewarding or even respectable.'

(Prof. J K Galbraith, 1908)

Work is the essence of self-identity and public image in our culture, and is closely tied to perceptions of status and lifestyle. The loss of paid work can lead to a loss of confidence of self-perception, routines, structures and time perspectives. Our society is highly regulated by work and work patterns.

Job loss is therefore a major life change, involving loss and the subsequent adjustments required after any bereavement. Unemployed people frequently pass through recognizable patterns of loss – an initial denial, with a sense of relief or holiday; increasing distress as they become aware of the seriousness of their situation and the prospects of poverty; earnest job seeking; resignation and decreased social interests; depression and isolation, and the related impacts on their family, partner and friends.

Unemployment raises basic concerns such as housing security, an inability to forward plan, indebtedness, financial dependence and social humiliation. The sheer lack of money prevents the unemployed person from participating in society. The length of unemployment has a direct negative effect on psychological functioning, as the impact of not fitting into an employment-based culture becomes increasingly felt. The change of role at home and in the community means a change in self-perception in which the ex-worker is now a social debit rather than a working credit. The unemployed person is trapped in a cycle of poverty and frustration which an income-based society does not accommodate. Unemployment benefits were designed for short-term relief, but in many instances are now serving as the only source of long-term sustenance.

The changing patterns of the demand for labour resulting from automation and other technological change have greatly increased the demand for highly educated and white-collar workers and decreased the demand for low-skilled, uneducated workers. At the same time many older middle-management workers are unemployed and many school leavers cannot find their first job. The issue of growing long-term unemployment is a serious and increasing problem for modern industrialized societies; and requires strategies for solutions which consider the human as well as the economic face of the problem.

Women's work

'Home is the girl's prison and the woman's workhouse.'

(George Bernard Shaw, 1903)

Not all work is formally renumerated and much of women's work traditionally falls into the category of unpaid work. Much discussion has taken place as to the desirability of changing this situation and the value of unpaid domestic work and child rearing to economic development. Equal-opportunity legislation and affirmative action practices have begun to address these issues in some countries, but there continues to be a recognition internationally that women as a group within and without the paid labour force tend to be disadvantaged by existing systems.

The problems women face within the labour force generally relate back to the impacts of the roles of child bearing and rearing on their working life – life-cycle issues exclusive to the female sex at this practical level. These issues and the related attitudinal problems are historical and impact on all women workers regardless of age and reproductive status. Until recently women in work were almost always unmarried and childless and becoming married or pregnant meant being forced to leave work in many occupations. However, patterns of employment are beginning to change.

The Impact of War

In most Western countries, prior to the Second World War the profile of employed women was those who were young and unmarried, now it is generally the older and the married. Since the Second World War the number of women in industry has dramatically increased, and over the last two decades, for example, women in the United States have taken two thirds of the millions of new jobs created in the information-based work explosion (Cox and Cox, 1984).

War has had a major impact on women's work as men have gone away, leaving women in employment as their substitutes. In July 1914 5,966,000 women were employed in industry in Britain. In July 1918 this had risen to 7,311,000. Estimates of women replacing men in this period in the metal industry were 704,000, a 16 per cent rise; in the chemical industry 35,000, a 19 per cent rise, and in the government establishments 197,000, a 44 per cent rise. Between the First and Second World Wars the number of women workers and their relative importance in the total labour force in Britain expanded in the engineering trades and the clerical, commercial and professional fields. The proportion of women working in factories returned to pre-war levels. The Second World War saw an increase in women's employment in the metal and chemical industries, agriculture and horticulture, transport and local and national government services. In June 1939 27 per cent of the total workforce was women, in June 1944 this had increased to 39.4 per cent. In agriculture over this period there was an increase of 10.2 per cent, in the metal and chemical industries 20.3 per cent and in national government work an increase of 45 per cent.

Female labour ceased to be considered as a marginal factor in industrial labour power, it played an essential and acknowledged part in the war effort. Women were given the opportunity and a taste for industrial work, often skilled industrial work. Women were admitted to apprenticeships, particularly in engineering and electrical trades. This led to some change in the mental attitude to the subject of women's work as the general public was now accustomed to seeing 'quite important' tasks entrusted to women (ILO, 1946).

Work opportunities

Traditionally, work opportunities for skilled women are few, and men receive more money than women in many industrial situations, despite the fact that they carry out the same quantity and quality of work (Game and Pringle, 1983).

Recruitment to positions is often governed by sex. Most women are recruited to service positions of a generalist nature, personal services; clerical and secretarial work; education; welfare and health. Some industries employ women, but in a narrow range of job opportunities compared with men, in repetitive process work and domestic jobs such as cleaners, cafeteria workers, nurses and child minders. Most of the work is in the food and clothing industries and is low paid, repetitive, low skilled and gives minimal job satisfaction. This pattern has persisted to a great extent despite changing work patterns and modes of production over the ages.

Today, in the United States, women without children are more likely to work than men, approximately 74 per cent of men and 67 per cent of women with children work, and 79 per cent of women under 18 years without children work. Women are starting new businesses twice as often as men; in Canada one third of small businesses are owned by women, in France one fifth; in Britain since 1980 self-employed women have increased in number three times as fast as self-employed men.

A bi-modal or two-phase pattern has developed for female workers in paid employment, fitting around child-rearing patterns. Research in industrialized countries shows that at around 25 years of age about 60 per cent of women are economically active, between 26 and 35 years, 45 per cent, and from 45 years to retirement economic activity peaks at around 60 per cent. This pattern is being largely driven by married women. All of these developments have occurred against a background of technological change and economic decline, and social and family-structural changes. However, women continue to face a lack of defined career structures and promotional prospects, though job mobility is increasing.

Health issues

Overall health trends in working women are not well documented though there is some evidence that their advantage over men of a lower incidence of stress-related disorders, cancer and cardiac-related illnesses is gradually reducing. There is limited information on sex differences in response to workplace hazards except in the extensive area of reproductive impacts or teratogenisis. The introduction of new technology continues to raise issues about risk exposure to hazards to child bearing, such as fear of radiation exposure from visual display units (VDUs), or visual display terminals (VDTs). These issues are usually dealt with at a regulatory level, tending to err on the side of caution even when there is no evidence of a problem. With regard to VDUs or VDTs, guidelines have been incorporated into many industrial awards allowing pregnant women to choose whether they continue to work with them or not, even though there is no evidence at this time to indicate they can have detrimental effects if the machine is manufactured and maintained within prescribed standards. One of the major issues with hazardous exposures and pregnancy is that the foetus is at its most vulnerable to damage in the first few weeks of development, when many women do not know, or do not want it known, that they are pregnant.

The move towards consideration of the particular issues of pregnant women is a big step from the recent past when marriage or pregnancy meant having to leave employment. This is illustrated well in discussion of the role of the pregnant flight attendant, a socially impossible entity even fifteen years ago in most countries. In developing guidelines for pregnant flight attendants the risks to the mother and the child were explored in terms of potential hypoxia, trauma and abortion; the changing body mechanics of size, shape and balance during the pregnancy, and the role requirements while flying.

Equal employment opportunity

Until the introduction of equal opportunity legislation, flight attendants (or hostesses) were selected for their single marital status, attractive physical appearance, youth, height requirements relevant to the planes, and weight to fit with a socially prescribed norm of desirability. The term 'hostess' was seen as derogatory by many of the attendants. Pregnancy, and even marriage in some companies, meant job termination in this role. With the introduction of equal opportunity much has been done to change the emphasis to one of focusing on the task and the task demands and the ability of the staff to fulfil their duties.

Work and family

Working women face opposing demands and constraints of work and family. Women often have a conflict between child bearing and career aspirations and expectations, and suffer guilt while working and paying for child care. Research shows that this is a quality-of-care issue rather than an issue of the frequency or length of contact, as children of working mothers generally have increased intellectual stimulation and financial advantages over children of non-working mothers. On the contrary, most employed women work a double work day, potentially causing strain, mental health problems, overload and exhaustion. Child care is an expensive and distressing issue for many working mothers, particularly with the decline of the extended family.

Work entitlements

Women usually work because they have to and because they are entitled to, and through work they have increased social support, self-esteem, and independence, and decreased isolation, loneliness and financial concerns. The dramatic increase in the number of women working is a major challenge to work organization and women's role in society. There are many issues which require addressing to improve the lot of single women, single mothers, supporting mothers and women with supportive partners and the provision of work which fits their particular needs. There is a need for alternative employment practices which allow job sharing and flexibility; alternative child care structures; retraining in new work practices and technologies; legislation to broaden the basis for equal opportunity and affirmative action and to encourage and support working families; positive initiatives to make people aware of existing 'prejudices' against women and remove them; and attitudinal changes in schools to broaden concepts of female work and encourage participation in new opportunities. At the work-floor level, there is an urgent need to address issues of poor working conditions and exploitation, the 'glass ceiling' effect, the continuing inequities in pay, sexual harassment, and other gender-related problems.

Child labour

> *'See saw, Margery Daw, Johnny shall have a new Master, Jacky must have but a penny a day, Because he can't work any faster.'*
>
> (Mother Goose Melody, 1765)

In 1959, the General Assembly of the United Nations issued the Declaration of the Rights of the Child including a statement that:

> The child shall no longer be admitted to employment before an appropriate minimum age; he shall in no case be caused or permitted to engage in any occupation or employment which would prejudice his health or education, or interfere with his physical, mental or moral development. (WHO, 1987)

The International Labour Organization (ILO) estimated that, at the beginning of the 1980s, the overall number of children who were 'economically active' internationally was around 50 million, other agencies estimating as high as 75 or 100 million.

In 1992, the ILO conservatively estimated that child workers constituted over 18 per cent of all children aged between 10 and 14 in developing countries; at least 7 per cent in Latin America; 18 per cent in Asia and 25 per cent in Africa. Many of these children have run away from their families, are orphaned or abandoned and are deprived of adequate nutrition, health care and education, and if they cannot work to be able to eat they are not likely to survive.

Current recessionary times and increased unemployment have led to traditional forms of child labour, such as sweatshop industries, re-emerging, even in some industrialized countries. In the United States in 1993 it was estimated that 5.5 million children of 12 to 17 years of age were 'economically active' (Badran, 1995).

Working conditions

The majority of child labourers are engaged in agriculture, others work in small-scale enterprises such as brick making, handicrafts, carpet manufacturing, or as waiters in bars and restaurants, domestic servants, sex workers and scavengers in large rubbish sites. Some work in dangerous industries such as glass manufacturing, construction and mining.

For many, the work is characterized by exploitation, excessively long hours, low pay and heavy physical loads, inadequate working conditions and exposure to occupational hazards, including, in some work, physical and psychological neglect, drugs and violence.

Paid child labour (persons under 15 years of age) is defined by the ILO as the systematic exploitation of children by employers outside the child's family. Children are not normally supposed to offer their labour in the labour-market and are not able to negotiate their terms of employment with trade-union backing, therefore child employment is quite different from adult employment. Children are, therefore, in a vulnerable position from which they can be readily exploited. Exploitation involves payment (much less than adults), abuse of health, and forced work in jobs unsafe to adults or with hazards to children in terms of growth, work capacity and development.

The minimum age for employment stipulated by the ILO is 15 years, between 15 and 18 years the person is considered to be a 'young person' and special work standards apply to this group. Children between the ages of 13–15 years are permitted to do 'light work', defined loosely as work that is not likely to be harmful to the children's health or development, and will not prejudice their attendance at school, participation in vocational orientation and approved training programmes, or their capacity to benefit from instruction received. No absolute minimum age is stipulated for children involved in public performances; employed in family undertakings provided the work is not harmful, prejudicial or dangerous; and when pupils in schools for vocational and technical education.

Health risks

It is presumed that children occupationally exposed to the same doses of toxic chemicals as adults are more readily affected because of their smaller body weights, but there is a paucity of epidemiological studies in this area because of the difficulty of studying situations where children are illegally exposed, and also because of the high turnover of labour in these situations.

There is little available data on work capacity or anthropometrics of children and most of the tools, equipment and work situations in which they are employed are designed for adults, the children having to compensate accordingly. This leads to situations such as respirators, when available, not worn because they do not fit; musculoskeletal problems from oversized adult seating or reaching to adult-height benches, and children suffering from heat exhaustion in conditions which do not affect adults.

Developmental issues

Work often competes with education, disadvantaging the child for future employment. For many children economically productive activity deprives the child of time and opportunity to go through the normal developmental stages, separates them and forces them into independence in daily life at a very early age.

At work the child is young, an employee, unlikely to assert their rights or needs, often subject to very rigid discipline, intimidation and even physical abuse. In many countries there is no protection legally for work injuries to children – particularly when they have been illegally employed.

Children are often forced to work by their parents or other adults. This is often done with an economic motive when families can see no other option for survival of the child or the family. Child prostitution is a form of child labour readily condemned (yet readily consumed) by the Western world while many families, particularly in some Asian countries, see it as the only opportunity for their child to have a future. Poverty, shortcomings in the educational systems, inadequate regulations to restrict child labour, ineffective enforcement of even basic controls, and a lack of international awareness of the scale of these problems, all contribute to the existence of child labour.

Migrant workers

> *'Which of us is to do the hard and dirty work for the rest – and for what pay?'*
>
> (John Ruskin, 1819–1900)

Slavery

The use of foreign labour has been a practice in societies with organized labour since the time of the slave used by the Ancient Greeks and the Roman Empire. In the sixteenth century many African people were born into slavery but sometimes free people submitted to slavery in order to avoid famine, work off debt, or as a punishment for crime. A purchased slave had few rights while the lot of a domestic slave was not notably worse than that of a free man.

The great increase in the slave trade and its abuses occurred after the first European settlement in America; in 1503 Africans were brought over by the Spaniards to work in Hispaniola; Sir Richard Hawkins took his first cargo of slaves to the West Indies in 1562.

Between 1680 and 1786 more than two million slaves were imported into the British-American colonies, including 600,000 to Jamaica within 80 years. Mortality rates were high in this trade – a shipment of 5000 may have cost as many as 30,000 lives due to disease, escape attempts and deaths in raids on the villages when slaves were being taken.

Slaves led a wretched life doing the work considered to be unsuitable for their captors and with little concern for their health or welfare.

Migrant labour

Migrant labour use by industrialized countries originated in the nineteenth century and expanded during the twentieth century, interrupted only by the two world wars. Foreign or migrant labour is used extensively because of an inadequate supply of national labour; difficulty filling arduous and low-paid jobs such as mining; and occasionally because particular skills of the migrants are useful in particular industries such as languages in the hospitality industry.

Many migrant workers or persons making up foreign labour numbers are involuntary in that although they are being exported under coercion, for their own and their family's survival, they are primarily under the control of another party who is exploiting cheap labour opportunities for their own gain – a common situation with domestic labour such as Filipinos working in other richer Asian countries and the Middle East.

The countries exporting labour generally have manpower surpluses relative to their level of national economic activity; few vocational skills and reduced economic activity and social opportunities. The importing country gains cheap and vulnerable labour – particularly when the migrants are illegal. It also gains workers at minimal cost as they do not generally have rights to local social security and welfare services. Some groups, such as the 'guest workers' in Western Europe, are now seen as a 'problem' as their children are native-born citizens of the country and expect to stay and have equal rights with other nationals.

The flow of labour is generally from a poorer, rural and agricultural economy to an industrial economy with supposedly better prospects.

Health and social issues

Migrant workers are generally young, unskilled, lacking the language of the new country and lacking the experience of the more complex and sophisticated culture. These factors alone raise health and social issues.

These workers tend to stay within the protection of their own cultural grouping for obvious reasons of support, a fact which can further limit their integration into the new culture. The migrant worker commonly lives in sub-standard accommodation, doing work the local population refuses to do, and often being exploited because of their lack of knowledge of local standards and conditions, or lack of local language skills. Often the threat of job loss and the impact this would have on their very survival (particularly when they have a dependent family in their former country), leads to the acceptance of working conditions which flagrantly ignore labour laws and safety standards.

Many contemporary migrant workers are refugees who were highly skilled and educated employees in their own country, now working in unfamiliar lowly paid and physically demanding jobs.

Language fluency in the chosen country of work is essential for both a basic level of understanding of instructions and safety issues, and for the movement of migrant workers to some level of social autonomy and control over their work and social conditions.

Development of labour regulation and law

> *'We in some unknown Power's employ, move on a rigorous line, can neither, when we will enjoy, nor when we will, resign.'*
>
> (Matthew Arnold, 1822–1888)

Labour law generally covers personal labour relations, contracts between the individual and the employer; collective labour relationships; conditions of work – hours, weekly rest, holidays, occupational health and safety, industrial accidents, occupational and non-occupational diseases.

Occupational health and safety issues form part of the working conditions, initially addressing issues such as guarding, protection from hazardous substances, first aid, and workers compensation; moving gradually into the field of injury prevention through medical monitoring and protection of the working environment including noise, dust, lighting and ventilation. Laws regarding health and safety have only been dealt with in a comprehensive manner in most industrialized countries in recent years. Laws have also been developed to protect particularly vulnerable groups, such as women, young persons, or those exposed to particular hazards, i.e. in mining, building and construction (see Chapter 5, Legislation).

The International Labour Organization

The International Labour Organization (ILO) has adopted many conventions and recommendations covering nearly every aspect of labour problems. A convention ratified by a member state of the ILO becomes legally binding when legislation is enacted in that member state to give effect to the convention. When this is done the state is bound to apply its terms throughout its national territory. Britain was one of the first countries to attempt to address labour regulation and its model and laws impacted on a number of other countries, particularly those in the British Commonwealth. Labour laws seek to perform three basic functions: rationalize the individual employment relationship; regulate the relations between organized labour and the employers and/or the government; and moderate the operation of the market in some circumstances.

The regulation of labour

In 1351 the British Statute of Labourers introduced a system of labour-market regulation which empowered local justices of the peace (often the local employers) to fix wages by reference to the price of bread, and made it a criminal offence for servants to leave their employment before the end of an agreed term without their master's consent or for a good cause.

In the late 1340s, the population of Europe was decimated by the Black Death, bubonic plague, which led to an acute shortage of labour. The remaining workers could therefore demand relatively high wages.

The 1351 Act provided that wages be held down to levels prevailing before the plague, and that all men and women under the age of 60 without income from property or merchandise must work for any master who wanted their services. The Act made withdrawal or withholding of labour a criminal offence, so collective action by workers to improve terms and conditions of employment was virtually impossible without individuals being prosecuted.

Typically, the servant performed menial tasks around the house or was a farm labourer – sometimes both depending on the time of the year. The master had extensive powers over the servant, over virtually every aspect of their lives, but also responsibility, i.e. a duty to employ continuously even if there was little work to be done. A few groups, such as the Luddites and the Arts and Crafts movement, were well known for their protests in defiance of the Act and against the movement from skill-based craft work to mass industrial production.

The emergence of unions

Until 1824, various acts were passed supporting the approach of using the law to suppress groups of workers, referred to as 'combinations', who were attempting to improve their collective lot in terms of work conditions. The 1824/5 acts constituted a recognition by parliament that it was neither equitable nor practicable to seek entirely to suppress 'combinations' of workers, but not until 1906 was criminal law excluded from the industrial arena and civil law attenuated.

The 1825 acts embodied a range of offences which could be committed in the course of industrial disputation including threats, molestation, intimidation and obstruction – this being often interpreted to maintain that it was unlawful to threaten to strike. However, the Master and Servant Act, which was based on the provisions of the Statute of Labourers of 1351, remained in force and exposed workers to criminal liability. As late as 1872, there were more than 17,000 prosecutions and 10,000 convictions under this legislation in a single year.

The 1825 acts were repealed in 1875 and since then criminal law has had little bearing on the individual employment relationship in Britain. Labour legislation is being based on civil rather than criminal law. Thereafter, unions began to develop legally.

Towards the end of the nineteenth century and beginning of the twentieth century, northwestern Europe and North America had developed labour legislation. These were whole bodies of laws concerning labour matters, such as regulations and similar statutory instruments adopted for the administration of laws – decrees, ordinances, orders, regulations, codes of practice, etc. Some isolated countries began the process earlier; many Asian and African countries still have only the basic enactments in force, these being promulgated in the 1960s and 1970s.

Issues for developing countries

Developing countries is a term generally used for those countries which are developing a Western model of industrial economy. The lack of development refers to their level of industrialization, not their human society. Many countries fit into this grouping, all having their own particular cultural and economic practices and issues. Variations between practice in developed and developing countries become particularly pertinent when developed countries are imposing their work systems. Cultural, religious, ethical, economic and other related social factors should always be considered. Any development should be implemented in response to local requirements and not from an agenda set by an external country. It should enhance work effectiveness while integrating local values.

Currently there is considerable movement of industry from Western countries to developing countries, often to exploit relatively cheap labour or to maintain production which is no longer acceptable in their own country. An example of this is the movement of some asbestos production, with its inherent safety problems, by Western-based companies to South Korea.

Many traditional work practices and tools are well designed for their particular work environment and found strange and unacceptable by Westerners. Vehicles such as rickshaws are very well designed for general carrying, and practices such as head load bearing are efficient if high speed is not required.

Postures such as sitting on floors, low seats or squatting are habitually practised from an early age in many developing countries and have considerable practical advantages, including the lower floor level air temperatures, increased venous return while working, the ability to use the legs to stabilize work, reduced work height and greater freedom for postural change. Workers in other cultures have different climatic tolerances, anthropometric build, and nutritional, organizational, physical and cognitive requirements.

In any work development the local context of tasks, jobs, skills, career, organization and environment must always be considered. Expectations of physical work capacity and workload may vary markedly, other countries' standards often considered by Westerners to be remarkably heavy in relation to body weight. Most workers in tropical countries prefer to work during the day, having acclimatized to the heat, while Westerners see the night as a cooler option.

Much of the existing industry in undeveloped countries uses old and poor technology and has related problems with noise, heat, bad postures, toxic chemicals and dust, heavy manual loads and lack of safety precautions. In many cultures where poverty is the motivation for work, deafness and early ill-health retirement bonuses are considered preferable to not working in noisy and unsafe environments.

Imposed industry

Workers who move from rural areas to industrial work in cities often have a considerable disadvantage in their new community and are prone to problems associated with changes in diet, disease and reproduction. Many industries impose disciplines and work practices which interfere with traditional daily life activities and local customs, such as shift work. Modern technology, such as office automation, is often imposed without the acclimatization process undergone in the West as the products gradually developed.

The international movement of industries between countries has many impacts aside from the obvious issues of potential exploitation. Authoritarian management styles are often irrelevant when the worker's experience has been one of autonomy and personal responsibility. Working systems are often imposed without sensitivity to the local resources. Many norms established in industrialized countries are either unsuitable or based on views of overall needs without recognizing the local practices.

Cognitive variables such as perceptions in traditionally non-pictorial cultures may lead to difficulty dealing with technical drawings. Cultural, educational and religious factors are often ignored. Communication and work performance are often dependent on verbal and written information, visual displays and control stereotypes, which are unknown to the local workers. Western colour perceptions, such as red for danger, may be confusing for other cultures: for the Chinese red is the colour of happiness and prosperity. Safety equipment and protective clothing often do not fit and are seen as unnecessary when local clothing is well adapted to the climate, and the wearing of shoes may be unknown.

Many of the existing industries rely on technology and raw materials from the former Eastern bloc and face issues of economic changes and high energy costs. Often cheap imported equipment and processes are used in dilapidated or dangerous conditions, i.e. missing guards and no instructions. Local resources for control and adaptation of technology are often inadequate and therefore any technological advantages are lost and other problems are created (Shahnavaz, 1992).

Anthropometrics

Comparative anthropometric studies and other anthropometric data from developing countries demonstrate differences in almost every part of the human body between industrialized and developing countries, racial groups and age groups. The data shows that generally there are taller people in North America, the European Continent and Scandinavia, medium-sized people in Africa and the Middle East and shorter people in Latin America, Asia and the Far East. Hand dimensions, which are crucial to machine and tool design and use, vary greatly: West-Indian female hands are significantly larger than West-European and Indian hands; and Hong Kong Chinese have smaller hands than the UK and USA populations and larger hands than the Japanese. Hand dimensions, however, follow a different pattern from that of standing and sitting heights between industrialized and developing countries. Body measurements differ significantly between urban and rural areas. People from rural areas are on average smaller than those in urban areas, possibly relating to nutrition and living standards (Kogi and Sen, 1987). Most available anthropometric data is based on Western sources, generally from a selected military population which has its own inherent biases.

Mismatches in anthropometrics have significant implications for the use of many items of equipment and machinery, such as driving vehicles, and using safety equipment. Most respirators currently used in developing countries are designed to fit American and European soldiers rather than for use by civilian workers, and fit has a major impact on function and acceptance.

The impact of rapid change

At a human and environmental level it is increasingly recognized that the combination of the impact of the mechanization of traditional industry and the introduction of new manufacturing are frequently having a detrimental impact. Factors relevant to this are the use of inappropriate, unsafe and poorly maintained equipment; the lack of qualified personnel; misfit issues; the lack of awareness of ergonomics and occupational health and safety issues; the lack of regulations and enforcement and proper inspection and supervision; and the shortages of resources. These often combine with short-term profit gains at the expense of long-term impacts, and all contribute to high accident rates, occupational diseases, low productivity, poor product quality and equipment deterioration, and environmental pollution.

These issues can be addressed by the use of appropriate person– machine–environment design based on local anthropometric data; the incorporation of traditional or ergonomically designed tools, appropriate work methods and work postures; the monitoring of physical workloads including lifting and carrying; and the control of emissions with sensitivity to the local environment.

Workload

Workload expectations vary within cultures and even within industries in one culture. The motivation for the work can impact markedly on the accepted workload, as can the duration of the task and the autonomy of the worker. Issues of survival, food, family, discipline; general well-being, nutrition and fitness, can all impact on work readiness and ability. Climatic influences, such as extreme cold or heat, and factors such as war and famine, can radically change workload perceptions and work motivation.

With changes in patterns of work, workload alters, the introduction of technology generally leading to a reduction in physical demands. The changes in methods used for ship loading is a dramatic illustration of this, where the introduction of computer-controlled container loading systems has moved most wharfies from dockside labouring to keyboard operation.

Workload is regulated to some extent, though there is little international uniformity, largely because of varied work practices and cultural expectations. Some countries have agreed maximum lifting limits, and temperature limits for hot and cold work, and the ILO has conventions and recommendations in a number of areas relating to workload limits.

Work mortality and morbidity

Workers continue to die at work despite occupational health and safety and related legislation. The number who die in some fields of work has markedly decreased, but work-related mortalities and injuries continue to be a cost to industrialized and undeveloped societies.

Life expectancy is increasing in many countries, and the number of workers available changes accordingly. Patterns of work, death and disability are all related and integral to societal functioning and attitudes. Attitudes to life and death, injury and disability, vary from culture to culture, influenced by experiences, expectations and beliefs.

The first phase of industrial and urban development (and a rapidly expanding urban population) is nearly always marked by a temporary increase in the death rate and injury rate, reflecting the disruption to familiar activities, the appearance of new occupational diseases, epidemics such as measles, smallpox and typhus; unsatisfactory housing and a lack of public health and support systems. This impact reduces as patterns are established as new norms, only to arise again with the next wave of development.

With increasing affluence, the expectations of work environments tend to be higher and the level of discomfort and perception of disability is reflected in the nature of reported conditions. Work practices which are tolerated in times of war, for example, would not be accepted in times of affluence and peace. When unemployment levels are high, many workers will tolerate levels of discomfort and stress they would not in times of ready job mobility.

Causes of deaths

Historically many occupational groupings died frequently from particular causes. Table 1.1 lists some of these occupational groupings.

The impact of social class and poverty on death rates has reduced in most industrialized countries because of improved control due to legislation and the increased management of hazardous work practices, and improved socioeconomic conditions generally.

Table 1.1 Groupings of occupation and disease

Disease	*Occupation*
Intestinal and infectious diseases	Pioneers, soldiers, miners
Tuberculosis (often with silicosis as underlying cause)	Miners, and workers in occupations involving brewing, delivering or selling alcoholic beverages; and many trades, i.e. knife grinding
Zoonotic bacterial diseases (diseases from animals)	Veterinarians, farmers, wool sorters, i.e. anthrax
Viral diseases including anthropoid-borne diseases	Occupations undertaken in tropical or forest regions, traditionally affected explorers, missionaries, international aid medical workers, soldiers and construction workers, i.e. malaria, yellow fever, typhus
Syphilis and other sexually transmitted diseases	Commercial sex workers, soldiers
Helminthiases	Schistosomiasis is an important occupational infection occurring usually in rice farmers in endemic areas; hookworm disease has caused much invalidity in farmers
Neoplasms	Many occupational groups unless exposure to toxins has been controlled, including chimney sweepers, asbestos workers, uranium miners, workers in contact with radiation
Respiratory system related disease	Workers exposed to great heat or to dusts are susceptible to diseases such as pneumonia, silicosis
Injury, poisonings and drowning	Watermen, fishermen and sailors; explosions, fires, electrical accidents, falls, spills and slips, due to poor design of equipment or work practices, possible in most areas of employment

Work-related disasters continue to occur, killing hundreds and thousands of people, commonly where there has been poor attention to equipment design and maintenance, and work practices. The Bhopal and Chernobyl disasters are two recent examples and historically it has been noted that activities such as the slave trade caused massive loss of life. It is estimated that in Africa in the seventeenth and eighteenth centuries there was a loss of half a million lives annually to the slave trade. During this period depopulation occurred in the Belgian Congo at a rate which reduced the population from 20 million to 8 million in only 15 years.

Table 1.2 Life expectancy

	Deaths by age, 1985–1990			
	0–4 years (%)	*5–14 years (%)*	*15–64 years (%)*	*65+ years (%)*
Developed regions	3	1	26	70
Undeveloped regions	34	8	30	28
World population	27	6	29	38
Africa	46	13	27	14

(Source: adapted from the Special Tabulations from the 1992 Revision, World Health Data.)

Life expectancy

Life expectancy has improved in many regions with better nutrition and living standards, but there continues to be marked international variability. This is demonstrated in the figures taken from World Health Organization data listed in Table 1.2

Impairment, disability and handicap

Impairment, disability and handicap have been defined by the World Health Organization (WHO, 1980) in a manner which assists in understanding the impact of work-related issues in varied cultural contexts.

Impairment is defined by the World Health Organization as any loss or abnormality of psychological, physiological or anatomical structure or function. These may be temporary or permanent, and include the existence or occurrence of an anomaly, defect or loss in a limb, organ, tissue, or other structure of the body, including the systems of mental function. Impairment represents exteriorization of a pathological state, and it reflects disturbances at the level of the organ.

Disability is defined as any restriction or lack (resulting from an impairment) of ability to perform an activity in the manner or within the range considered normal for a human being. It is characterized by excesses or deficiencies of customarily expected activity, performance and behaviour, which may be temporary or permanent, reversible or irreversible, and progressive or regressive. They may arise as a direct consequence of impairment or as a response by the individual, particularly psychologically, to a physical, sensory or other impairment. Disability represents objectification of an impairment, and reflects disturbances at the level of the person. Disability is concerned with abilities, in the form of activities and behaviours, that are generally accepted as essential components of everyday life, such as excretory control or the ability to walk.

Handicap is defined as a disadvantage for a given individual, resulting from an impairment or a disability, that limits or prevents the fulfillment of a role that is normal (depending on age, sex, and social and cultural factors) for that individual. It is concerned with the value attached to an individual's situation or experience when it departs from the norm. It is characterized by a discordance between the individual's performance or status and the expectations of the individual themselves, or of the particular group of which he/she is a member. Handicap thus represents socialization of an impairment or disability, and as such it reflects the consequences for the individual – cultural, social, economic and environmental – that stem from the presence of impairment and disability. Disadvantage arises from failure or inability to conform to the expectations or norms of the individual's universe.

Handicap thus occurs when there is interference with the ability to sustain what might be designated as 'survival roles'. A soft-tissue back injury in a Nepalese labourer may have the same impairment as that of an Australian office worker, but the disability and handicap factors are likely to be very different. A fractured ring finger on his non-dominant hand may have no impact in terms of disability or handicap for a truck driver but cause many problems for a professional pianist.

Factors influencing mortality, work-related impairment and resulting disability will be fundamentally influenced by cultural attitudes, patterns and expectations. Most industrialized countries are rarely exposed to and (properly) horrified by work-related death and accidents, and continue to enforce regulations which assist in their reduction. In some other countries, work is primarily related to efforts towards basic survival and death is a commonplace and accepted part of everyday life. Until basic living and health conditions improve and other poverty-related issues are better managed, these contrasts will continue to exist.

Social and political implications of changing work patterns

> *'It takes centuries 'ere the free labourer agrees to sell the whole of his active life, his very capacity for work, for the price of the necessities of life, his birthright for a pottage.'*
>
> (Karl Marx, 1818–1883)

Increasingly, people face decisions about their involvement in employment or self-employment and their attitude to work and its importance to life. Marx said, 'To give all of one's labour power in return for a wage was seen as grievous loss of independence, security and liberty.' (Marx, 1976). Contemporary humans have embraced industry and work and our life is neatly divided into industrial and domestic compartments.

In non-industrialized societies workers had some control over their own means of production. Externally imposed work practices (outside slavery) were rare before the feudal system. Work hours were not distinguishable from leisure time, work was done for the sake of the produce.

Agricultural workers entered an exchange economy which led to the social division of labour, the division between producers and consumers. Industry became increasingly mechanized and technology increasingly sophisticated. Towns grew and people moved from primary production to secondary then tertiary industries. Industrialized work disciplines and ethics were inculcated, work became machine paced. Work took place away from home, changing family and social dynamics. Mass production methods led to reduced knowledge requirements and more recent automation to the development of increasingly high skill and specific knowledge occupations.

Modern merchandizing methods and consumer credit systems exploit mass markets, and presume continuing income therefore continuous work. Most workers consume beyond subsistence levels and see themselves as a consumer and producer.

In the 1990s we have a society which functions at a global level in which technology increasingly impacts on both our work and leisure activities. With increasing long-term unemployment there is an ever widening gap between the rich and the poor. Employment structures are changing with the development of job-sharing systems, increased flexibility, consultancy work, employment contracts, opportunities for early retirement, and home-based work. Working hours are reducing and industry is operating within the 'global village'. New technology is rapidly being integrated into manufacturing, service industries and everyday life as we move to an automated currency and information technology work base.

People are increasingly searching for intrinsic non-economic motivations and demanding more interesting and satisfying work. The line between work and leisure is again beginning to blur and systems such as the Internet offer work opportunities which are only beginning to be realized. We are experiencing the development of a new age and a new work pattern.

Acknowledgments

Thanks to Chris Fitzgerald for permission to use his photograph; Paul Gardiner for photographic assistance; Philip Meyer for his advice regarding content; and Technisearch for their invaluable administration support.

References and further reading

Ahlburg, D. A. (1986). The social costs of unemployment. In *Work Leisure and Technology*, (Castle, R., Lewis, D., Mangan, J. eds) Cheshire: Longman.

Anonymous (1987). *Children at Work: Special Health Risks*. World Health Organization Technical Report Series, Geneva, Switzerland, World Health Organization, No. 756.

Arendt, Hannah (1958). *The Human Condition*, University of Chicago Press.

Argyle, M. (1989). The history of work. In *The Social Psychology of Work*, 2nd edn, Penguin Books.

Badran, Hoda, Chairperson, International Committee of the Rights of the Child (1995). Children pay a high price for cheap labour. *Report to the Progress of Nations*, Child Rights Section, UNICEF.

Barnes, R. M. (1963). *Motion and Time Study; Design and Measurement of Work*, 5th edn, John Wiley and Sons.

Butler, F. and Roberts, C. (1984). Women's employment and unemployment. *Ergonomics*, **27**, 585–595.

Chamberlain, G. (1983). Pregnant women at work. *Lancet*, **1** (8313), 228–230.

Cox, S. and Cox, T. (1984). Women at work: summary and overview. *Ergonomics*, **27**, 597–605.

Creighton, B. and Stewart, A. (1990). *Labor Law: An Introduction*. The Federation Press.

Game, A. and Pringle, R. (1983). *Gender at Work*. Sydney: Allen and Unwin.

Grandjean, E. (1988). *Fitting the Task to the Man*. Taylor and Francis.

Herzberg, F. (1966). *Work and the Nature of Man*. World Publishing.

Herzberg, F., Mausner, B. and Snyderman, B. (1959). *The Motivation to Work*, Wiley.

I.L.O. (1946) *The War and Women's Employment, the experience of the United Kingdom and the United States*. Montreal: International labor office.

Jones, B. (1982). *Sleepers, Wake!* Oxford: Oxford University Press.

Kogi, K., Sen, R.N. (1987). Third World Ergonomics. *International Reviews in Ergonomics*. Current Trends in Human Factors Research and Practice, Vol. 1, (D.J. Oborne, ed.) Taylor and Francis.

Marx, K. (1961). *Economic and Philosophic Manuscripts of 1844*. New York.

Marx, K. (1976). *Capital, vol. 1*. [1867], (tr. Ben Fowkes), London: Penguin.

Shahnavaz, H. (1992). Ergonomics in Vietnam. In *Ergonomics in Action*, Vol.2, April, pp. 133–135. Oxford: Butterworth-Heinemann.

Taylor, F.W. (1964). *The Principles of Scientific Management [1911]*, Harper and Row.

Thompson, E.P. (1967). Time, Work-Discipline and Industrial Capitalism. *Past and Present*, No. 38, pp. 56–97.

World Health Organization. (1980). *International Classification of Impairment, Disability and Handicap*. World Health Organization, Geneva.

2

An Historical Perspective of Work Practice Services

Catherine Paterson

Learning objectives

At the end of this chapter the reader should be able to:

1 Discuss how sociological, political, economic and technological factors have both stimulated and deterred the development of rehabilitation services.
2 Recognize the importance of the international exchange of information and experience in the development of rehabilitation services.
3 Trace the events which have affected the development of work-related occupational therapy.
4 Outline the relationship of scientific management and ergonomics to the role of the occupational therapist.

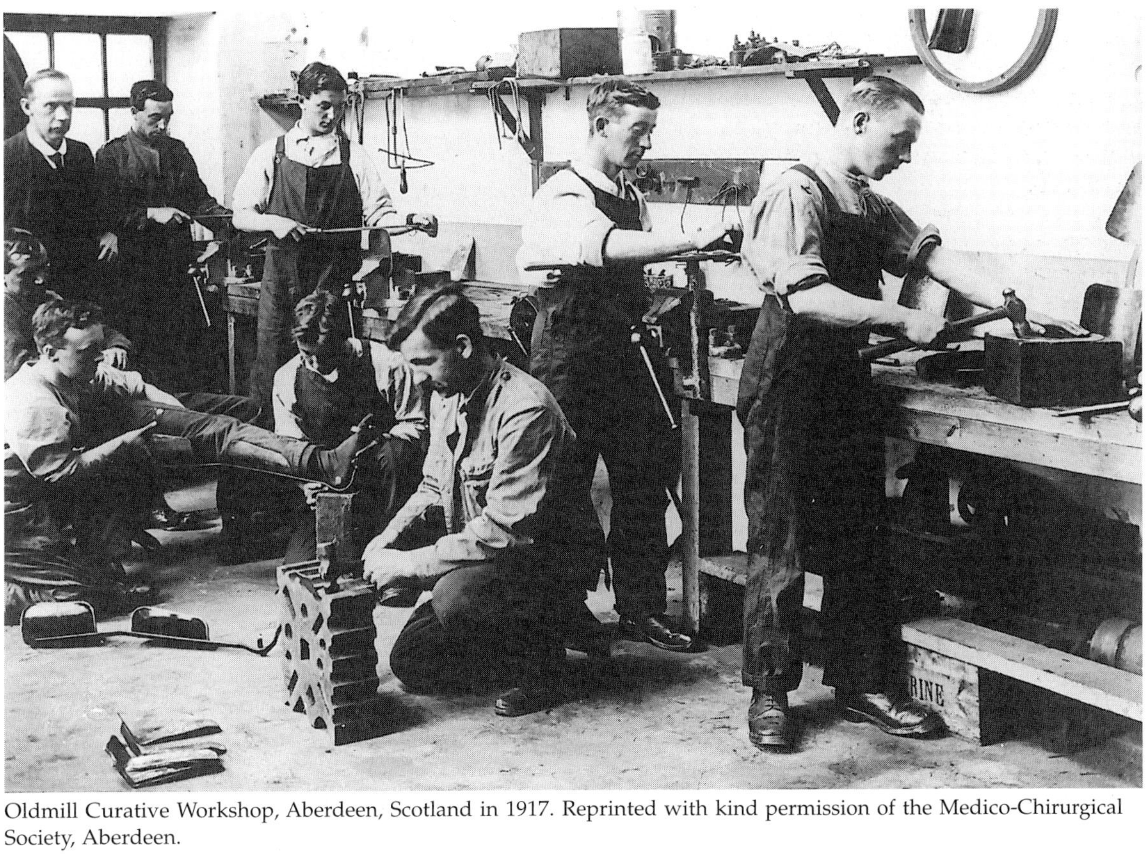

Oldmill Curative Workshop, Aberdeen, Scotland in 1917. Reprinted with kind permission of the Medico-Chirurgical Society, Aberdeen.

Abstract

Work, especially remunerative employment, has been both an integral part of the treatment process and the aim of rehabilitation during the past two centuries in many countries.

In this chapter vocational rehabilitation is explored in relation to: moral treatment in nineteenth-century asylums; work cures in sanatoria; curative workshops for the war-wounded; and, finally, the rehabilitation services for the civilian and service casualties of the Second World War. These were essentially medical-led developments. However the profession of occupational therapy has also been influenced by industrial practice, particularly through the study of scientific management, industrial psychology and physiology, and ergonomics.

The history of work-based practice and the emergence of the profession of occupational therapy is discussed with reference to many complex sociological, political, economic and technological factors.

Introduction

This chapter aims to demonstrate, through significant events during the past two centuries, how sociological, political, economic and technological factors have influenced work practice services in general and work-related occupational therapy in particular. It also demonstrates how the role of the occupational therapist has been limited by lack of numbers, and has been both encouraged and restricted by other professionals.

The nature of work has changed dramatically over the past two centuries. The Industrial Revolution resulted in agricultural workers seeking employment in towns in the new factories dominated by machines. Scientific management with its time-and-motion study, fragmentation of tasks, conveyor belts and production lines further restricted the worker's control over his or her own work pattern; and, more recently, computer-based technology has replaced many manual and clerical jobs. These technological changes have all influenced the types of illness and injury affecting workers–from the tuberculosis of the cotton factories to the repetitive strain injury of the VDU operator. Changes in transport and the technology of war have had similar effects.

Advances in medicine have influenced survival, level of permanent disability, and length of convalescence and rehabilitation. An open fracture in the nineteenth century could lead to death, in the First World War to amputation and prolonged rehabilitation, and in the latter part of the twentieth century to internal fixation and minimal disruption of function.

The demand for labour and society's attitude to disability, particularly during war, has stimulated the development of both the services for injured workers and service personnel and the underpinning theory; conversely rehabilitation services have declined during times of high unemployment. The terminology related to those with disability and the services provided for them have constantly changed, as words have developed negative connotations, e.g. cripple, or when new terms have been required to describe new services.

However during the two centuries some principles have remained relatively constant. The acknowledgement, at least by some, that poor working conditions can lead to illness and injury; that work, which is meaningful, rewarding and not overly fatiguing, contributes to human happiness; that there is a relationship between psychosocial and physical health; and that work can be the means as well as the end of the process of rehabilitation. A recurrent theme, also, has been the international exchange of information and experience, which has influenced developments throughout the world.

These principles have been specifically explored, in this chapter, in relation to: moral treatment in nineteenth-century asylums; work cures in sanatoria for tuberculosis; curative workshops for the war-wounded in the First World War, and the rehabilitation services for the civilian and service casualties of the Second World War. The literature relating to these topics provides a rich source of material, through which the fundamental principles of vocational rehabilitation and resettlement and the origins of the emergent profession of occupational therapy can be traced.

Moral treatment

Work as a therapeutic agent was first introduced as an aspect of moral treatment of the insane in the late eighteenth and early nineteenth centuries, a reform which Bockhoven (1971), Bing (1981) and Peloquin (1988, 1993) have associated with the development of occupational therapy. The names most associated with moral treatment are Phillipe Pinel (1745–1826) and William Tuke (1732–1822), although others, particularly Sir William Ellis (1780–1839), were especially interested in the role of work.

Pinel is renowned for 'striking off the chains' of the patients of the Bicêtre during the French Revolution. He advocated the use of occupation and recorded in 1806 that 'it was pleasing to observe the silence and tranquillity which prevailed in the asylum at Bicêtre, when nearly all the patients were supplied by the tradesmen of Paris with employments which fixed their attention, and allured them to exertion by the prospect of a trifling gain' (Pinel, 1806: 193) Tuke, a tea merchant, founded the Retreat at York, England, in 1796 for the care of mentally ill Quakers. From the start the patients were encouraged to be involved in domestic activities and outdoor exercise, however an attempt in the 1830s to extend casual gardening to 'spade husbandry' was not wholly successful probably because the patients were mainly from a trading, artisan or professional background, which made them consider such work as unappealing if not degrading (Digby, 1985). However Pinel and Tuke were more concerned with reforming regimes of care within asylums than a return to employment of those discharged.

On the contrary, Ellis, who was medical superintendent of county lunatic asylums for pauper patients at Wakefield and later at Hanwell in England, was concerned that poverty and unemployment lead to insanity and that insanity in turn aggravated poverty. Ellis successfully introduced means to enable patients to gain employment on discharge. During their time in hospital the men were encouraged either to follow their own trade or to learn a new one from the keepers or tradesmen employed about the institution (Ellis, 1838).

The success of these developments, particularly at the Retreat, greatly influenced psychiatry in North America, particularly in the establishment of Friend's Asylums for the Insane at Frankford in 1817 and the Bloomingdale Asylum in New York in 1821 (Licht, 1948). Occupation was advocated by such influential psychiatrists as Thomas Kirkbride (1809–1883), the organizer and first secretary of the American Psychiatric Association, and Benjamin Rush (1745–1813), who wrote the first textbook on psychiatry in the United States (Licht, 1948). A direct descendant of Dr Benjamin Rush was Dr William Rush Dunton (1893–1966), medical superintendent of the Sheppard and Enoch Pratt Hospital, who became one of the founders of the profession of occupational therapy (Licht, 1967).

The use of occupation in the treatment and management of the mentally ill in the nineteenth century greatly influenced the development of the profession of occupational therapy especially during the first half of the twentieth century, however parallel and complementary developments were taking place for patients with physical conditions.

Development of work cures in tuberculosis

As well as asylums for the mentally ill, the Victorian reformers of the nineteenth century were concerned with public health measures to control infectious diseases such as typhus, cholera and smallpox. They also built fever hospitals for the isolation of people with infectious diseases, including open-air sanatoria for patients with tuberculosis. Up until the middle of the twentieth century, tuberculosis was a major cause of death and disability, and even when the patient did recover, other workers' fear of infection often led to prolonged unemployment.

Open-air sanatoria for rest and sunshine were established from the 1850s, however in 1888 the sanatorium at Nordrach-Baden in Germany was successfully founded on the additional principle of subjecting the patient to absolute rest until his fever had subsided, and then exercising the body very gradually until he could go through a day involving light work without adverse reaction. This regime was adopted by Marcus Patterson (1870–1932) in England, who developed the theory of 'autoinoculation', that is the patient inoculated himself with small doses of toxins produced by the graduated exercise to stimulate antibodies. Patterson's theory, though later discredited, was widely acclaimed at the time (Singer and Underwood, 1962).

Also influential was the Papworth Village Settlement which was founded in 1917 by P.C. (later Sir Pendrill) Varrier-Jones (1883–1941). It consisted of a hospital, sanatorium, and village settlement with industries attached. After the acute phase, the patients would live in the village settlement with their families and work in the industries at trade-union pay. These industries included carpentry, joinery, cabinet making, boot making, tailoring, portmanteau and attaché-case making, printing, sign writing and jewellery making. For psychological as well as economic reasons, Varrier-Jones aimed to make the industries at Papworth a commercial enterprise and not dependent on charity. Papworth Industries was to become a very successful enterprise indeed, expanding from a turnover of £400 in 1928 to over £130,000 in 1937 (Bryder, 1988).

This segregation of the tuberculous family from the rest of society was controversial, and the commercial aspects were daunting. In any case doctors preferred more medical rather than occupational regimes of treatment, and Bryder has argued that the challenge to work therapy from surgical intervention during the 1930s was due as much to professional interests and economic and social pressures as to any superiority of surgery over conservative treatment (Bryder, 1988).

The use of work as an integral part of treatment did not appear to be a feature of sanatoria in North America. J. R. Dingley, medical superintendent of a sanatorium in Sussex, toured the United States and Canada in 1930, where he found no patients doing 'grade work' and only one facility for 'aftercare', which was at the Altro Workshop in New York. Dingley reported that the Altro managers considered that patients turned out of American sanatoria were too nervous to work, and it took the Altro management a long time to convince the patients of the curative value of regular employment (Bryder, 1988).

However, in 1914, George E. Barton (1871–1923) had opened Consolation House in Clifton Springs, New York, a school, workshop and vocational bureau for convalescents. Barton, an architect, contracted tuberculosis in 1901 and was obliged to rest, as he did periodically for recurrent attacks. In 1912, his left foot was amputated after frost bite, and he developed a hysterical paralysis of the left side of his body. He helped his own recovery in Clifton Springs by manual work, primarily carpentry and gardening, and was so successful that he decided to devote the rest of his life to the reclamation of the sick and disabled. Barton was one of the six founder members who assembled in Consolation House on 15 March 1917 to sign the certificate of incorporation of the National Society for the Promotion of Occupational Therapy, renamed the American Association of Occupational Therapists in 1923 (Licht, 1967).

Of the signatories, two others, Thomas B. Kidner and Dr William Rush Dunton were interested in the 'reconstruction' or 're-education' of the 'cripple', and the lessons to be learned from scientific management in that process, especially since Kidner was already involved in the re-education of Canadian soldiers and the United States was about to join the allies in the First World War.

Scientific management and the First World War 1914–1918

In the late nineteenth century, industrial processes began to be studied in an organized fashion, using time-and-motion studies, and what was termed 'scientific management' was developed by two American engineers, Frederick W. Taylor (1856–1915) and Frank B. Gilbreth (1868–1924). Scientific management not only revolutionized industry, but influenced both the practice of surgery and the re-education of the crippled. As Cooter (1993) has demonstrated, 'concerns with efficiency and economy in the military were becoming analogous to those of modern industry', at a time when the casualties of the First World War were causing a manpower crisis.

Taylor worked in the Midvale steelworks of Philadelphia where, in the early 1880s, he began a series of time studies designed to increase the productivity of the machine shop. He then turned his attention to the workers and introduced time- and-motion study as an aid to efficient management. In *The Principles of Scientific Management* (1911) Taylor demonstrated the analysis of the work process around the machines. By sub-dividing tasks into their component parts, and timing the components, unnecessary movements could be eliminated and the whole job could be completed more efficiently (Merkle, 1980).

Pheasant (1991) maintained that Taylorism – the fragmentation of the production process into discrete short-cycle tasks, led to work tasks which were unsatisfactory. Not only were they psychologically unrewarding and socially alienating, they frequently involved fixed working postures or the repetitive loading of isolated muscle groups.

Gilbreth, a disciple of Taylor, worked with his wife Lillian (1879–1972), a teacher and industrial psychologist. They made detailed laboratory studies in motion, which included using cinematography, with a specially devised clock and a cross-sectioned background, to analyse activity. From the film, the basic elements involved in the work could be identified and recorded on a Simultaneous Cycle Motion Chart, using 'therbligs' ('Gilbreth' reversed) which were symbols to depict actions such as: find, select, grasp, position and assemble (Gilbreth, 1915).

Lillian, in particular, was a pioneer in making the environment easier for the physically handicapped, while her husband was greatly concerned with the re-education of the industrial worker, interests which naturally embraced the re-education of crippled soldiers during and after the First World War. At a time of great shortage of workers, Gilbreth maintained that: 'the world needs the work of every person existing and able to be a producer, but most important of all is the cripple's own need for constructive activity, and for feeling that he is still able to do "a man's job" in the world' (Gilbreth, 1917: 278). Gilbreth considered that this was best achieved by using a simultaneous-motion cycle chart and by providing some change that would adapt the work to the man. He maintained that this change: 'may consist principally of rearranging the surroundings, equipment and tools. It may consist of slight modifications of machinery. It may consist of changing the method by which the work is done, that is, of allowing some other work member of the worker's body to perform the motions that formerly were made by the member that is now maimed or missing. In any case the need is for invention' (Gilbreth, 1915: 282).

Gilbreth visited hospitals in Europe in 1914 and 1915 to analyse surgeons' work. He also met with disabled veterans and learned of the ground-breaking research of Professor Jules Amar. On his return, the Gilbreths presented papers to several professional groups on 'the re-education of the crippled soldier', including the founding conference of the National Society for the Promotion of Occupational Therapy. During the conference, Frank Gilbreth and Jules Amar were elected honorary members of the Society, and they met with Barton and Dunton (Creighton, 1992). Gilbreth later recommended Barton's book *Re-education* in relation to the need for psychotherapy for the crippled soldier (Gilbreth, 1918).

Professor Jules Amar, a French physiologist, and Dr Jean Camus, a French fracture expert, were influenced by Taylor and applied his principles to medicine. The work of both was translated into English at the end of the war (Cooter, 1993). Amar was appointed by his government to investigate scientific management and apply its principles to the training and re-employment of wounded soldiers (Creighton, 1992). In his book *The Physiology of Industrial Organisation and the Re-employment of the Disabled* (1918) Amar discussed his research on the physiology of work, and how he used his extensive apparatus, e.g. the ergometric cycle, for the measurement and graphic recording of muscular activity, expenditure of energy, respiration and biochemical indications of fatigue. He also demonstrated how these measurements were used in the assessment and in the 'professional education' of amputees by giving what is now known as biofeedback. Amar outlined three stages in re-education:

> During the first period, that of functional re-education, it is necessary to analyse the movements of the subject, in order to determine his functional condition, to restore, as far as possible, his former work capacity, and finally, to make sure that prolonged exertion does not threaten to impair the resistance of the organism (Amar, 1918: 230)

The second stage was the fitting of a prothetic appliance 'not to replace the lost limb or segment of a limb, but to supplement or replace a lost or badly impaired function'

(Amar, 1918: 257). Amar developed his 'Worker's arm' with Parade Hand and universal grip or pliers. The final stage, which led directly to re-employment was the stage of 'professional re-education' in special workshops.

Dunton compared Gilbreth's method with that of Professor Amar:

> Mr Gilbreth believes in fitting the machine to the man, making whatever additions or adaptations are necessary to enable the cripple to do efficient work. Professor Amar on the other hand makes his prosthetic apparatus in such a way that the man is adapted to the machine. It would seem that Mr. Gilbreth's is the better principle. (Dunton, 1919: 107–8)

Gilbreth's adaptations of machines were probably best suited to the production lines of North-American industry, but the methods adopted by Amar were probably more suited to the majority of the amputees in France who worked on the land and required strength in the stump and a simple prosthesis to grip or steady tools and materials. However Amar's use of scientific measurement during re-education, due to its complexity, was not used extensively, although the use of curative workshops under medical direction was developed throughout France, Britain, Canada and the United States.

Curative workshops in the First World War 1914–1918

Early in the First World War, the large numbers of casualties in the German and Allied armies, combined with the shortage of civilian manpower, forced the European governments to develop services for vocational rehabilitation, particularly for amputees. In Britain, the two most significant people in this vocational rehabilitation of the war wounded, through the establishment of curative workshops, were Sir Robert Jones (1857–1933), founder of orthopaedic surgery, and King Manuel (1889–1932), the deposed king of Portugal, who lived in exile in England.

At the beginning of the war, Jones developed an orthopaedic service at the Alder Hey Hospital outside Liverpool, to eliminate military 'wastage'. The success of his treatment, based on continuity of care, with the emphasis on the restoration of physical function, led to his appointment as Military Director of Orthopaedics in March 1916. By the end of the war, under Jones' direction, twenty special military hospitals with some 20 000 beds had been established in Britain, the first of which was at Shepherd's Bush, London (Cooter, 1993).

Manuel became preoccupied with the plight of the disabled after establishing a private officers' hospital at Brighton in 1914 (Cooter, 1993). In late 1915, under the auspices of the Joint War Committee of the Red Cross and Order of St John, he visited French and Belgium hospitals and was particularly impressed by the workshops at the Anglo-Belgian Hospital at Rouen. He was also influenced by the Canadian Hospital at Ramsgate (Manuel, 1918). Manuel and Jones became allies, and Manuel persuaded the War Office to establish the first curative workshop at Shepherd's Bush in 1916, having induced the Joint Committee to provide the first £1000 (Cooter, 1993). Ten further curative workshops were set up attached to special military hospitals throughout Britain (Manuel, 1918).

Jones considered that the governing principle in regard to curative work was founded on the knowledge that voluntary movements were of much more value than passive movements:

> The exercises practised in the curative workshop are of two kinds – the direct and indirect – a screwdriver may be employed to supinate the arm, a saw to exercise the elbow, painting to move the shoulder – but with an ingenious instructor, special ways are constantly devised in order to directly affect the joint involved. The indirect method of attack is often employed. For example, when a man with a stiff ankle is set to plane or saw wood, he unconsciously uses the ankle as he gets interested in the work which his hand is doing. (Jones, 1921: x)

Of equal importance was the psychological benefit of meaningful occupation to men who could have spent as long as eighteen months in hospital (Manuel, 1918). As Jones observed in the Preface to *Notes on Military Orthopaedics*:

> Those of us who have any imagination cannot fail to realize the difference in atmosphere and *morale* in hospitals where the patients have nothing to do but smoke, play cards, or be entertained, from that found in those where for part of every day they have regular, useful and productive work. (Jones, 1917: iii)

However Cooter concluded that:

> Perhaps the most important feature of the workshops to win the favour of the War Office was their very considerable economy to the State. In the name of occupational therapy, ... they manufactured all the splints, surgical boots, and other appliances required ... At Shepherd's Bush, those assigned to the workshops also performed all the maintenance work for the hospital, and carried out the wiring and plumbing for the installation of the electrotherapeutic and hydrotherapeutic departments. (Cooter, 1993: 118)

Canada was also developing services for disabled soldiers. Thomas B. Kidner (1866–1932), a London-born architect and Director of Technical Education for Calgary, was appointed in 1915 as Vocational Secretary of the Canadian Military Hospitals Commission. During his tenure he developed a system of vocational rehabilitation for disabled veterans in Canada (Reed and Sanderson, 1980). Dunton recorded that this included 'teachers giving instruction in various crafts, stenography and typewriting, drawing, shop arithmetic, and in fact, anything which will aid the patient to fit himself to earn a living' (1919: 108).

Because of his position and expertise, Barton invited Kidner to become a founder member of the Society for the Promotion of Occupational Therapy in 1917, and early in 1918, Winifred Brainerd, who was in charge of occupations at the Sanatorium at Clifton Springs (adjacent to Barton's Consolation House), went to Toronto to help plan and participate in the first course for 'instructors in bed-side occupation'. When these emergency courses were discontinued in the summer of 1919, over 350 young women had been trained and posted to military hospitals throughout Canada (Robinson, 1981).

In 1918, Kidner accepted the position of Special Advisor on Rehabilitation to the United States Federal Board of Vocational Education (Reed and Sanderson, 1980). In the States the system of orthopaedic surgery, restoration of function and vocational rehabilitation developed by Jones and Manuel was adopted by two orthopaedists, Joel Goldthwait and Elliott Brackett, who were responsible for creating the Division of Orthopaedic Surgery within the Medical Department of the Army and for organizing a reconstruction programme for soldiers who had been disabled (Gutman, 1995). A letter from Dr Herbert Hall of Devereaux Mansions, Marblehead, Mass., written early in 1918 to one of the committees starting a school of occupational therapy, outlined the process of rehabilitation to be followed in the United States:

> The government plan divides the rehabilitation of the crippled soldiers into three parts, which may merge into each other. First, the bedside occupations such as weaving, wood-working, etc. The effect of these is purely medical and not commercial. The next step is the curative workshop where the patient has opportunities to use tools in the machine shop. This stage is intended to restore the functions of the nerves and muscles. The patient can make splints and orthopaedic apparatus. This stage is not intended to be vocation, the aim being still medical. The third stage is reached when the workshop has accomplished its purpose. The soldier then comes under the Bureau of Vocational Education where the individual is studied with the view of giving him training in technical schools, from this the man is placed in a trade or profession. (Spackman, 1968: 68–9)

In order to carry out the first two stages, 'reconstruction aides' of two kinds – physiotherapy and occupational therapy – were recruited (Gutman, 1995). Approximately 1685 reconstruction aids were eventually in service, of whom about 460 served abroad (Low, 1992). The occupational therapy aides were 'to teach various forms of simple handcraft to patients in military hospitals and other sanitary formations of the Army, especially to those patients in the orthopaedic wards as well as to the patients suffering from nervous and mental diseases' (Low, 1992: 38).

At first there was no training, the occupational therapy aides were skilled teachers of craft or commercial subjects with no medical background. However initial intensive courses, lasting from six to twelve weeks were run in Chicago, New York and Boston, and eventually at twenty three other schools (Hopkins, 1988). The National Society for the Promotion of Occupational Therapy approved the war courses in both the States and Canada. Many of the schools for the training of reconstruction aides were expanded and continued as approved training programmes, however most closed permanently at the end of the war (Low, 1992).

Gutman (1995) argued that the development of occupational therapy was heavily influenced by the relationship that evolved early between orthopaedists and reconstruction aides, this affiliation marking an early willingness by occupational therapists to accept the medical model as one guide for clinical practice. As Low has demonstrated, the occupational therapy aides performed their duties in settings that were under the strict supervision of physicians:

> To maintain a connection with medicine and the curative aspects of activity, the aides relied on physicians to direct the selection of activity. The physicians accepted and supported the aides as technical assistants. The female aides were nurturers who provided diversional activity that, while very important to successful convalescence, was not to be considered on a par with vocational training that was handled by men. (1992: 42)

It was to be some considerable time before there was a body of professional, qualified occupational therapists who could challenge this situation.

Developments during interwar period

Although the First World War had given the impetus to the new field of occupational therapy in the States, its development after the war was slow. Occupational therapy programmes and personnel in all US army hospitals were reduced until there were only three employed occupational therapists (Hopkins, 1988). However, the needs of disabled ex-servicemen also focused attention on the infinitely greater number of handicapped civilians. This led to the Vocational Rehabilitation Act of 1920, which defined rehabilitation as 'return to remunerative employment'. By 1938, all 48 states were engaged in rehabilitation of the physically disabled. However most occupational therapists at this time were primarily working with the mentally ill (Cromwell, 1985).

In Canada, the demobilized occupational therapy reconstruction aides were involved in the opening of the Curative Workshop in Toronto in 1920, and another in Winnipeg in 1922, as a place where 'men (veterans) of reduced capacity for work can make a living still, if sheltered means of work is provided for them' (Driver, 1968). The Ontario Society of Occupational Therapy was formed in 1921, and it was instrumental in persuading the University of Toronto to introduce a two-year diploma course, which was started in 1926, the same year in which the Canadian Association of Occupational Therapists was established. However the Depression severely restricted developments: from 1929 unemployment in Canada was devastating, and the out of work included occupational therapists (Driver, 1968).

In 1933 Miss Amy de Brisay, a graduate of the Toronto emergency course in 1919, and head of the occupational therapy department at the Toronto General Hospital, was invited to go to Edinburgh for a year to establish a physical occupational therapy department at the Astley Ainslie Hospital in Edinburgh (Driver, 1968). Several Canadians served after her in Edinburgh, and in 1937 Miss Gloria Langmaid helped to establish the first school of occupational therapy in Scotland, based on the course at the University of Toronto (Groundes Peace, 1957).

Meantime in England, occupational therapy was introduced by Dr Elizabeth Casson (1881–1954), a physician with a diploma in psychological medicine. While on holiday in 1926, she visited Bloomingdale Hospital, New York, and the Boston School of Occupational Therapy, and the idea of an English school took shape in her mind. She opened a residential psychiatric clinic in Bristol in 1929 and the Dorset House School of Occupational Therapy in 1930, with Miss Constance Tebbit, who had trained in Philadelphia, as its first principal. In 1939, Dr Casson opened the Allendale Curative Workshop for outpatients suffering from varying forms of physical disease or disability, which had an important role to play during the Second World War (Casson, 1955).

Rehabilitation in the Second World War 1939–1945

Like the First World War, the Second World War necessitated the development of emergency hospitals and rehabilitation services for the wounded, thus providing the stimulus for the further development of occupational therapy. The Official Medical History of the Second World War in the UK includes this account:

> After 1918 the orthopaedic centres were dismantled and occupational therapy again reverted, for the most part, to the mental hospital service. On the outbreak of the Second World War, however, the need for providing the best means of rehabilitation after injury assumed a new significance, for not only were there the Service personnel to be considered but also the large numbers of members of the civilian community who were in danger of being incapacitated by air raids. It was accordingly decided that at all the special centres provided under the Emergency Medical Services for the reception and treatment of disabling injuries – orthopaedic centres, long-term fracture hospitals, spinal and head injury centres, neurosis centres, etc. – occupational therapy departments should be built and equipped as an integral part of the scheme. . . .
>
> Male handicap instructors and members of the Educational Corps were chiefly responsible for this work, together with a few trained occupational therapists who had joined the Women's Auxiliary Services. . . . The chief difficulty in developing occupational therapy was not the shortage of accommodation nor lack of materials, but the great scarcity of trained therapists. (Balme, 1953: 730–1)

In 1940, the Allendale Curative Workshop was moved from Bristol, away from the bombing, to Barnsley Hall Hospital, Bromsgrove, Worcestershire and became the model for occupational therapy departments in the Emergency Medical Services hospitals throughout England. The Dorset House School was also relocated and over 200 candidates were trained on emergency courses (Peto, 1955).

The impact of the war was soon felt throughout the Commonwealth. From 1943 to 1946 over 82 Canadian occupational therapists served in the Army, Navy and British Emergency Medical Service, of whom about 47 served overseas, some in Scotland (Robinson, 1981). Miss Amy de Brisay returned with other Canadians to help the newly qualified Scottish occupational therapists staff the emergency hospitals, and to set up a rehabilitation centre for miners (Groundes Peace, 1957).

In Australia, there were only three qualified occupational therapists at the start of the war – Ethil Francis, who graduated from the Philadelphia School in 1933; Sylvia Docker, who was already a physiotherapist and who trained in London in 1934; and Joyce Keam, who trained in London in 1937. An emergency course was set up in 1942 in Sydney with Sylvia Docker as its director, and by 1945, 54 students – both civilian and military – had gained their diplomas. Major Joyce Keam became the first occupational therapy advisor to the Australian Army. She concluded in the *Bulletin* the newsletter of the club which was the precursor of the Australian Association of Occupational Therapists, in June 1949, that:

> Occupational therapy in military hospitals suffered from the inevitable disadvantages attendant upon the pioneering of a new profession in an emergency situation. The ignorance of many medical men regarding the specific prescribing of occupational therapy and the inexperience of newly qualified therapists, were perhaps the greatest handicaps. Added to these were the difficulties in the early days of obtaining adequate accommodation, equipment and supplies.
>
> On the other hand, military hospitals provided the field for an Australian wide demonstration of occupational therapy on a scale which would have been impossible in civilian hospitals for many years to come. (Anderson and Bell, 1988: 10)

Work went on until twelve months after the war ended when the military hospitals were gradually taken over by the Repatriation Department. Keam then worked with the Department of Post-War Reconstruction to set up rehabilitation centres in each state to cater for ex-service personnel, whose illness or injuries were not attributed to war service, a scheme which was eventually taken over by the Commonwealth Department of Social Services (Anderson and Bell, 1988).

Parallel developments took place in the United States when it entered the war. A reconditioning programme in the Armed Forces was established according to the War Department Training Manual, 8–291 on 'Occupational Therapy':

> To accelerate the return of convalescent patients in the highest state of physical and mental efficiency consistent with the capabilities and the type of duty to which they are being returned . . .

> or to provide for their return to civilian life in the highest possible degree of physical fitness, well orientated in the responsibilities of citizenship and prepared to adjust successfully to social and vocational pursuits. (1944: 1)

However not all UK surgeons approved of this model. Particularly in plastic surgery, real war work was considered more appropriate. Between reparative operations the men were placed in factories.

> The officer in charge of this made contact with the war factories from which many of the civilian casualties had come. Rehabilitation workshops were set up in these factories with which the surgeon kept closely in touch. Injured workmen and others were enabled to work on machines producing war materials, and modifications were made to assist in the re-education of damaged hands and legs, and the value of such adjuvant to the usual post-operative procedures was immediately apparent. The scheme was enlarged to bring real work to those men in the wards who could not immediately go to the factory. The result was that the patient was able to do remunerative and useful work from a day or two after his injury; production was increased; and best of all, the duration of the disability was materially shortened. (Cope, 1953: 334)

Occupational therapists themselves would have preferred to use more realistic activities, but their choice was limited.

> In the physical field the choice was controlled largely by the materials made available through the special government priority system. These were mainly those for 'handicrafts' – in some cases almost too light and diversional in the eyes of keen therapists. A second controlling factor was that the occupations were deliberately limited by the government authorities to 'crafts' and excursions into the realms of 'trade' were not permitted. (MacDonald, 1957: 30)

It was during this period that textbooks primarily by occupational therapists for occupational therapists were first published. E. Mary MacDonald, principal of the Dorset School of Occupational Therapy, in collaboration with a medical colleague Norah Haworth, produced the *Theory of Occupational Therapy* in 1940. John H. C. Colson, a physiotherapist as well as an occupational therapist, published *The Rehabilitation of the Injured – Occupational Therapy* in 1945. Both texts included sections on resettlement in industry, stressed the grading of activities from light to very heavy and placed much emphais on the analysis of activities for their biomechanical effects, a process which Licht later termed 'kinetic analysis' (Licht, 1958).

Post-war development

Just as after the First World War, when the desire to provide integrated services for injured workers was thwarted by the economic depression of the 1920s and 1930s, so the stimulus for rehabilitation services could not be maintained immediately after the Second World War, but as countries have recovered economically the profession of occupational therapy has shown steady growth worldwide.

The political climate in post-war Britain led to further development of the Welfare State. In 1948 most occupational therapists found themselves working within the National Health Service, when it took over the hospitals, particularly the mental hospitals and those general hospitals which had been part of the Emergency Medical Services during the war. However there was little money in post-war Britain for major investments in the new health service.

In the United States the 1943 amendments to the Vocational Rehabilitation Act of 1920 had precipitated a whole wave of rehabilitation activity in health-care settings reinforcing the concept of returning people to 'remunerative employment' as the original definition of rehabilitation decreed. However according to Cromwell (1985) occupational therapists largely abandoned their interest in work-related programming. Instead the essential purpose and focus of programming was on the reduction of disability from acute illness or injury. This included the use of crafts as a communication process in psychiatry and the development of assistive devises for activities of daily living programmes. Spackman (1968) considered that this fragmentation of the occupational therapist's role was directly related to the lack of occupational therapists, and later writers viewed this period as one of professional derailment, when the profession moved away from the values of the founders to more reductionist practice (Shannon, 1977).

In Australia the development of the profession was greatly influenced by the appointment of two American Directors of Training – Marjorie Fish in Sydney in 1948 and Doris Wilkins in Melbourne in 1950 (Anderson and Bell, 1988). Sadie Philcox pointed out in her 1968 Sylvia Docker lecture that:

> When the Victorian [Melbourne] School commenced in 1948, there was a distinctly new concept of training brought to bear on its organisation due, most probably, to the influence of new procedures required for the practice of rehabilitation medicine. There was more emphasis on an understanding of work demands and trade practices. (Anderson and Bell, 1988: 106)

The slow but steady expansion in the numbers of occupational therapists worldwide throughout the 1940s created the desire for the establishment of a formal network for the international exchange of information and experience.

World Federation of Occupational Therapists

The idea of the World Federation of Occupational Therapists was conceived in Sweden in 1951, when a number of occupational therapists were attending a conference of the International Society for the Welfare of Cripples – now Rehabilitation International. A preparatory commission met in 1952 with representatives or letters of support from the founders: Australia, Canada, Denmark, India, Israel, New Zealand, South Africa, the United Kingdom and the United States of America. The Federation was launched at the First International Congress in Edinburgh in 1954 (Mendez, 1986).

The conference was attended by over 200 delegates from 21 countries. There were five major themes reflecting the interests of the time: tuberculosis, poliomyelitis, psychiatry, cerebral palsy, and rehabilitation and resettlement. Speakers from the UK, Canada and the USA discussed rehabilitation services in their countries (WFOT, 1964), although this does not imply that services were not developed elsewhere.

The World Federation of Occupational Therapists has grown since 1954 from nine to 44 member countries, and an international congress takes place every four years. In this way the international influences, which were so evident in the spread of moral treatment on both sides of the Atlantic in the nineteenth century, can be carried on worldwide into the twenty-first century.

Development of ergonomics

Even before the Industrial Revolution, the relationship between what is now termed ergonomic factors and health was recognized. For example Bernardino Ramazzini (1633–1714) of Modena, who is generally recognized as the father of occupational medicine, described a range of occupational diseases, including repetitive strain injury in scribes and notaries. He wrote in 1713:

> The maladies that afflict the clerks aforesaid arise from three causes: first, constant sitting, secondly the incessant movement of the hand and always in the same direction, thirdly the strain on the mind from the effort not to disfigure the books. (Pheasant, 1991: 7)

However adapting 'man to work' and 'work to man' has been mainly a feature of the twentieth century, through the study of scientific management, industrial psychology and physiology and through the multiprofessional applied discipline of human-factors engineering or ergonomics.

The work of Amar on industrial physiology – the study of human energy expenditure and fatigue – and the work of Taylor and Gilbreth on scientific management – the elimination of waste in industry – has already been discussed. The manpower shortages of the First World War ensured their international recognition by both industry and the rehabilitation services.

After the First World War, the Industrial Fatigue Research Board and the National Institute of Industrial Psychology were founded in the UK. These bodies collaborated on the scientific investigation into human performance in industry and many studies were published in the 1920s (Murrel, 1965). However, the Wall Street Crash (1929) and the worldwide economic depression of the 1930s resulted in high levels of unemployment and therefore a supply of cheap labour. Industry was no longer interested in research into human performance.

However the climate again changed with the outbreak of yet another war. In the Second World War military equipment became so complex and operating speeds so high, that men either failed to get the best out of the equipment or suffered complete operational breakdown (Murrel, 1965). The study of man–machine interaction again became a high priority. Roebuck (1975) recounted that, among the many problems, it was found that cockpits were too small for many pilots, thus hampering or even preventing certain pilot movements, so that interest in the study of body dimensions (anthropometry) was stimulated.

After the war, the emphasis on fitting the machine to the man became more fully developed as both commercial, governmental and military agencies continued the study of body dimensions, work-space requirements and physiological and psychological factors (Roebuck, 1975). However, the research was primarily within individual disciplines until 1949, when an interdisciplinary society was formed and the term ergonomics coined (Murrel, 1965). The Ergonomics Research Society with its anatomists, physiologists, industrial medical officers, design engineers and architects aimed to facilitate the exchange of ideas and expertise between the many disciplines which had made a contribution to the increase of human performance during the Second World War and to extend the application of the principles beyond the military sphere (Singleton, 1982).

In 1957, the Human Factors Society was formed in the United States, where the terms 'human factors engineering', 'human engineering', 'engineering psychology' and 'human factors' have been used interchangeably, although the term 'ergonomics' is becoming more recognized (Berg Rice, 1995). The International Ergonomics Association was formed in 1961 (Murrel, 1965).

Just as Scientific Management provided the tools for task analysis at the beginning of the century, so the discipline of ergonomics has much to offer occupational therapists in the design of environments for people with disabilities both in the home and at work. Ergonomics is also important in the emergent field of health promotion. Just as Ramazzini in the seventeenth century knew why scribes and notaries developed repetitive strain injury, so ergonomics provides the method for the design work stations and equipment which could prevent many chronic and painful disorders.

Conclusion

History is interesting for its own sake, but also facilitates understanding of contemporary roles and relationships. Just as our sense of personal identity demands roots in the past from family history, our professional identity and understanding of the contexts in which we work are enhanced by knowledge of their development. There is also the myth that past occupational-therapy practice lacked rational theoretical underpinning and was essentially diversional. What the history of occupational therapy in work practice services demonstrates is that the humanistic concern for the well-being of workers incapacitated through disease or injury has always been accompanied by genuine efforts to understand biomechanical, physiological and psychological processes.

Multiple choice questions

1 The description of which European asylum particularly influenced the development of psychiatry in North America in the nineteenth century?
   (a) Bicêtre Asylum in Paris
   (b) the Retreat near York
   (c) Wakefield County Lunatic Asylum
   (d) Hanwell County Lunatic Asylum.

2 What main political or economic event affected the development of work-based services for the disabled in the first half of the twentieth century?
   (a) shortage of manpower during the First World War (1914–1918)
   (b) number of disabled veterans of the First World War (1914–1918)
   (c) the Depression of the 1930s
   (d) all of the above.

3 Consolation House, Clifton Springs, New York was one of the first vocational rehabilitation centres and the venue for the founding of the National Society for the Promotion of Occupational Therapy (later the American Association of Occupational Therapists). Who founded Consolation House?
(a) George E. Barton
(b) William Rush Dunton
(c) Eleanor Clarke Slagle
(d) Thomas B. Kidner.

4 In which year was the National Society for the Promotion of Occupational Therapy founded?
(a) 1907
(b) 1917
(c) 1923
(d) 1954

5 Whose work stimulated the development of adaptation to the work environment and machines for disabled workers?
(a) Robert Jones
(b) Frederick W. Taylor
(c) Frank B. Gilbreth
(d) Professor Jules Amar.

For answers to multiple choice questions see p. 309

References

Amar, J. (1918). *The Physiology of Industrial Organisation and the Re-employment of the Disabled.* The Library Press Limited.

Anderson, B. and Bell, J. (1988). *Occupational Therapy: its Place in Australia's History.* NSW Association of Occupational Therapists.

Balme, H. (1953). Organisation of occupational therapy. In *Surgery,* (Z. Cope, ed.) p. 730, HMSO.

Berg Rice, V. J. (1995). Ergonomics: an introduction. In *Ergonomics for Therapists,* (K. Jacobs and C. M. Bettencourt, eds) pp. 3–12, Butterworth-Heinemann.

Bing, R. K. (1981). Occupational therapy revisited: a paraphrastic journey. *The American Journal of Occupational Therapy,* **8**, 499–518.

Bockhoven, J. S. (1971). Occupational therapy – a historical perspective. *The American Journal of Occupational Therapy,* **5**, 223–225.

Bryder, L. (1988). *Below the Magic Mountain: a Short History of Tuberculosis in Twentieth-century Britain,* Clarendon Press.

Casson, E. (1955). How the Dorset House School of Occupational Therapy came into being. *Occupational Therapy,* **3**, 92–94.

Colson, J. H. C. (1945). *The Rehabilitation of the Injured: Occupational Therapy.* Cassell & Company, Ltd.

Cooter, R. (1993). *Surgery and Society in Peace and War. Orthopaedics and the Organization of Modern Medicine, 1880–1948.* The MacMillan Press Ltd.

Cope, Z. (1953). Organisation and work of plastics units. In *Surgery* (Z. Cope, ed.) pp. 334–335, HMSO.

Creighton, C. (1992). The origin and evolution of activity analysis. *The American Journal of Occupational Therapy,* **1**, 45–48.

Cromwell, F. S. (1985). Work-related programming in occupational therapy: its roots, course and prognosis. *Occupational Therapy in Health Care,* **4**, 9–23.

Digby, A. (1985). Moral treatment at the Retreat. In *The Anatomy of Madness* (W. F. Bynum, R. Porter and M. Shepherd, eds), Tavistock publications.

Driver, M. F. (1968). A philosophic view of the history of occupational therapy in Canada. *Canadian Journal of Occupational Therapy,* **2**, 53–60.

Dunton, W. R. (1919). *Reconstruction Therapy.* W. B. Saunders Company.

Ellis, W. C. (1838). *A treatise on the nature, symptoms, causes, and treatment of insanity.* Reprinted in *Three Hundred Years of Psychiatry 1535–1860* (R. Hunter and I. MacAlpine, 1963) Oxford University Press.

Gilbreth, F. B. (1915). Motion study for crippled soliders. Reprinted in *The Writings of the Gilbreths* (1953) (W. R. Spriegel and C. E. Myers, eds), Richard D. Irwin, Inc.

Gilbreth, F. B. (1917). The re-education of the crippled solider. Reprinted in *The Writings of the Gilbreths* (1953) (W. R. Spriegel and C. E. Myers, eds), Richard D. Irwin, Inc.

Gilbreth, F. B. (1918). First steps on the solution of the problem of crippled soliders. Reprinted in *The Writings of the Gilbreths* (1953) (W. R. Spriegel and C. E. Myers, eds), Richard D. Irwin, Inc.

Groundes Peace, Z. (1957). An outline of the development of O. T. in Scotland. *Scottish Journal of Occupational Therapy,* **30**, 16–43.

Gutman, S. A. (1995). Influence of the US military and occupational therapy reconstruction aides in World War I on the development of occupational therapy. *The American Journal of Occupational Therapy,* **3**, 256–262.

Haworth, N. and MacDonald, E. M. (1940). *The Theory of Occupational Therapy.* Baillière, Tindall & Cox.

Hopkins, H. L. (1988). An historical perspective on occupational therapy. In *Willard and Spackman's Occupational Therapy,* (H. L. Hopkins and H. Smith, eds), Lippencott Co.

Jones, R. (1917). *Notes on Military Orthopaedics.* Cassell & Company Ltd.

Jones, R. (ed) (1921). *Orthopaedic Surgery of Injuries.* Henry Frowde & Hodder & Stoughton.

Licht, S. (1948). *Occupational Therapy Source Book.* The Williams & Wilkins Company.

Licht, S. (1958). *Therapeutic Exercise*. Elizabeth Licht.

Licht, S. (1967). The founding and founders of the American Occupational Therapy Association. *American Journal of Occupational Therapy*, **5**, 269–277.

Low, J. F. (1992). The reconstruction aides. *The American Journal of Occupational Therapy*, **1**, 38–43.

MacDonald, E. M. (1957). History of the Association. *Occupational Therapy*, June, 30–33.

Manuel, King (1918). The scheme of curative workshops in the orthopaedic centres of the United Kingdom. *The American Journal of Orthopaedic Surgery*, **3**, 149–156.

Mendez, M. A. (1986). *A Chronicle of the World Federation of Occupational Therapists: the first thirty year 1952–1982*. WFOT.

Merkle, J. A. (1980). *Management and Ideology: The legacy of the international Scientific Management Movement*. University of California Press.

Murrel, K. F. H. (1965). *Ergonomics: Man in his working environment*. Chapman & Hall.

Peloquin, S. M. (1988). Moral treatment: contexts considered. *The American Journal of Occupational Therapy*, **8**, 537–544.

Peloquin, S. M. (1993). Moral treatment: how a caring practice lost its rationale. *The American Journal of Occupational Therapy*, **2**, 167–173.

Peto, G. (1955). Dr Elizabeth Casson, OBE, MD, DPM. A tribute to her work. *Occupational Therapy*, **3**, 107–109.

Pheasant, S. (1991). *Ergonomics, Work and Health*. Macmillian.

Pinel, P. (1806). *A Treatise on Insanity*. Translated from the French by D. D. Davis (1962) Hafner Publishing Co.

Ramazzini, B. (1713). *De Morbis Artificum*. Translated by W. C. Wright (1940) as *Diseases of Workers*, Ch. 30, University of Chicago.

Reed, K. L. and Sanderson, R. S. (1980). *Concepts of Occupational Therapy*. Williams & Wilkins.

Robinson, I. M. (1981). Muriel Driver Memorial Lecture – The mists of time. *The Canadian Journal of Occupational Therapy*, **4**, 145–152.

Roebuck, J. A., Kroemer, K. H. E. and Thomson, W. G. (1975). *Engineering Anthropometry Methods*. John Wiley & Sons.

Shannon, P. D. (1977). The derailment of occupational therapy. *The American Journal of Occupational Therapy*, **31**(4), 229–234.

Singleton, W. T. (1982). *The Body at Work*. Cambridge University Press.

Singer, C. and Underwood, E. A. (1962). *A Short History of Medicine*. Clarendon Press.

Spackman, C. S. (1968). A history of the practice of occupational therapy for restoration of physical function: 1917–1967. *The American Journal of Occupational Therapy*, **2**, 67–71.

War Department Training Manual, 8–291 (1944). *Occupational Therapy*. US Government Printing Office.

World Federation of Occupational Therapists (1954). *Proceedings of the First International Congress*. WFOT.

3

Current Models and Trends in Work Practice Service Delivery

Jeraldine Perron and Margaret McKay

Learning objectives

By the end of this chapter the reader should be able to:

1 Describe the range and diversity of work programmes.
2 Identify how models of service provision are shaped in response to funding sources.
3 Compare service provisions in two contrasting health and social care environments.

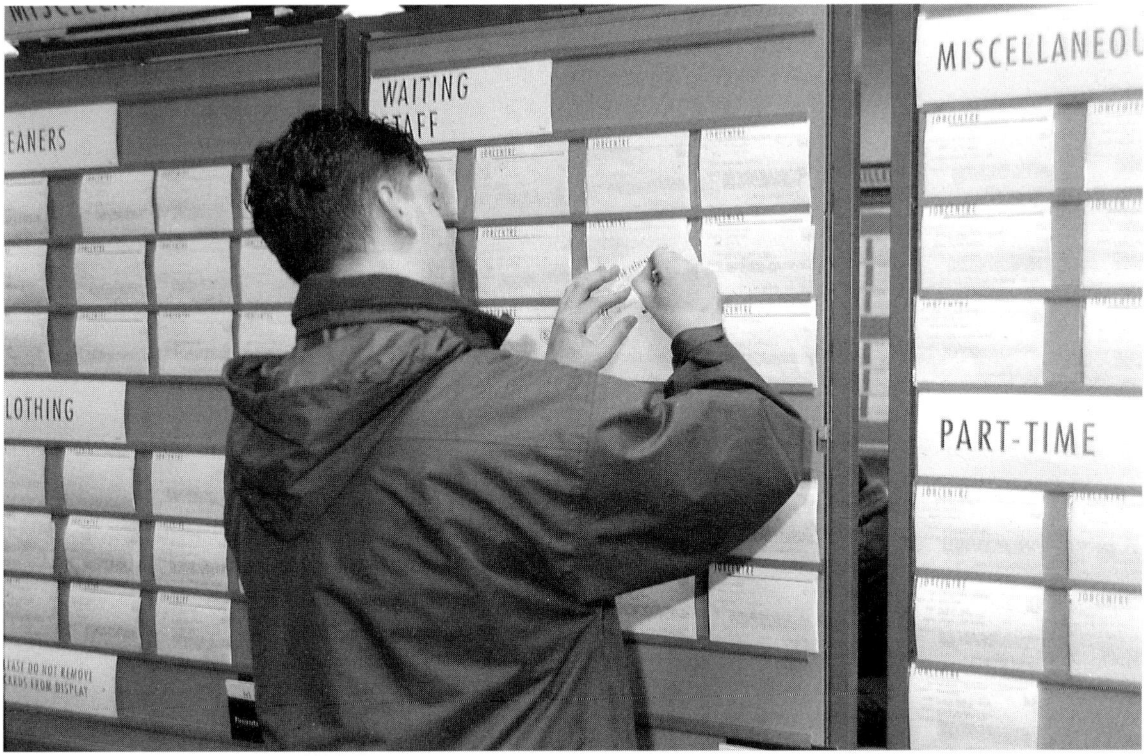

Introduction

The services offered within a country to assist workers to both gain access to and maintain employment are affected by diverse environmental influences. These include funding sources, social and cultural perceptions of disability, and professional expertise. This chapter explores the models of service provision in two countries, the USA and the UK, which have markedly contrasting health and social care environments.

A USA perspective

After a period of explosive growth in the late 1980s and early 1990s, work programmes in occupational therapy in the United States entered a period of increased demands for outcome efficacy and efficiency and for tighter financial accountability. Multiple forces influenced the direction of work programmes. They included changes that began to take place in workforce characteristics, in workplace characteristics, in the economy, in funding models, and in international competition (Johnston, 1988: 1–16). Deregulation of some industries such as the California utility industry thrust them for the first time into a competitive environment and promoted them to look seriously at medical costs, especially those associated with work-injury rehabilitation and prevention (Aron, 1995: October/November, 94). Additional forces included implementation of the 1990 Americans with Disabilities Act (ADA) (P. L. 101–336), Title VI–C Amendments to the Rehabilitation Act of 1973 (P. L. 99–506) and the Occupational Safety and Health Administration (OSHA) laws of the 1980s (Richardson, 1994: 92; Daus, 1995: April/May, 29).

The United States workforce is growing while the demographics of the labour pool are changing. According to the Bureau of Labor projections of participation, between 1992 and 2005 the workforce is expected to increase almost 19 per cent to total 151 million people (Fullerton, 1994: 29). With individuals born between 1946 and 1954 expected to comprise an increasing proportion of the workforce, the average age of workers will rise, and nearly half of them will be women. Ethnic minority workers, many of them immigrants from Asia, Africa and Central and South America, will increase from approximately 20 per cent to nearly 30 per cent of the workforce (Arriaga, 1994: 99). Eleven per cent of workers are expected to be Hispanic, 11 per cent black, and 5 per cent Asian and other non-Hispanic (Fullerton, 1994: 30). Additionally, disabled students are transitioning into the community, and individuals with HIV/AIDS or chronic illnesses, individuals with mental illness or cognitive impairment, and individuals with work injuries or illnesses are all entering the workplace in a more timely way than ever before. Successful employers will welcome and accommodate the diversity of their employees' cultures and languages, ages and education, and physical and cognitive status. They will provide training and retraining programmes, work-station modifications, health insurance, and other investments in these rich resources of human capital (US Merit Systems Protection Board, 1993: 40).

The United States workplace is changing. Computerization, mechanization and other technological improvements streamline the workplace and facilitate increased production of manufactured goods. However, this increased technology reduces the number of needed workers and the cost, or value, of the manufactured goods. In fact, the manufacturing industry, once at the economic core of the United States and an enormous job resource for the entry-level, blue-collar and immigrant labour pool, is not keeping up with increases in other areas of society and in the gross national product. Service industries, which do not produce a tangible product, such as product research and design, engineering, retailing and advertising, will continue to contribute a greater portion of the value of manufactured products. Companies seeking the bottom line are merging, downsizing, re-engineering and redefining jobs. While labour unions are becoming weaker, foreign competition is becoming stronger (Olson, 1994: 7). Growth jobs are predicted to be in the service sector and include law, natural, computer and mathematical science, health care, social science, and technical positions. Companies have already begun to control their costs by contracting for limited periods with independent consultants for specialized information and expertise, rather than incurring the costs of salaries and benefit packages for employees whose skills are needed only intermittently.

Largely due to increased technological sophistication, by 2005 more than half the new jobs will require some education beyond high school, and many will require a college education (Fullerton, 1988: 13). In the mid 1990s, 7 per cent of the population have fourth grade or lower skills and are usually able to find jobs in the unskilled market. However, by the turn of the century, only 4 per cent of jobs will be unskilled. It will become more difficult to find low-level jobs. Furthermore, even those jobs will require the basic skills of being able to read and understand written directions, add and subtract, and express oneself clearly (Richardson, 1994: 14).

Individuals entering or re-entering the workforce will need to alter their work behaviour, contend with increased workplace stress, and continually update and adapt their skills. At the same time, successful employers will appreciate these workers' experience and adaptability, and will reward their efforts to transfer their skills and broaden the application of their knowledge. As Robert Reich, US Secretary of Labour asserts, companies should 'treat their workers as assets to be developed rather than costs to be cut,' and they should 'invest in their workers' skills, not just in machines to replace them' (Lehigh, 1995: 69).

As more Americans provide services instead of produce goods, and OSHA continues to regulate industrial environment and equipment safety, the types and numbers of injuries and illnesses they encounter in the workplace will continue to change (Burchman, 1994: 3). As a result, vocational and rehabilitation professionals will need to adapt their services to both the changing needs of workers and the changing health-care reimbursement arena. For example, with the increased proliferation of computer jobs in the last ten years, the incidence of cumulative trauma disorders has risen (Abeln, 1995: 131). Meanwhile manufacturing jobs and the occurrence of back and traumatic hand injuries have declined (Daus, 1995: October/November, 31; Joe, 1995: 12). Between 1970 and 1992, the incidence rate for workplace injuries dropped from 10.9 to 8.9 per 100 employees, while the average days lost rose from 4.4 to 6.0 days per injury (US Department of Labor, Occupational Injuries, 1995: 5). During that same period, health-care costs quadrupled, and if they continue to double every five years, they will exceed $140 billion by the year 2000 (Daus, 1995: October/November, 3). With health-care costs accounting for 40–50 per cent of workers' compensation claims and eating into increasing portions of industry profits, employers have begun to scrutinize and demand a halt to their rising health-care and associated injured-worker costs, such as work rehabilitation programmes. Attempts to implement national health-care reform legislation early in the Clinton administration were unsuccessful. However, the potential threat of external regulation constraints prompted the health-care industry to enter rapidly into significant efforts to reduce costs by offering capitated and competitive managed care reimbursement packages to selected providers. The result has been 'the wholesale conversion of our health care system from a patchwork of profit centers into a network of cost centers and, thus, the muscling up of the hitherto flaccid demand side of the health care market' (Reinhardt, 1995: 26). Work programmes responded to new programme evaluation and fiscal monitoring activities by revising extended prevocational exploration activities and extensive medical rehabilitation programmes to emphasize quality service and efficient and effective outcomes (Wiklund, 1994: 9; Olson, 1994: 7). Former facility-based service delivery became characterized by industry-based job training and work-injury rehabilitation, transitional work programmes, job coaches, job accommodations, early return to work, and injury prevention activities (Dumas, 1994: 5–6). Managed care, capitation, work-injury management, case management, preauthorization, and utilization review replaced traditional programme administration and fee-for-service funding. The transition is not complete; diverse environmental influences continue to impact on work programmes in the United States.

Funding sources of work programmes in the United States

Payors are requiring work programmes to demonstrate successful, meaningful outcomes for their clients. Thus, in turn, work programmes have set assessment of potential restoration of function as the criteria for access to their programmes. According to a developer of medical disability assessment programmes, the 1992 US Task Force on Improving Medical Criteria for Disability Determination, comprised of government medical policy makers, reported the following finding:

> As functional status measures become more accepted by practitioners and researchers in the field, it is expected that they will become increasingly incorporated into the policies of government and private insurers. It is likely that they will ultimately become an alternative to the medical criteria now being used in SSI (Social Security Insurance) and SSDI (Social Security Disability Insurance) programs. They will be used in vocational rehabilitation programs at the State level to help determine rehabilitation and employment potential. They will be used in workers' compensation programs to determine appropriate compensation and the potential for rehabilitation and employment. They will be used in Medicare and Medicaid for purposes of payment, quality assurance and discharge planning. They will be used in the private sector, which has long had disability programs and is starting to develop long-term care programs. (M. Coupland, unpublished observation, 1995)

Despite the similarity of criteria for work programme access, for-profit and not-for-profit funding sources for work programmes influence the type, extent and location of services. Major sources include: workers' compensation, health insurance, public funds and community resources.

Workers' compensation (WC)

Workers' compensation is mandated in all states and is the major payor of industrial claims. It is a financial benefits programme purchased by employers through private insurance companies. Fee schedules, billing codes, and access to rehabilitation services vary by individual state laws and are overseen by a regulatory agency appointed by the state legislature (Pinson, 1991: 2). Workers' compensation began in the 1930s as a way to reimburse workers fairly for injuries and illnesses sustained in the course of their work and to reduce the costly legal avenues employees previously sought. Regardless of state, the common goal is to provide for medical expenses required to return the worker to gainful employment. A number of states are exerting efforts to control its out-of-bounds growth through reform legislation and changes in programme administration (Larson, 1994: 1).

Companies are also seeking to control WC costs. In fact, attempts to reduce WC costs is viewed at the third recent major attempt of companies to increase productivity and remain competitive with both national and global markets. In the 1960s, manufacturers sought to standardize mass production, while in the 1980s they focused on quality issues (Devlin, 1995: December–b, 8). Note: after a period following a work injury or illness, a disabled worker may elect to receive Social Security Disability Insurance (SSDI) disability benefits. Eligibility is re-evaluated every three years. If the individual is aged, blind or disabled and does not have work experience, he may be eligible for Social Security Insurance (SSI) benefits. An individual electing to receive SSDI or SSI benefits may be precluded from bringing action under the ADA or from receiving workers' compensation benefits. A person with a physical or mental disability cannot simultaneously be certified 'unable to work' and 'qualified to perform work' (Richardson, 1994: 92). The SSI is seeking to reduce disincentives for workers over 65 years of age to continue working by raising the amount older workers can earn and still collect benefits. It is also exploring the possibility of transferring rehabilitation services, including case management and physical capacity evaluation for work readiness into the private sector; if so, these funding changes could revise eligibility requirements for services.

Health insurance

Medical liability insurance

Automobile, homeowner, and business liability policies have historically paid for the second largest group of industrial claims. The liability carrier is billed directly and handles the coverage and claims payments through a case manager or claims adjuster who coordinates, negotiates fees for, and preauthorizes services and providers for monetarily limited medical care (Pinson, 1991: 2).

Fee for service indemnity insurance

The insured has free choice of health-care provider and will have his or her health-care bills submitted for payment according to cost or the insurer's schedule, i.e. usual and customary, or reasonable costs, traditionally without deductibles or co-payments. Most have now incorporated some case management such as utilization review and/or precertification to control costs. Although it occurs less often than in past years, some employers still question the work relatedness of cumulative trauma disorder and other work associated claims and encourage employees to use their general medical liability health insurance to pay for medical bills (Beckley, 1995: 26).

Private insurance

Coverage varies considerably as defined in individual policies. Services are usually billed by the individual service such as occupational or physical therapy, and often there is a deductible and a co-payment for each session. Many insurance companies require preauthorization and/or limit the amount, or charges, or number of treatment sessions (Pinson, 1991: 2).

Self-insurance

The employer sets aside funds to pay for work-related injuries and illnesses. Programmes can be self-administered or third-party administered (TPA) and can take almost any form, including an indemnity programme, HMO, PPO, etc. Because the employer assumes direct risk for costs, self-insured programmes can be less costly than if contracted with an insurance company, especially when the company implements proactive workplace safety activities. The number of self-insured companies is growing.

Public funds

Vocational rehabilitation legislation

The Federal Vocational Rehabilitation Act of 1973, Sections 503 and 504, provides federal funds, with state participation, to state vocational rehabilitation agencies and employer programmes, prohibits participants from employment discrimination on the basis of physical or mental handicap and requires 'reasonable accommodation' to handicapped employees and job applicants. Legislative proposals are under consideration which would revise and coordinate vocational rehabilitation services to allow individuals to access assistive technology using a voucher system 'in a linked system of sites designed to provide "multiple doors" for disabled and nondisabled people seeking employment' (Pfaff, 1995: 9).

Vocational education legislation

The federal government has passed a number of laws concerning vocational transition for students with moderate to severe disabilities with federal monies augmented by state and local funds. Special education and related services, including occupational therapy, have been available through the public school system since passage of Public Law 94–142, the Education for All Handicapped Children Act of 1975 (EHA). However, follow-up studies revealed that relatively few programme participants attained competitive employment or were involved in community activities, but large numbers were dependent upon public entitlement programmes (Spencer, 1995: 80). 1986 amendments to the law funded supported employment services in all states. In 1990, amendments were made to the EHA, and the law was renamed the 'individuals with Disabilities Act' or IDEA (Public Law 101–476, 1990). IDEA requires that all special-education students receive functionally oriented school-to-life transition services by age 16, including assistive technology, based on individual need (Brollier *et al.*, 1994: 347). However, the future of IDEA is unclear; concerns about high administrative costs are the focus as the bill makes its way through Congress for reauthorization in 1995 (Stahl, 1995: 13).

According to the US Department of Labor, as of 1995, all 50 states have been awarded federal school-to-work grants to develop programmes to bring the workplace into the classroom and to transform workplaces into places of learning for all secondary students. Eight states (KY, ME, MA, MI, NJ, NY, OR, WI) have been awarded implementation grants. Anticipating that all states will be awarded implementation grants by 1997, Requests for Information (RFI) have been sent out to invite 'qualified experts', including occupational therapists, to serve as potential contractors to assist with programme development (Personal observation, Lorraine Saunders, DOL, 1995: 202–219–8698).

Medicaid and Medicare

Federal and federal/state-funded coverage is very limited due to strict guidelines that are often tied to capitation or HMO arrangements that require existing contracts with the facility through which services are provided. However, the Tax Equity Fiscal Responsibility Act (TEFRA) rate for Medicare reimbursement methodology can also be used to develop a break-even price for rehabilitation programmes and thus a 'high ratio of cost to charges when these costs are also used in pro forma development with managed care and commercial patients for the purpose of determining profitability' (Beckley, 1995: 26). If anticipated federal reform legislation passes, it will shift health-care costs to private insurers, increase the numbers of uninsured Americans and, with the resulting lower wages and higher cost-sharing of health insurance contributions, disproportionately affect lower-income workers (Knox, 1995: 20).

Community resources

Community, religious and charity groups have traditionally sponsored and supported work programmes for various groups, often times in sheltered workshops. Some of these groups include Easter Seals, The Salvation Army, Catholic Charities, immigrant associations, Association for the Blind, United Cerebral Palsy, and local departments of mental health and mental retardation. Like other programmes, they have expanded their efforts into the community with vocational rehabilitation, supported, and competitive employment. Some have teamed up with groups, such as Independent Living programmes to provide technology and support for at-home computer jobs (Montagno, 1994: 35).

The history of Goodwill Industries demonstrates how one programme changed as community needs changed. In 1885, Rev. Edgar J. Helms went through Boston's elite neighborhoods collecting unwanted clothing and household items for his impoverished immigrant congregation. When his parish repaired and began reselling the items in the Morgan Chapel in the South End, the first Goodwill store was established. Through the years, Goodwill responded to meet the community's changing needs. These have included a home for homeless, the Fresh Air Camp, schools for troubled teenagers, Bargain Basement stores, and more recently, job training and placement programmes (Walsh, 1995: 21).

Types of funding agreements

A product of activities to contain spiralling health-care costs, managed care and its variations are pervasive in work programmes. And, as the funding agreements vary, so do the type, extent and location of rehabilitation and work-related services.

Managed care

Managed care is a term used both to denote all types of integrated delivery systems, such as HMOs, PPOs, and Medicare, that incorporate management of care received by consumers. The term is also used to denote the utilization tools, such as preadmission certification, utilization review, and the use of case managers to monitor the care of clients, that are applied to manage the practices of health-care providers. Generally viewed as less interested in the process and structure of the services provided and more interested in value for money spent, effective managed-care arrangements support competent, effective clinicians, stringent clinical documentation, standardization of treatment, and successful work-related rehabilitation programme outcomes (Framoze, 1995: 54; Weiner and de Lissovy, 1993).

Case management

Case management is such an integral component of managed care, it is sometimes used interchangeably with the term managed care. Definitions vary subtly, depending upon the position the case manager holds in the health-care delivery system. As defined by the Certification of Insurance Rehabilitation Specialists Commission in 1993, case management is 'a collaborative process that assesses, plans, implements, coordinates, monitors, and evaluates the options and services required to meet an individual's health needs, using communication and available resources to promote quality and cost effective outcomes'. (Fisher, 1995: 4). The definition of case management by the National Coalition of Associations for the Advancement of Case Management also describes the need for quality care and cost-effective outcomes, but it focuses on client health as it defines case management as 'a collaborative process that promotes quality care and cost-effective outcomes that enhance the physical, psychological and vocational health of individuals' (Beckley, 1995: 25). The case management specialist, or disability manager, serves clients and their families through provider programmes, and increasingly, through insurance-based arrangements (Devlin, 1995: November–b, 7). Case managers or disability managers determine conditions under which an individual can work, assist the individual in managing a disability so they can continue to work or return to work with a disability, and direct individuals to services which are both cost effective and have optimal functional outcomes. They are becoming an essential component of health care delivery (Habeck, 1994: 2; Richardson, 1994: 98).

24-hour managed care

Also called managed care for workers' compensation, 24-hour managed care involves the management, by an HMO, PPO, etc., of a group of employees or a particular employer for the worker's compensation, health, and perhaps any liability such as auto claims. As information is managed and processed at the same time as the delivery of medical care, health claims are administered faster and more efficiently, the quality of care is improved, and costs are reduced. The merger of insurance plans is a logical outcome of company reorganizations, whereby they now have singular reporting relationships for the managers of voluntary-group health benefits and of statutory workers' compensation. The employer's goals are to reduce costs and to return the injured speedily to the workplace, regardless of whether the injury occurred on the ski slopes or on the job (Aron, 1995: 95). Health-care practitioners thus must serve payors, employers and patients all as their customers (Framroze, 1995: 52). Florida and especially California are early states moving into this form of managed care.

Capitation

An increasing number of payors are replacing fee discounts and preferred provider arrangements with capitated fee arrangements with selected rehabilitation providers (Abeln, 1995: February/March, 110). A capitated agreement or contract is considered to be true managed care, as it involves the integration of clinical and financial components of health care into one arrangement. Providers operate within a fixed budget and are strongly motivated to provide cost-effective care and prevention strategies that keep the group members healthy. The risk is shared between the payor and the provider, the latter of whom is thus strongly motivated to provide cost-effective care (Rausch, 1995: 137). For sound business practice, the provider should try to ballpark the potential number of referrals by becoming knowledgeable about the company's history of injury utilization data, such as per cent of injuries per 100 employees. As the provider does not bill for services in either of the two types of capitated contracts, each type involves the need to provide quality care optimally within pre-determined guidelines (Apker, 1994: 60), a fixed monthly reimbursement rate for an identified group of individuals. The group may be arbitrarily defined as all the employees of a company or all residents of a certain catchment area, all persons on Medicare who sign up for the programme, or another group of individuals, such as an agreed-upon dollar rate for individuals with a specific diagnosis. Examples include cumulative trauma disorders or back injury. The provider's risk involves the fact that if the ICD9 system (International Classification of Disease) is used, there is no adjustment for severity, gender, age or comorbidity, and therefore there may be a significant variation in treatment costs.

Health Maintenance Organization (HMO)

An HMO is a legislatively regulated, prepaid, organized health-care delivery system for enrolled clients that incorporates a shared financial risk by the organization and by primary care physicians who coordinate care with providers within the system. There are four basic HMO models: staff, group, network and IPA (Weiner and de Lissovy, 1993).

- *Staff model.* Most members of the HMO receive care from physicians who are employed as staff and receive a salary.
- *Group model.* A single area multispecialty group practice with an exclusive contract only with the one HMO.
- *Network model.* A network of two or more group practices and sometimes individual providers who contract to provide care for the majority of members of an HMO, but who may also provide services for non-member clients.
- *Independent (or individual) practice association.* Individual physicians or small group practices contract to provide care to members of an HMO.

Preferred Provider Organization (PPO)

Member clients are free to obtain health care from 'preferred' providers within the plan either by incentives such as lack of co-payments or by encountering disincentives such as limited benefits if they receive care from out-of-plan providers. In return for client referrals, providers usually agree to discounted payments and case management of their care (Weiner and de Lissovy, 1993). EPOs are a type of PPO where the rehabilitation provider contracts with a managed care insurer for an agreed-upon price reduction, called a discount, in exchange for which the insurer allows the provider exclusive access to the insurer's clients. In order to enter into a realistic agreement, the provider must have a very good awareness of her fixed and variable costs, although a payor/provider risk-sharing agreement can be arranged (Weiner and de Lissovy, 1993). However, in what may become a trend, one major Californian PPO claims cost reduction tools such as discounts are inadequate to control total costs in WC cases; instead they employ case management to ensure claim early diagnosis, treatment and return to work as cost saving strategies (Devlin, 1995: December–a, 6).

Work programme models

Vocational and rehabilitation occupational therapy practitioners have responded to the need to become more cost effective by revising extended prevocational exploration and extensive medical rehabilitation programmes to become short-term programmes that are focused on quality, efficiency and effective outcomes (Wiklund, 1994: 5). Service delivery has become characterized by industry-based job training and work-injury rehabilitation, transitional work programmes, job coaches, job accommodations, early return to work and injury prevention activities. Job-site analysis, supported employment, work-injury management, preauthorization and utilization reviews have largely replaced traditional facility-based therapy, work hardening programmes, and fee for service reimbursement.

Acute care rehabilitation

An early post-surgery or injury programme of occupational and/or physical therapy to help the injured worker use the injured body part with less pain, and may then be followed by a work conditioning programme with an emphasis on flexibility, strengthening, endurance, and coordination and/or cardiovascular fitness (Fisher, 1993: 3). Depending upon the injured worker's situation, he may return to work, proceed to a work-hardening programme, continue in another work programme, or consider other options (Litke *et al.*, 1995: 19). With workers returning to their jobs early in the rehabilitation process, sometimes they begin work-hardening programmes and other return-to-work strategies during the acute stage of the rehabilitation programme (Zezina, 1995: 22).

Work hardening

In 1988, the Commission on Accreditation of Rehabilitation Facilities (CARF) defined work hardening as:

> interdisciplinary in nature, use of conditioning tasks that are graded to progressively improve the biomechanical, neuromuscular, cardiovascular, metabolic and psychosocial functions of the client in conjunction with real or simulated work activities. Work hardening provides a transition between acute care and return to work, while addressing the issues of productivity, safety, physical tolerances, and worker behaviors. Work hardening is a highly structured, goal-oriented, individualized treatment program designed to maximize the individual's ability to return to work. (Ogden-Niemeyer and Jacobs, 1989: 13)

Despite some respectable outcome studies and an attempt by the Commission on Accreditation of Rehabilitation Facilities (CARF) to set standards and control their development, clinic-based work-hardening programmes have largely had limited return-to-work outcomes, and have disillusioned many third-party payors (Lacerte, 1992: 19; Niemeyer, Jacobs, *et al.*, 1994: 327; King, P., 1993: 596; Dumont and Vance, 1992: 1; Wyrick *et al.*, 1991: 109; Jacobs, 1991: 1; Felix, 1992: 19). Facility-based work-hardening occupational therapy practitioners and other rehabilitation professionals neglected to consider the occupational bonding between the workers and employers, to utilize employer resources in job accommodations, to utilize practical situational assessments appropriately and to simulate and approximate work adequately in a facility-based setting (Shrey, 1992: 4). Furthermore, they may have overestimated the usefulness of new treatment technology for work hardening programmes and underestimated their lack of awareness of employer/employee labour relations (Lacerte, 1992: 19). Although the concept of an organized programme to physically prepare the injured worker to return to the job was recognized, its facility-based programmes had limited success. Then, in the early 1990s, managed-care entered into the workers' compensation process and propelled work-hardening programmes into new and more successful directions. Workers began to return to the workplace to continue their rehabilitation programme, rehabilitation providers began to see employers as advocates, and employers began to invest in workplace ergonomic assessments and injury-prevention programmes (Zezima, 1995: 58; Burles, 1993: 1).

On-site work injury management programmes (WIM)

During the early 1990s, rehabilitation professionals found faster and better outcomes when they worked closely with employers. Industrial rehabilitation professionals began to design their programmes as win–win partnerships with employers for disability management as well as medical rehabilitation. They worked together to have the injured worker attain a reasonable capacity to return to his original job or to begin a new job and then to keep that worker back at work. This employer/provider partnership between rehabilitation professions and employers created an environment where rehabilitation professionals began to view employers as potential customers with whom to develop relationships, to understand their needs, and to provide the services to meet those needs on an ongoing basis while focusing on long-term successful outcomes. For example, after the worker re-entered the worksite, the therapist as job coach assisted with problem solving, with suggestions for symptom control techniques, and with reassurance that returning to work is a reactivation process (Priebe, 1995: 5). Rehabilitation professionals also began to develop injury prevention programmes and ergonomic interventions. Each partner in the relationship has complementary expertise, knowledge and skill to contribute to a successful WIM programme (Hunter, 1994: 2). Provider expertise, knowledge and skill contribute:

- Medical literature
- Human anatomy and physiology
- Healing processes and successful treatments
- Medical protocols and procedures
- Medical community contacts and relationships
- Availability of other health-care resources
- Teaching resources, i.e. slides, handouts, models, etc.
- 24-hour hotlines for injury prevention, identification and questions.

Employer expertise, knowledge and skill contribute:

- Corporate/plant operations and procedures
- Production/assembly processes
- Practical application of safety programmes
- Industrial hygiene experience
- Company resources
- Other business contacts/referrals
- Work-site culture
- Union management relationships
- Job descriptions and role delineation.

Instead of providing care in the clinic, WIM programmes have moved almost entirely into the workplace. Borrowing from the home health model, rehabilitation professionals provide services to the individual at the workplace that are 'critical to enhancing functional outcomes in an economical fashion' (Devlin, 1994: B1). Even during demanding company growth periods, implementation of a proactive WIM programme can provide a safer workplace and effectively reduce claims and costs (Devlin, 1995: July/August/September, 1). On-site work programmes maximize employees abilities and skills for a safe and functional work re-entry because they combine 'the physical, social, and cultural factors affecting the injured worker with the performance of activities, tasks, and roles related to job achievement' (Christiansen, 1991: 18). Employer/provider programmes that are entirely on site gain the following advantages:

- Early medical intervention
- Reduced lost work time
- Convenience for worker
- Easy accessibility of professional consultations
- Support of ongoing warm-up and stretches prevention programme
- Timely work-site inspections, job modifications, and worker education
- Increased employee self-esteem and satisfaction in gainful employment
- Increased employee ownership of their responsibilities in the work re-entry process.

(Dumont and Vance, 1992: 3–4; Larson, 1994: 1–2)

On-site work injury management programmes have already demonstrated industry acceptance and financial success. In one example, an independent-therapist-owned private practice in Maine has provided on-site physical therapy services and injury prevention programmes to a large shipyard, paper mills, work products manufacturing and a retail clothing and sporting goods company for six years. Services included basic modalities, work conditioning, and functional assessments with a primary therapeutic focus on an active early mobility, patient education and the resumption of normal function. Then, because of significant reductions in their serviced companies' medical and indemnity costs and lost work days, Granite Hill Physical Therapy in Brunswick developed a reputation for success and expanded its sites and services to other companies (Dumont and Vance, 1992: 4).

Early return-to-work programmes

In an attempt to reduce their rising workers' compensation costs of wage replacement and their medical costs associated with claims by employees injured in the workplace, companies are instituting early return-to-work programmes (ERTW), also called transitional work or modified work (Devlin, 1994: B1). In ERTW programmes, employers and rehabilitation professionals shifted from looking at the workers' impairments and what they cannot do, to focusing on what they can do, and respecting their limitations, how soon they can enter or return to the workplace during or after their rehabilitation programme (Dumas, 1994: 5; Shoemaker, 1992: 18). The American with Disabilities Act (ADA), which has limited pre-employment physicals and other common employment practices that restricted access to the workplace for workers with a disability, also contributed to the shift and to easier access to the workplace. Under the ADA, an injured worker who is a 'qualified individual with a disability' may need individualized reasonable accommodations, worksite modification, reduced work hours, absences and leaves without pay, and other ADA considerations (Growick, 1993: 9; Canelon, 1995: 461; Larson, 1995: 4). The ADA can serve all workers with a disability; however, only workers who have been injured on the job are eligible for workers' compensation benefits (Growick, 1993: July/August, 7). In order to avoid any misunderstandings among their employees, knowledgeable employers address both the workers' compensation system and the ADA Provision Title I, Employment, in collective bargaining agreements that specify job duties, pay, seniority rights, and job bidding provisions (Devlin, 1992: 5). Thus, proactive employers manage an effective formalized ERTW programme in coordination with the injured worker, multidisciplinary health-care specialists, and as appropriate, the workers' compensation carrier (Richardson, 1994: 95). Yet, early-to-work cannot be the only goal; a well-coordinated ERTW programme ensures that the employee has made sufficient recovery and does not re-enter the workplace prematurely, only to reinjure himself. A strong, trusting working relationship between all members of the team ensures that the worker receives appropriate care and safely returns to the workplace and productivity (Daus, 1995: April/May, 26; Simental, 1994: 105).

There are two main forms of ERTW programmes. In the individual model, following receipt of a medical evaluation of the injured worker's abilities, the employer may negotiate with the worker and the worker's compensation carrier to have the worker return for a predetermined period in a less demanding alternative duty position, at a lower rate of pay that is supplemented by worker's compensation to a higher rate than if the worker remained unemployed at home.

Another form of an ERTW involves a transitional work centre which provides individually designed programmes, in a separated area within a company's environs, to assist medically approved employees with acute or chronic disabilities to enter the workplace, whether the precipitating injury or illness occurred on or off the job. Initially an outgrowth of disability management committees, they are usually run by a rehabilitation case manager with joint cooperation of labour and management. Selected jobs that are not already being done are gradually modified until the employee's strength, function and confidence enable him, with his supervisor's support, to return fully to his normal duties or to a new position. The programme is time limited, goal directed, and group oriented to provide social support and encouragement to return to work. Mutual employee/employer programme advantages include the prevention of lost work time, the protection of employee benefits, and the timely return to a normal lifestyle (Tweed, 1994: 56).

The successes of ERTW or transitional programmes are documented. A study conducted in 1993 by the W. E. Upjohn Institute for Employment Research found that proactive return-to-work programmes resulted in fewer lost-work-day cases per 100 employees. One company in the study, Steelcase Inc., found that their average number of lost work days due to injury is one third the national average in light metal industry. Additionally, Steelcase's coordinated team approach, which includes the medical department, the workers' compensation department, safety, the manufacturing supervisor, and the employee, saves them about $4 million per year or about one third of their projected costs (Child, 1995: 7).

In either form of ERTW or transitional programme, proactive suggestions to create a can-do environment include: developing a safety committee with representation from both management and labour, conducting essential function job analyses, pre-determining alternate duty jobs, making job accommodations, implementing assistive technology as indicated, and creating temporary positions if necessary to bring the worker into the workplace. 'Workers with impairment who participate in transitional work are able to minimize the economic, physical, psychological, social and domestic losses related to work disruptions caused by injury or illness' (Shrey, 1992: October/November, 6). Only lawyers, who benefit from the adversarial employer–worker relationships, and health-care providers who fail to see employers as allies and who hold onto the old medical model rehabilitation programmes do not benefit from ERTW or transitional programmes for injured workers.

Rural programmes

Work rehabilitation services to the rural population present unique challenges. Rehabilitation personnel are limited and must travel long distances, job opportunities and insurance and workers' compensation benefits are limited, the proportion of poor and older workers is growing, and the occupations are often dangerous (Smith, 1995: 3). However, rehabilitation personnel in rural programmes have successfully encountered issues that will ensure their viability and perhaps even serve as models for future health-care delivery programmes in other areas (Lavergne, 1995: 72). One such issue involves the self-employed injured workers who are loath to take time off work because of their strong work ethic and because of their limited financial resources. Many of these workers are blue-collar workers or farmers who are likely to try to work through their pain and become more injured by the time they see a health-care provider. Many are poorly educated, but highly skilled. Others are educated, but working at jobs that provide them with more money than the jobs they were trained for. Rehabilitation providers, including occupational therapy practitioners, have found they must provide programmes that make sense to the work-focused lifestyle of these injured workers. Much success has been possible by utilizing assistive technology to modify equipment and worksites (Paiva, 1995: 67; Torres-Davis and Crowl, 1995: 29).

It is anticipated that rural work programmes will benefit from increased access to the Internet promised by the Telecommunications and Information Infrastructure Assistance Program (TIIAP). In November 1995, Larry Irving, the assistant secretary for commerce, announced that grants were made 'to health care providers, schools, libraries, public safety organizations, and state and local governments. . .to give children in farming communities and inner cities access to the Internet, bring improved health care to the elderly . . ., provide on-line workers' training and job opportunity information . . . and improve public safety.' (For more information: Paige Darden, NTIA Office of Public Affairs, at 202–482–1551.)

Vocational rehabilitation (VR)

Vocational rehabilitation (VR) growth has been fuelled by implementation of the federal Vocational Rehabilitation Act of 1973, by the ADA in 1992, and then by the need to reduce workers' compensation costs. VR services can be initiated at any stage of the rehabilitation process and within any model (Braddom, 1992: 507). Furthermore, advances in technology and improved rehabilitation outcomes have increased the number of individuals with disabilities who, with ergonomic and job modifications, could return to the workplace, or with vocational habilitation special training, could obtain their first job. The quadriplegic adolescent can plan to utilize her intellectual capabilities, technological mobility and communication equipment, and vocational school or college training to enter the workforce. Also, people with chronic diseases, including HIV/AIDS, 'can work quite well' with vocational rehabilitation services (Caulfield *et al.*, 1994: 13).

Some individual companies have begun to implement internal vocational rehabilitation programmes to help employees with work injuries and illnesses returning to the job to learn new job skills. For example, one Californian utility company increased job placement by 31 per cent in its first year of implementation (Aron, 1995: October/November, 95). Other companies have implemented vocational rehabilitation services for injured workers, including those with chronic pain, who have not been able to manage transition programmes for their pre-injury jobs successfully. Traditionally, vocational rehabilitation programmes have used an 'evaluate, train, then place' model with limited success. Recently, VR programmes have had anecdotal success with a supported employment model of 'evaluate, place and train, then support'. Occupational therapy practitioners have the training and skill to expand their services in VR programmes for clients with a wide range of disabilities.

Supported employment (SE)

Considered as a component of vocational rehabilitation, supported employment is defined as 'individualized support on and off the job site, initial and ongoing employment services, and assistance from a skilled job coach' (Parent, 1994: 2). SE owes its record of success in achieving employment for individuals with a variety of severe disabilities to providing them with individualized supports, such as identification of skills and interests, helping them find a job and with the hiring process, providing job-site training, and a job coach who serves as a trainer, advocate and facilitator in providing and coordinating the various ongoing supports, such as transportation, employer relations, and independent living arrangements (Mason, 1995: 55). Increased survival rates for seriously injured individuals, advances in medical and assistive technology, implementation of the ADA and Titles III and VI-C of the Rehabilitation Act Amendments, and improved rehabilitation outcomes have supported the implementation of supported employment (SE) programmes. Individuals with traumatic brain injuries, mental retardation, HIV/AIDS, or mental illness – even when severe and persistent – and who were previously served in sheltered workshops and day treatment programmes, began to seek first-time entrance into competitive employment (Yaffee *et al.*, 1994: 20; Flynn, 1995: 65–6; Harvey, 1994: 2–3; Marmer, 1995: April 24, 16; Shafer *et al.*, 1991: 15; Jackson, 1994: 251).

Sheltered employment

Sheltered workshops are often sponsored by community and charity agencies for individuals with severe cognitive and/or physical limitations. In recent years, there has been a strong move away from sheltered employment towards supportive and competitive community arrangements for those clients who are able to move into the community with support services, assistive technology, and other workplace accommodations. Goodwill Industries and United Cerebral Palsy are organizations that continue to maintain sheltered workshops (Sax, 1995: 16).

Home-based employment

The numbers of disabled and non-disabled individuals who are choosing to work at home either part or full time are growing. Home workers include married women with children, long-distance commuters and consultants, individuals with computer modems connected to their offices, and individuals with mobility or cognitive impairment who are able to accomplish their job tasks with assistive and office technology, and support services. Disability managers or vocational counsellors provide services to home workers in need much as they do to work-site clients. Common options for home employment include computer utilization, telemarketing, clerical, business and professional services, and light manufacturing. Home workers must be able to tolerate social isolation and limited intellectual stimulation, and be able to work with minimal supervision (Breen *et al.*, 1991: 383–4).

Health and wellness promotion programmes

> Health promotion: 'systematic efforts by an organization to enhance the wellness of its members through education, behavior change, and cultural support.' (Johnson, 1986: 13)
>
> Wellness: 'the process of adapting patterns of behavior that lead to improved health and heightened life satisfaction.' (Danches, 1989: 215)

Rehabilitation professionals, including occupational therapy practitioners, teach employers how to prevent work injuries and illnesses and teach injured workers how to regain their ability to return to the workplace. However, employers have come to recognize that keeping their workers on the job and productive entails more than promoting occupational safety. They have determined that lost work time and medical costs incurred by employees are due to unhealthy lifestyles and their resultant preventable illnesses. In attempts to keep employees and their families healthy, employers are instituting insurance premium disincentive for poor health habits, and are engaging health-care and rehabilitation professionals often in managed care to provide health and wellness programmes. As early as the early 1980s, employers instituted stress management programmes in a health promotion context and as a preventive measure to healthy, asymptomatic workers to teach them skills for recognizing and coping with stress (Murphy and Shoenborn, 1987: vii). In addition to providing the programmes, Hershey Foods Corporation reduces employee health insurance fees for acceptable results for each of five risk factor measures: tobacco use, blood pressure, weight, exercise and cholesterol. Companies are unusual that do not provide smoking cessation or weight reduction programmes. In fact, 81 per cent of 1507 worksites reviewed in a 1992 study by the US Department of Health and Human Services had at least one health promotion activity (Murphy, 1995: 3).

Health promotion activities in the workplace are supported at the federal level. In December 1995, a federal advisory panel at the National Institute of Health called for fundamental societal lifestyle modifications that help prevent heart disease, diabetes, osteoporosis and certain cancers. Saying that physical activity is both a personal and societal responsibility, they called for schools and worksites to enable students and workers to exercise at least 30 minutes a day (The Boston Globe, 1995: 12).

Occupational therapy practitioners have a tradition of holistically approaching their client's health problems and potential problems by evaluating and modifying their clients occupations (Spencer, 1989: 217). The Representative Assembly of the American Occupational Therapy Association articulated that tradition when they adopted a formal statement on 'The Role of the Occupational Therapist in the Promotion of Health and the Prevention of Disabilities' in 1978. Cost-effective health and wellness promotion programmes are becoming a primary mode of service by all health care providers, including occupational therapists.

School-to-work transitions

Robert Reich, US Secretary of Labor, reports that today's workers are being challenged by workplace requirements and demands that are continuously evolving in response to technological advances and environmental impacts. Preparation for the next generation of workers needs to begin in schools where young people will obtain both classroom and real-life apprenticeship experiences and where, rather than recite facts, future workers will learn to identify and solve problems and to work together in teams that utilize each other's skills to innovate together (R. Reich, on the NPR radio programme 'The Connection', 27 November 1995). A federally sponsored school-to-work initiative with grants to all states will enable implementation of cooperative programmes between schools and industry to help prepare todays' students to be successful in tomorrow's workplace. These student groups, these future workers of tomorrow, need to value all members, including their fellow students with disabilities. Workers with disabilities have a poorer record of being employed than the general population; they especially need to develop work skills and to have real-life apprenticeship experiences if they are to participate in tomorrow's work teams.

Passage of the Education for All Handicapped Children Act (EHA) of 1975 mandated occupational therapy services in school systems. At that time, many occupational therapy practitioners reoriented from a medical to an education-based practice and developed community and work readiness programmes to help children and youth with disabilities develop gross and fine motor skills and improve their sensory perception processing as pre-readiness skills in preparation for entry into community and work life (Carrasco, 1993: 1; Barber *et al.*, 1993: 1; Spencer, 1989: 162). Follow-up studies however revealed that handicapped high-school graduates were not entering the workplace, but were more likely to be 'characterized by segregation, dependency, and non-productivity' (Spencer, 1995: 80). Several amendments were then made to the EHA which was renamed the Individuals with Disabilities Act (IDEA) (Public Law 101–476, 1990). IDEA emphasized an outcome-driven process. It shifted away from standardized and development-referenced assessments and from discipline-specific programme planning and goal setting to a coordinated multidisciplinary team intervention in terms of the student's actual performance in work, community living and socialization (Spencer, 1989: 162). Occupational therapy practitioners' assessments and interventions related to occupational performance in daily living activities, work and recreation, in both temporal and environmental performance contexts, are complementary to the work of other professionals on the team, and an essential component of effective transition planning and service delivery (American Occupational Therapy Association, 1994: 1047; Spencer, 1995: 80).

Preparation for the world of work begins early. Young children observe and model their behaviour after their parents, teachers, therapists and others in their homes, communities and schools. Playing with peers offers children opportunities to develop the roles, values and sensorimotor, cognitive and psychosocial competencies essential for school and work preparation (Brollier *et al.*, 1994: 346; Carrasco, 1993: 2).

The formal school-to-work programmes for children with disabilities begin by age 16. These school- and community-based education and occupational therapy programmes, along with parental and adult service agencies' involvement, enable students with disabilities to develop and practise competence in the work habits, interpersonal skills, self-awareness, and functional, environmentally based abilities in essential life occupations. With the support of both IDEA and the ADA, students with disabilities have the legal supports to integrate into the community and to maintain employment (Barber, 1993: 2; Brollier *et al.*, 1994: 347–8).

Occupational therapy practitioners focus on the individual's ability to participate in productive occupations throughout their lifespan (Jacobs *et al.*, 1992: 1086). Their training enables them to help parents and teachers prepare the next generation of workers. Federally initiated school-to-work transition programmes for children with and without disabilities will provide the means for them to implement their services.

Integrated service networks

In order to contain health-care costs, health-care organizations are not only looking at funding agreements, but are restructuring and positioning themselves in order to provide quality, yet cost-effective services. Thus, health-care organizations are merging, right-sizing and forming horizontal associations with other similar providers, or vertical associations with services offered along the continuum from acute-care to long-term services.

Rehabilitation network

A rehabilitation network is a form of managed competition in which the organizers of a network of rehabilitation providers set the rules for structured competition whereby member providers are selected based upon established criteria, including timely and effective delivery of services. Continued participation in the network is determined on an annual basis, based upon overall performance. One current programme exists in Ohio where the Bureau of Workers' Compensation developed criteria for such networks with the Ohio Chapter of the National Association of Rehabilitation Professionals in the Private Sector (NARPPS) (Growick and Finch, 1994: 1).

Continuum of care

A continuum of care is a vertical continuum of rehabilitation services affiliated in a single system in which services are provided at multiple points of client entry, from acute care through work rehabilitation. Such systems are becoming more common and are frequently a result of a merger or affiliation of previously competitive and/or nearby entities which allows it to position itself very competitively over other more limited programmes. For example, one medical centre in Los Angeles consists of a 40-bed acute rehabilitation unit, a transitional care centre (TCC), a range of typical and atypical outpatient services, including a CARF accredited outpatient programme, and a number of standard and innovative community-based programmes (Sullivan, 1995: 98).

Managed competition

Managed competition is a term for a health-care organizational structure where organized group-capitated health plans, rather than individual services, are managed by government regulations. In contrast to external cost containment by government-set prices and budgets, providers engage in price competition. Increased client cost-consciousness, and hopefully judicious utilization of services, is facilitated by requiring participation in insurance premium payments, health service deductibles and co-payments, and by receiving care only from those providers in their group-capitated plans (Reinhardt, 1995: 29). Although this attempt at health-care reform and cost containment during the Clinton administration was not successful, payors have responded to its concepts in subsequent plans.

Current quality assurance methods

TQM – Total Quality Management

Also referred to as QI or Quality Improvement, and more recently as CQI or Continuous Quality Improvement, TQM is a systems approach to quality imported in concept from Japanese industry, and involves attention to the work process in which the goal is continually to meet the increasing expectations (outcomes) of the business community and external referral sources (customers). It is customer focused and value driven in that standards are defined by quality measures such as effectiveness, reliability and efficiency. When the defined quality standards are not attained, the organization examines and revises the process. As work rehabilitation becomes more standardized, TQM will become a more common means of outcomes measurement (Wiklund, 1994: 5, 9).

Utilization review

Utilization review involves the process of looking at the documentation of care provided to the client either retrospectively (after the care has been provided) or, more frequently, concurrently (while under care of the provider) to determine if care met defined guidelines. This process is usually implemented either to validate or deny a claim for payment.

Outcomes evaluation and management

Outcomes evaluation and management is the system implemented by rehabilitation providers to track and monitor programme objectives, demographics and outcome measurements that enable the management of cost-effective, quality-focused programmes with successful outcome track records. The growing emphasis on quality-based continuous improvement and statistical process measuring has enabled organizations to move from crisis management to process improvement. Measurement of quality may be in terms of the perceptions of the recipients of the services. According to Craig Veloso, PhD, OTR/L, assistant professor at the University of Chicago, Department of Occupational Therapy, the 'worker's perceptions about the workplace may be more predictive of successful return to work than traditional work capacity measurements' (Apker, 1994: 61).

Anticipated trends

In response to changes in workforce characteristics, in workplace characteristics in the economy, in funding models, in international

Related terms

Any willing provider (AWP) AWP laws serve to extend the access of a rehabilitation provider to clients who may not have an insurance plan which has a contract with that provider. The guarantee of 'the right of a provider to contract with a managed care plan, provided that it meets the price, quality and credentialing standard that the plan has established' (Lindberg, 1995: 79). As a result of a groundswell of legislation by independent providers and consumer groups, by the mid 1990s, 26 states had some form of AWP laws which are a competitive challenge to managed care plans.

Catchment area The catchment area is the area served by a health-care provider or programme.

Case rate The case rate is the set amount of money per client, which usually includes a discount, that a payor agrees to pay for a package of care that guarantees defined outcomes as determined by utilization review (Framroze, 1995: 56).

Cost avoidance Cost avoidance involves the utilization by an employer of prevention and other programmes as an attempt to reduce accidents and illnesses and their associated costs, such as wage replacement, medical care, replacement training, and productivity losses. Self-insured employers are likely to implement cost avoidance measures (Dumas, 1994: 5).

Cost containment Cost containment describes the cooperative efforts by the employer, insurer and rehabilitation provider, such as case management and on-site rehabilitation programmes, to control the cost of an injury or illness. In a workers' compensation case, reducing the two primary costs, including replacing the workers' wages (indemnity costs) and paying the medical costs associated wth the illness or injury, greatly assist in cost containment efforts (Dumas, 1994: 5).

Cost per case The cost per case is a measurement standard payors use for provider selection, whereby facilities are compared to determine efficiency and effectiveness of their rehabilitation programmes. It is not a consistently acceptable means of comparison as some quality providers may have costs, such as a labour costs, that are not entirely within their control (Dumas, 1994: 5).

Indifference point The indifference point is a term borrowed from microeconomics price theory whereby the payor decides to select a provider based on price, such as case rate or group rate, when the provider's quality is determined to be equivalent to that of another provider (Beckley, 1995: 28). The payor's definition and perception of quality may include the patient's perceptions of such things as the speed of the admissions process, or the courtesy of housekeeping personnel! Such facilities find therefore they must be service oriented and promote their programmes not only by their effectiveness and efficiency, but by such things as the courtesy of their personnel.

Product-line management Product-line management describes the process of developing a cost effective way to provide a particular service by assigning licence requiring duties to licensed personnel and assigning other tasks to non-licensed personnel. Administrative reporting lines are not necessarily by profession. However, clinical standards are clearly defined and monitored.

competition, and in legislative changes, work programming in the USA has undergone drastic but exciting changes. Work rehabilitation programmes for factory workers, farm workers, home workers, and even children, have moved out of the facility or clinic and into the workplace. Individuals with HIV/AIDS or chronic illnesses, individuals with mental illness or cognitive impairment, individuals with work injuries or illnesses, and students with disabilities are all entering the workplace in a more timely way than ever before. Managed care pervades funding sources which are demanding cost containment and successful programme outcomes. But, the changes have only begun.

Industrial rehabilitation

Industrial rehabilitation programmes will implement defined treatment protocols and will expand loss-prevention consultation and evaluation services. Rehabilitation professionals, including occupational therapists, will provide ergonomics consultation, job-site analyses, ADA functional job and accessibility analyses, pre-employment and work-tolerance assessments, functional capacity evaluations, cumulative trauma and back-injury prevention programmes, and set up transitional modified duty programmes as well as rehabilitate the worker to be able to do the essential tasks. On-site therapy will be common in offices, manufacturing companies and in rural areas. Rehabilitation professionals will assist payors to evaluate therapy costs at various access points, including home care, and compare providers (Apker, 1994: 60; Ellexson, 1994: 42). As the number of older employees increases, rehabilitation providers will develop focused programmes for this cohort.

Supported employment

Supported employment services, along with assistive technology and protected by the ADA, will be expanded for persons with HIV/AIDS, mental illness, substance abuse and severe physical disabilities. As adolescents with HIV/AIDS and others with long-term illnesses successfully grow into young adults, they will need appropriate support services and other work programmes to increase empowerment and informed choice. With continued federal financial support, supported employment with assistive technology aids will be the primary form of support and training for the increasing numbers of individuals who work at home (Shafer *et al.*, 1991: 16).

School-to-work transitioning

Work preparation training for students with and without disabilities will involve classroom education and real-life community and work experiences.

Home-based employment

More than seven million workers 'commuted' to their offices via fax machines, telephones and e-mail in the mid 1990s. That number is expected to grow tremendously (Gates, 1996: 35).

Job training

At a meeting at the Massachusetts Institute of Technology in December 1995, called 'Job Training in the 21st Century', a group of economists, policy makers and community representatives noted that job-training programmes, which now consist of a lot of short-term classroom training, are not keeping pace with employers' high skill needs. Some of their ideas to improve job training in Massachusetts included teaching incarcerated men and women social values and job skills, seeking philanthropic and state funds for successful programmes, improving the public schools and redirecting some worker's compensation expenditures into company worker training programmes (Lewis, 1995: 50).

Marketing

Rehabilitation professionals with diversified skills will join with other providers formally or in networking to service multi-state employers and insurers.

Accreditation

Programme providers who have consistently high standards, good outcome measures, shared risks, and direct dialogues with payors are likely to be strong and profitable and thus have less need for accreditation. Furthermore, accreditation is familiar to public entities, but not to the growing number of self-insurers. Some programmes may seek CARF (Committee on Accreditation of Rehabilitation Facilities) in order to assist with improving outcome measures and becoming more efficient, in order to remain viable (Pinson, 1991: 2; Croteau, 1991: 6).

Utilization management

Rehabilitation professionals will increase services that include functional-capacity evaluations, second opinions, expert testimony, and specialized assessments for dysfunction.

Outcomes evaluation and management

Rehabilitation providers will increasingly implement systems to track and monitor programme objectives, demographics and outcome measurements that enable the management of cost-effective and clinically proficient programmes that meet community and referral source needs (Wilkerson, 1995: 115). According to a developer of medical disability assessment programmes, the 1992 US Task Force on Improving Medical Criteria for Disability Determination, comprised of government medical policy makers, reported the following finding:

> As functional status measures become more accepted by practitioners and researchers in the field, it is expected that they will become increasingly incorporated into the policies of government and private insurers. It is likely that they will ultimately become an alternative to the medical criteria now being used in SSI (Social Security Insurance) and SSDI (Social Security Disability Insurance) programs. They will be used in vocational rehabilitation programs at the State level to help determine rehabilitation and employment potential. They will be used in workers' compensation programs to determine appropriate compensation and the potential for rehabilitation and employment. They will be used in Medicare and Medicaid for purposes of payment, quality assurance and discharge planning. They will be used in the private sector, which has long had disability programs and is starting to develop long-term care programs. (M. Coupland, unpublished observation, 1995)

Funding arrangements

There will be an expansion of managed care that will result in: an increase in competition resulting in a reduction in the number of insurance companies, due to mergers and acquisitions; 24-hour managed care for workers' compensation will proliferate as employers note the reduced costs and increased employee productivity.

> Payors who insist on quality care at reasonable fees will recognize the value of the rehabilitation industry.
>
> Treatment algorithms will not represent 'cookbook medicine' but rather a long overdue standardization of techniques. Provider credentialing and benchmarking will assure that only competent, effective clinicians are hired. Stringent clinical documentation requirements will serve in a risk management (lower malpractice rate) capacity. Ineffective procedures and modalities will be removed from the clinician's arsenal, while new ones will be added. More hospitals will become 'health care systems', diversify their services, and start their own managed care plans. Insurers will interact more directly in the provision of health care services. (Clifton, 1995: 52)

Older workers

In a study of over 400 companies, the American Association of Retired Persons (AARP) identified eight trends:

1 Cost cutting has become a top priority for senior management.
2 Technology is a key to competitiveness.
3 Health-care costs are rising, with no end in sight.
4 Retirement is being redefined.
5 The American workforce is in the midst of a massive restructuring.
6 There is an emerging mismatch between employee needs and the way jobs are organized.
7 The 50-plus age group has begun to attract attention.
8 The federal government is beginning to assume a greater role in the business world. (Mann, 1992: 40)

Additionally, the AARP identified the following six points:

1 Positive attitudes toward older workers remain high.
2 Despite these positive attitudes, there are two obstacles that appear to impede the full utilization of older workers in American business:
   (a) the untested willingness and ability of older workers to adapt to new technology;

(b) the relative cost of employing older persons, particularly in salary requirements and health insurance.

3 The perspective of older workers themselves closely mirrors gatekeepers' attitudes.
4 Companies have made little or no progress in implementing programmes to utilize older workers more fully.
5 The largest companies (1000 or more employees) continue to display the least positive attitudes toward older workers.
6 There is an increased role for third-party institutions other than the employers and older employees themselves.

(Mann, 1992: 40–1)

Role of occupational therapy practitioners

Despite the ongoing changes in the workforce and workplace, occupational therapy practitioners are uniquely skilled to maintain a significant place in the work practice system.

> Occupational therapy practitioners focus on the individual's ability to participate in productive occupations throughout their life span. Through prevention, assessment, and intervention strategies, occupational therapy practitioners often collaborate with other members of the health team and assist persons to optimize their ability to engage in purposeful occupation while facilitating a safe and successful entry into or return to work. (American Occupational Therapy Association, 1992: 1088)

Multiple choice questions

1 The major payor of industrial claims is:
(a) managed care
(b) disability insurance
(c) workers' compensation
(d) vocational rehabilitation
(e) the federal government.

2 Work-hardening programmes:
(a) have been replaced by work conditioning
(b) are an essential component of work rehabilitation
(c) are not feasible in rural programmes
(d) have moved out of the clinic and into the workplace.
(e) are always covered by worker's compensation insurance.

3 Depending upon the setting, work programme goals may include:
(a) general endurance and cardiac conditioning
(b) increases in muscle strength and joint range of motion
(c) ability to do the essential tasks of the job
(d) training in specific skills such as lifting 50-pound boxes, learning to follow written directions, developing computer skills, or using a forklift
(e) all of the above.

4 Future work programming trends in the USA include:
(a) 24-hour managed care for workers' compensation and treatment standardization
(b) increased federal and state funding
(c) the demise of supported and sheltered employment programmes
(d) less emphasis on technical and service industry skills
(e) a lowering of the retirement age as the number of older workers increases.

For answer to multiple choice questions see p. 309.

References

Abeln, S. H. (1995, February/March). Managing risk under capitation. *Rehab. Management*, 110–11.

Abeln, S. H. and Alpert, (1995, June/July). Reducing the risk of CTDs. *Rehab. Management*, 131–132.

American Occupational Therapy Association (1992). Statement: occupational therapy services in work practice. *Am. J. of Occ. Therapy*, 1086–8.

American Occupational Therapy Association (1994). Uniform terminology for occupational therapy, 3rd edn. *Am. J. of Occ. Therapy*, 1047–59.

Apker, C. (1994, August, September). New payment for industrial medicine. *Rehab. Management*, 59–62.

Aron, L. J. (1995, August/September). The payor–provider partnership. *Rehab. Management*, 109–10, 127.

Aron, L. J. (1995, October/November). Return to work: the employer perspective. *Rehab. Management*, 94–5.

Arriaga, R. L. (1994, August/September). Cross-cultural considerations. *Rehab. Management*, 99–101.

Barber, M., McIrney, C. and Struck, M. (1993, June). Training for transition from school to work. *Work Programs SIS Newsletter*, 3–4.

Beckley, N. J. (1995, June/July). *Rehab Case Management. Rehab. Management*, 25–8.

Boston Globe, The (1995) Tying sloth to heart disease, panel seeks changes. 21 December, p. 12.

Braddom, R. (1992, August). Industrial rehabilitation: an overview. Rehabilitation of the Injured Worker. *Phys. Med. and Rehab. Clinics. of No. Am.*, 499–510.

Breen, T. L., Clark, K. L. and Moran, M. (1991). Home based employment. In Occupational Therapy Work-Related Programs and Assessments, (K. Jacobs, ed.) pp. 383–91, Boston: Little, Brown.

Brollier, C., Shepherd, K., Markley, F. (1994). Transition from school to community living. *Am. J. Occup. Ther.*, **8**(4), 346–53.

Burchman, P. (1994, December). Bureau of labor statistics study sheds light on workplace injuries and hazards. *Work Programs SIS Newsletter*, 3–4.

Burles, B. (1993, March/April). Oregon workers' comp reform relies on managed care organizations. *Work Injury Management*, 1–5.

Canelon, M. F. (1995). Job site analysis facilitates work reintegration. *Am. J. Occup. Ther.*, **49**(5), 461–70.

Carrasco, R. C. (1993, March). Work-related programs for children and adults: part I. *Work Programs SIS Newsletter*, 1–4.

Caulfield, M., Carey, C. and Mason, C. (1994, Autumn). Project employ: rehabilitation services facilitating employment of individuals with HIV/AIDS. *American Rehabilitation*, 12–16.

Child, L. (1995, June). Workers compensation: managing a healthier bottom line. *Work Injury Management*, 6–7.

Christiansen, C. (1991). Occupational therapy: Intervention for life performance. In *Occupational Therapy, Overcoming Human Performance Deficits* (C. Baum and C. Christiansen, eds), pp. 18–19, Thorofare, NJ: Slack.

Clifton, D. W. (1995, April/May). Diversifying for success in the '90s. *Rehab Management*, 52–60.

Conley, S. (1995). Health-related disabilities, pain, and employment: initial impact of the Americans with disabilities act of 1990. *Journal of Vocational Rehabilitation*, **51**, 43–54.

Croteau, B. (1991, March). Does CARF accreditation make a difference in reimbursement? *Work Programs SIS Newsletter*, **5**(1), 3, 6.

Danches, J. W. (1989). Prevention. In *Work In Progress*. (S. Hertfelder and C. Gwin, eds), pp. 213–46, Rockville, MD: Am. Occ. Ther. Assoc.

Daus, C. (1995, April/May). Onsite rehab. *Rehab. Management*, 25–9, 132.

Daus, C. (1995, October/November). Traumatic hand injuries. *Rehab. Management*, 31–4.

Devlin, P. (1992, July/August). Anatomy of successful early return to work programs: inception, operation and measures of effectiveness. *Work Injury Management*, 5–9.

Devlin, P. (1994, June). Onsite work hardening. *Work Injury Management*, **3**, B1–B2.

Devlin, P. (1995, June). Briefs. *Work Injury Management*, B1–B4.

Devlin, P. (1995, July/August/September). Case study shows key elements in a work injury management partnership that effectively reduced claims and costs. *Work Injury Management*, 1–3.

Devlin, P. (1995, November). Disability managers: profile of an emerging specialist. *Work Injury Management*, 6–7.

Devlin, P. (1995, December-a). PPO gives therapy major role, avoids discounting. *Work Injury Management*, 6–7.

Devlin, P. (1995, December-b). Industrial rehabilitation: what clients look for in a provider partnership. *Work Injury Management*, 7–9, 15.

Dumas, M. (1994, November). Coordinating workers' compensation, ADA, and early return-to-work programs. *Work Injury Management*, 5–8.

Dumont, D. and Vance, S. R. (1992, July/August). Industrial physical therapy: a model of onsite intervention. *Work Injury Management*, 1, 3–4.

Ellexson, M. (1994, April/May). One-stop shopping – developing an industrial rehabilitation service to meet consumer demand and competition. *Rehab. Management*, 42–4.

Felix, D. C. (1992, September/October). Where is work hardening going? *Work Injury Management*, 19.

Feuerstein, M. (1991). A multidisciplinary approach to the prevention, evaluation, and management of work disability. *J. of Occup. Rehab.*, **1**(1), 5–12.

Fisher, T. (1993, December). Work conditioning is not work hardening. *Work Programs SIS Newsletter*, 3.

Fisher, T. (1995, October 6). Case management: the key to successful return to work or case closure. *Occupational Therapy Forum*, 4–5.

Flynn, C. (1995, June). A closer look at VR service delivery. *TeamRehab*, 65–6.

Framroze, A. (1995, February/March). 24 hour managed care. *Rehab Management*, 51–57, 131.

Frederick, C. (1994, December 15). The rigors and rewards of rural practice. *OT Week*, 16–19.

Fullerton, H. (1994, April). Another look at the work force. *The American Work Force: 1992–2005*, pp. 29–38, Washington, D.C.: U.S. Department of Labor.

Gates, B. (1996, January). The road ahead. *Working Woman*, 33–40.

Growick, B. (1993, July/August). ADA and workers' compensation: what are the critical issues? *Work Injury Management*, 7–9.

Growick, B. and Finch, J. (1994, June). Managed competition in rehabilitation. *Work Injury Management*, 1–4.

Habeck, R. (1994, December). Examining the disability management model for rehabilitation service delivery. *Work Injury Management*, 1–6.

Hallam, R. (1995). Mental health work rehabilitation services in the United States – innovation and good practice. *Work*, **5**, 41–50.

Harvey, R. (1994, Summer). Enhancing employment outcomes for individuals with serious and persistent mental illnesses. *American Rehabilitation*, 2–8.

Hettinger, J. (1995, August 24). The portals PARTNERS project. *OT Week*, 18–19.

Hunter, S. and McCallister, D. (1994, November). Employer/provider partnership: a case example. *Work Injury Management*, 1–4.

Jackson, J. D. (1993). After rehabilitation: meeting the long-term needs of persons with traumatic brain injury. *Am. J. Occup. Ther.*, **48**(3), 251–5.

Jacobs, K. (1991). *Occupational Therapy Work-Related Programs and Assessments*. Boston: Little, Brown.

Joe, B. E. (1995, November 30). Effective work programs. *OT Week*, 12–13.

Johnson, J. A. (1986). *Wellness: A Context for Living*. New Jersey: Slack.

Johnston, W. B. and Packer, A. E. (1987). *Workforce 2000: Work and Workers for the 21st Century*. Indianapolis, IN: Hudson Institute.

Johnston, W. B. and Packer A. E. (1988). *Opportunity 2000: Creative Affirmative Action Strategies for a Changing Workforce*. Indianapolis, IN: Hudson Institute.

King, J. W. (1995, February/March). Repetitive strain injuries. *Rehab. Management*, 51–8.

King, P. (1993). Outcome analysis of work-hardening programs. *Am. J. Occup. Ther.*, **47**(7), 595–603.

Knox, R. A. (1995, December 6). Cutbacks to shift health costs to workers. *The Boston Globe*, 20.

Lacerte, M. (1992, July, August). The downfall of work hardening. *Work Injury Management*, 19.

Larson, B. (1994, December). On-site work rehabilitation: the employer, insurer, and provider connection. *Work Programs SIS Newsletter*, 1–2.

Larson, B. A. (1995, December). On-site work rehabilitation: the employer, insurer, and provider connection. *Work Programs SIS Newsletter*, 1–2.

Lavergne, O. J. (1995, December/January). Rural rehab. *Rehab. Management*, 72–4.

Lehigh, S. (1995). Vicious circle. *The Boston Globe*, 3 September, pp. 65, 69.

Lewis, D. E. (1995). Group eyes ways to upgrade job training. *The Boston Globe*, 14 December, p. 50.

Lindberg, G. E. (1995, October/November). The any-willing-provider controversy. *Rehab. Management*, 79–81.

Litke, C., Scott, D. and Smetler, K. (1995, November/December). Back to work with a team of therapists. *Workplace Ergonomics*, 18–20.

Mann, W. C. (1992, Fall). Older workers with disabilities. *Technology and Disability*, 37–46.

Marmer, L. (1995, April 24). For-profit supported employment site spurs on workers. *Advance for Occupational Therapists*, 16.

Mason, C., Carey, C. and Jaskulski, T. *et al.* (1995). Providing supported employment and other vocational rehabilitation services to individuals with HIV/AIDS. *J. of Voc. Rehab.*, **5**, 55–64.

Milne, J. (1995). State gets mental health patients out of institutions, and into jobs. *The Boston Sunday Globe*, 22 January, p. 26–7.

Mitchell, K., Leclair, S. (1992, August). Building a working alliance with employers. Rehabilitation of the Injured Worker. *Phys. Med. & Rehab.* Clinics of No. Am., pp. 647–63.

Montagano, T. (1994, Spring). Bringing the rehabilitation family together: an independent living-vocational rehabilitation partnership. *American Rehabilitation*, pp. 35–36.

Murphy, J. (1995, May 8). Wellness programs gather steam. *Advance for Occupational Therapists*, 3, 16.

Murphy, L. R. and Schoenborn, T. F. (1987). *Stress Management in Work Settings*. Washington, DC: National Institute for Occupational Safety and Health.

Niemeyer, L. O. and Foto, M. (1994, June/July). Partnering in workers' compensation. *Rehab. Management*, 138–41.

Niemeyer, L. O., Jacobs, K. and Reynolds-Lynch *et al.* (1994). Work hardening: past, present, and future – the work programs special interest section national work-hardening outcome study. *Am. J. Occ. Ther.*, **48**(4), 327–39.

Ogden-Niemeyer, L. and Jacobs, K. (1989). *Work Hardening State of the Art*. Thorofare, NJ: Slack.

Olson, S. (1994, December). Some psychological aspects of industrial injury. *Work Injury Management*, 7–9, 14.

Parent, W., Unger, D. and Gibson, K. (1994, Autumn). The role of job coach: orchestrating community and workplace supports. *American Rehabilitation*, 2–11.

Paiva, R. (1995, March). Logging with a disability. *Technology and Disability*, 67–71.

Pfaff, K. (1995, August). Bills propose VR overhaul. *TeamRehab Report*, 9.

Pinson, C. C. (1991, March) Work programs reimbursement: what is happening across the nation? *Work Programs SIS Newsletter*, **5**, 1–3.

Priebe, J. and Bierle, D. (1995, June). Industrial rehabilitation: practical aspects in developing partnerships. *Work Injury Management*, 1–5.

Rausch, R. W. (1995, June/July). Succeeding under capitation. *Rehab. Management*, 135–7, 164.

Reinhardt, U. E. (1995, February/March). Managed competition and Technical innovation. *Rehab. Management*, 25–31.

Richardson, M. (1994). The impact of the Americans with Disabilities Act on employment opportunity for people with disabilities. *Annu. Rev. Public Health*, **15**, 91–105.

Sax, C. (1995, May). Change of life. *TeamRehab Report*, 16–20.

Shafer, M., Revell, W. G. and Isbister, F. (1991). The national supported employment initiative: a three-year longitudinal analysis of 50 states. *J. of Voc. Rehab.*, **1**(1), 1–17.

Shoemaker, R. J. (1992, July/August). Reaction to disability. *Journal of Rehabilitation*, 18–24, 28.

Shrey, D. E. (1992, September/October). Employer-based work return transition programs and the deinstitutionalization of America's injured workers. *Work Injury Management*, 4–6.

Simental, S., Niemeyer, L. O. and Foto, M. (1994, October/November). The workers' comp team. *Rehab Management*, 105–7.

Smith, T. S. and Alexander, I. (1995) Issues and practices accross rural rehabilitation in the United States. *Technology and Disability*, **4**, 3–10.

Spencer, K. C. (1989). The transition from school to adult life. In *Work in Progress* (S. Hertfelder and C. Gwin, eds), pp. 157–80, Rockville, MD: American Occupational Therapy Association.

Spencer, K. C. (1995). Transitions: from school to adult life. *Work*, **5**, 79–84.

Stahl, C. (1995, June 26). Idea: will it still fly? *Advance for Occupational Therapists*, 13, 54.

Sudimack, J. and Cooper, A. M. (1992, August). A broad view of rehabilitation of the industrially injured worker. Rehabilitation of the Injured Worker. *Phys. Med. & Rehab. Clinics of No. Am.*, 589–97.

Sullivan, T. L. (1995, April/May). St Jude's continuum of care. *Rehab. Management*, 98–101, 131.

Torres-Davis, A. and Crowl, B. (1995). Assistive technology legislation applications for rural populations. *Technology and Disability*, **4**, 29–34.

Tweed, V. (1994, June/July). Transitions to success. *Rehab. Management*, 56–61.

US Department of Labor. Bureau of Labor Statistics. (1995, April). *Occupational Injuries and Illnesses: counts, rates, and characteristics*, 1992.

US Merit Systems Protection Board, (1993). *Evolving workforce demographics: federal agency action and reaction.* Washington, DC: Erdreich, BL.

Walsh, P. M. (1995). Goodwill: more than old clothes. *The Boston Globe*, 21 April, pp. 21, 25.

Weiner and de Lissovy, (1993, Spring). Raising a tower of Babel – a taxonomy of managed care and health insurance plans. From *The Journal of Health Politics, Policy, and Law*, **18**(1), NC: Duke University Press. In a reprint distributed by the American Occupational Therapy Association for the Government Relations Department Update for the Managed Care Forum, April 11, 1995.

Wiklund, M. (1994, June). TQM: An investment for the future. *Work Injury Management*, 5–9.

Wilkerson, D. (1995, December/January). Developing outcomes management tools. *Rehab. Management*, 114–117, 129.

Wyrick, J. M., Niemeyer, L. O., Ellexson, M., Jacobs, K. (1991). Occupational therapy work-hardening programs: a demographic study. *Am. J. Occup. Ther.*, **45**(2) 109–12.

Yaffe, H., Fitzgerald, R., Dunfee, M., Weatley, E. and Wurzbacher, M., (1994, Summer). Project CIRCLE: strategies for increasing the choice, control, and competence of survivors of brain injuries in the vocational rehabilitation process. *American Rehabilitation*, 20–31.

Yankowitz, R. and Muscante, S. (1994, Autumn). The use of cognitive functional assessment in a psychiatric vocational rehabilitation program. *American Rehabilitation*, 32–7.

Zezima, M. (1995, 14 November). How work hardening works in the managed care era. *Advance For Occupational Therapists*, 22, 58.

A UK perspective

Abstract

Historical, political, social and cultural factors influence work practice services. This chapter identifies the major influencing factors affecting service provision as a direct result of the current changes in health and social service development in the UK. These changes challenge the occupational therapy professions to take a wider view of service delivery and to look to the voluntary and private sectors as potential areas of service delivery in addition to traditional practice areas within health care and local authority provisions.

Introduction

Historical and political factors have shaped and directed past and present vocational services for people with disabilities in the UK who wish to access training and return to, or gain employment. The Disabled Persons Employment Acts 1944 and 1958 provided the basis for the services on offer today. The Department of Education and Employment, a branch of the UK civil service structure, has the statutory remit to implement the provision of these Acts. The initial Acts of 1944 and 1958 were initiated to respond to the needs of war veterans returning from military service. Currently the acts' main provisions include legislative support for the assessment and training of people with disabilities. As described by Pratt (1995), it places a duty on employers to adhere to a Quota Scheme, and to hire a quota of registered disabled people. This quota currently stands at 3 per cent, and only businesses of 20 or more employees are subject to the Act.

The consultative document Employment and Training for People with Disabilities, published in 1990 by the Employment Department Group, marked an important point in the development of services to assist people returning to employment. It followed a comprehensive review of existing provision. The review considered the demographic changes in the UK and influences on the labour market, considering views suggested to the government by the Public Accounts Committee and the National Advisory Council on Employment of Disabled People.

The consultative document offers the following considerations:

1 That the effectiveness of present provision for assisting individuals with disabilities should be questioned about its continued effectiveness, and that people have a right to be treated as individual people and not categorized, to be served and not managed by services.
2 The full commitment of employers must be secured. It is employers who, through their policies and practices, will primarily determine how far disabled people are able to find, keep and advance in work. This may suggest that there requires to be a review of the efficiency of the present Quota system in Britain which is considered to have been redundant and impossible to enforce for many years.
3 Services must be relevant to changing structures of the changing labour market in the 1990s.
4 The contribution to public services which voluntary organizations and others in the community can make must be utilized, to tap sources of expertise and knowledge, and to bear particular commitment, sensitivity and flexibility.
5 Services must be coherent in working together and where necessary to meet ends.
6 People with disabilities must have appropriate incentives to work. (Employment Department Group, 1990)

All the issues pointed out in the consultative document should be considered when planning services for job seekers with disabilities. The Department of Employment, who amalgamated in summer 1995 to become the Departments of Education and Employment, has consulted with specialist groups and service providers to ensure that job seekers have equal access to appropriate training opportunities, and are not being slotted into existing services where they have to adapt to the training environment, or compromise some elements of their training in order to meet the strict criteria established by some funding bodies, although many believe that this consultation should be more comprehensive. Renfrewshire Employment Liaison Initiative (RELI), a multi-agency pressure group, published a resume of the government white paper (January 1995) on Anti-Discrimination Legislation. It suggested intentions to:

- Place a duty on employers to make 'reasonable adjustment' within the workplace.
- Replace the present Quota scheme which has been in place since 1944 and is considered by many as redundant and impossible to enforce.
- Promote statutory right of access to goods and services to people with disabilities.
- Create a National Disability Council to advise the government on employment-related issues to be addressed and measures to be taken.
- Influence and strengthen local authority guidance to the Ministry of Transport on low-floor buses and right of access to buses/railway stations
- Offer guidance on access standards for new schools.

Current models used in the delivery of work programmes in the UK

Vocational/Employment
Educational
Social
Rehabilitative
Occupational therapy model

Current work rehabilitation services are delivered via a diversity of models and approaches, and these have developed in response to statutory requirements and access to the particular funding available at specific periods in time.

Vocational/employment

This model focuses on the provision of services which lead directly and specifically to employment and job readiness. Intervention is coordinated by government agencies and offers specific funding that provides access to employers and training providers.

Employment service

One branch of the government, the Department of Education and Employment, manages the Employment Service and has the responsibility of administering and delivering support services for those entering employment.

Through the Employment Services' national network of job centres and Placement Assessment and Counselling Teams (PACT), it is committed to accessing career opportunities for people with disabilities, and to help employers recruit, retain and develop opportunities for job seekers. The specialist provision offered by this service includes input from occupational psychologists, physiotherapists and technical consultants. Whilst this has never been a traditional area of employment for occupational therapists, it would seem that there is an obvious role enhancing the present service with their unique combination of skill and knowledge in the area of occupational performance.

Placement assessment and counselling teams (PACT)

PACT teams aim to provide a coherent employment advice and assessment service for both employers and those seeking employment. They advise on the following:

- Good working practice
- Recruiting people with disabilities
- Retaining employees who have become disabled
- Providing financial assistance to employ people with disabilities
- Adapting working environments
- Job assessment and restructuring
- Work preparation and employment rehabilitation
- Provision of equipment and ergonomics in the workplace
- Accessibility to premises
- Developing disability awareness
- Providing advice regarding legal obligation under the Disabled Person Employment Acts of 1944 and 1958.

(Employment Service, 1992b)

Ability development centres (ADCs)

There is a national network of nine ADCs in the UK providing a service which aims to work in partnership with the PACT teams by providing professional and technical staff who assess job seekers' functional capacity and identify suitable equipment that would enable individuals to achieve independence in the workplace. The ADC staff also provide a technical advice service to employers, quality training to employers, short-term rehabilitation and training for job seekers and offer disability awareness training for job centres. (Employment Service (1992) Ability Development Centre Scotland.)

Disability employment advisors (DEAs)

DEAs are members of PACT teams and are based in local job centres, working closely with mainstream services. DEAs help individuals to access employment and assist employers to recruit or maintain employees with disabilities by providing advice and access to funds, equipment or other services such as ADCs (Employment Service, 1992b).

Sheltered workshops/sheltered placements

Sheltered workshops

The majority of sheltered workshops in the UK are managed by one organization called Remploy, who provide 14 000 out of a possible 20 000 sheltered placements in the country. These workshops function as small business entities. The factories and workshops compete in the open market and provide a range of quality goods and services such as packaging, assembly, engineering clothing and furniture, all at competitive prices. Sheltered employment caters for those who require more substantial and longer-term support and offers a protected and supportive working environment as well as an income. Local authorities and voluntary organizations also provide services, and these are offered in conjunction with the Employment Service, with contracts lasting three years.

Sheltered placements

Sheltered placements enable people to work in mainstream employment and the employee is paid the full rate for the job. The salary is negotiated between the employer, who pays for the percentage of the work actually carried out, and any top up is provided by the sponsoring agency, usually a voluntary organization, local authority or Remploy, and will be funded by the Department of Education and Employment (Employment Service, 1994a).

Access to work

This service is for people who are unemployed in work or self-employed, and who need to get a job, keep a job, or make progress in their career. Employees do not have to be registered disabled to apply or to be eligible for assistance, but should have a health problem which affects the kind of work they can do, and this health problem would be likely to last twelve months or more. Through Access to Work, potential employees with disabilities are eligible for assistance to the value of £21 000 over five years paid by the Employment Service. This funding will assist in adapting work premises or providing specialist equipment. Employers do not have to pay unless the assistance brings general business benefit, such as making buildings more accessible to customers and others. In this case the employers would be expected to share the cost.

Work preparation

This service provides an opportunity for disabled job seekers to address specific issues/problems that they might meet in the workplace. Organizations selected by the Employment Service provide the specialist programmes offering skill and expertise in assisting the clients to meet the requirements to be job ready. Work preparation enables individuals to identify and assess abilities, assisting people to understand the effects of their health problem on work-related activities, increasing the person's confidence to pursue work opportunities effectively, and to establish realistic employment aims (Employment Service, 1994a).

Job introduction scheme (JIS)

This scheme enables an individual with a disability to try employment for an introductory period. This scheme is useful for employers who may have practical concerns about whether to employ a candidate with a disability. The JIS enables them to offer potential candidates a trial period at £45 per week for a period of six weeks. During the period of the JIS, the employer is expected to pay the candidate the normal rate for their job during the trial period. The job can be full time or part time but it must be expected to last for at least six months after the trial ends. It has to be a genuine job offer and not specifically created to take advantage of the scheme. The JIS cannot be used for jobs within government departments and does not apply to placements in supported employment or in any other government-funded training scheme (Employment Service, 1994c).

Training for work (TFW)

This provision also bases its philosophy on the vocational/employment model, focuses on liaison with employers and offers training programmes which are directly related to the acquisition of specific vocational skills. In Scotland, TFW is managed by a government body known as Local Enterprise Companies (LECs). Renfrewshire Enterprise represents the Renfrewshire area of the West of Scotland. The LECs in Scotland are responsible for providing Training for Work schemes in conjunction with the Department of Education and Employment to provide a training service for unemployed job seekers between 18 and 60 years. Many voluntary organizations are contracting with the LECs to provide training to specific client groups, particularly people with disabilities. Some examples include The Scottish Association for Mental Health and Enable (formerly Scottish Society for Mental Handicap). Unfortunately there is no specialist provision for trainees with disabilities within Training for Work, or no particular pathways for special needs groups which would permit a flexible approach to training, and funding that would allow for the delivery of graded training. Organizations like Scottish Association for Mental Health are negotiating with LECs throughout Scotland to establish policies for flexibility in accessing special needs funding.

The TFW funding is output related, and projects funded under this scheme strive to achieve the agreed outcome measures as directed by each LEC. These are directed towards the achievement of clearly identified positive outcomes. Many training providers involved with trainees with mental health problems or learning disabilities, for example, find that there is little opportunity for flexibility in working towards these outcomes. The main emphasis is on identifying 'hard' or structured outcomes indicators, such as trainees entering full-time employment, full-time further education or vocational qualifications at levels 1, 2 or 3. An example of a level 1 is the Business Administration level 1 certificate administered by City & Guilds of London. This is one of the most basic levels of vocational qualification offered, and encompasses nine units covering several practical and theoretical aspects of business administration, including information technology, receiving callers and colleagues, reprographics, filing, mail handling, and petty cash.

Training providers, many of whom are voluntary organizations, negotiate with each LEC to attempt to reach the most suitable level of outcome for their specific client group. In this situation, many occupational therapists are being employed as training managers within these services and are also involved in reaching balanced and appropriate outcome measures for the prospective trainees. For many service providers, it is difficult to assist clients to achieve the levels identified by the LECs due to psychological, cognitive or intellectual constraints, particularly for those with learning disabilities or mental health problems.

For many trainees who enter into training, employment may only be one of many goals, it may be unrealistic for clients to be able to return to employment or the trainee may feel that they cannot afford to enter full-time education, replacing benefits with temporary bursaries. Many in fact do choose part-time education, where they can remain on benefits, and this offers trainees an opportunity to grade and develop their learning gradually and at an appropriate pace. Training providers are striving to encourage LECs to adopt a more flexible approach to the recognition of a range of positive outcomes, e.g. returning to part-time education, entering voluntary work to develop work skills, or pursuing further training with mainstream training providers. The LECs are also being encouraged to recognize more flexible indicators of success, such as personal and social development, and progress in areas that do not lead directly to employment. The difficulty for many training providers is that they feel compromised by a conflict between the outcomes set by funding bodies and the aim of meeting the more holistic needs of the trainees.

TFW is primarily employer based and training would be contracted to take place within an industrial environment, with the trainee seconded to an employer base. Special needs training has been mainly project based and training takes place within supported and simulated training environments, mainly on organized sites or within a health-care base. These areas are usually accredited by a formal training body such as Scotvec or City & Guilds, and trainees are offered employer placements if they feel able to undertake training within an industrial environment. The TFW service offers training for one full year, although it is widely recognized that, for many trainees, one year may simply be the inauguration of a long process towards job readiness. Whilst on TFW, the trainee cannot claim Incapacity Benefit from the Department of Social Security, but instead receives a training allowance paid by the Department of Education and Employment. This causes concern for many individuals who consider TFW as an option since the trainee has to reapply and make a fresh claim for their state benefit on completion of their training, and even though the trainee may not feel job ready, the fact that they have engaged in training may jeopardize their benefit status. A trainee may be refused a return to their previous benefit on the basis that if they are capable of sustaining attendance on a full-time course, evidence may suggest that they are well enough to undertake work. This likelihood acts as a disincentive to trainees with disabilities (Royal Association for Disability and Rehabilitation, 1994).

European social fund

This service is funded from the European Union and although it focuses on the vocational model, it offers flexibility and adaptability in its delivery, recognizing the special needs of disabled trainees and offering recognition of personal and social as well as vocational development. This service straddles the vocational and the rehabilitative model. European Social Fund projects are primarily accessed by voluntary organizations. Funding comes direct from Europe and is allocated to government departments who in turn contract it out to other agencies to allocate. In Scotland, the Scottish Office advocates responsibility to the Scottish Council for Voluntary Organizations to distribute funds to specific projects. Voluntary organizations are invited to apply, and compete for allocation of funds. This funding is accessed via specified pathways and there is a discreet allocation of funding for trainees with disabilities; this allows for training to be tailored to suit specific needs. The training can only be accessed if the trainee has been unemployed for a period of six months or more and the training can last from eighteen months to three years. Outcome measures identify educational and vocational developments, but there is also recognition of personal, social development and of health-care needs which should be addressed during the period of training. Training is primarily project based and many voluntary organizations apply for this money in partnership with traditional health-care providers. Training usually takes place on the simulated training site, and job transition and employer placements are offered in industrial settings if appropriate. Community and life-skills training is offered as part of the course and clients are encouraged to return to employment or education if they wish, but consideration is given to alternatives to employment and training, such as preparation for unemployment and constructive use of leisure time. Trainees are paid a training allowance and travel/subsistence, and allowances do not alter or influence training.

Educational model

The educational model is focused on the individual as learner/student. Services are concentrated primarily in educational establishments, schools and colleges of further/higher education offering services specifically for students with extended learning needs. Services are offered throughout the education system and career guidance services. It strives to offer students with disabilities the opportunity to participate in their educational development within the environs of primary, secondary and further/higher education. The following represent services offered by many colleges of education. Many colleges of further and higher education provide specialist services for students with disabilities. These departments are commonly known Support for Learning Departments and Extended Learning Support services and teams are available to offer discreet services. Extended learning support offers students support planning and assessment of needs, offering specialist advice regarding the physical and psychological learning environment. Support for learning offers students a wide range of educational opportunities, usually in liaison with mainstream departments within the college, and also more specific courses in adult basic education, independent living skills, and personal and life-skills training. Many occupational therapists introduce students to the services as a process of rehabilitation, to promote links with community services and to introduce clients to the concept of utilizing community-based provisions. Support for learning is a useful method of introducing clients to a supported and flexible educational resource, and this is a potential area where the occupational therapist could become involved in developing the concept of occupational performance into the educational environment.

Social model

This model is adopted by many services provided by the Social Work Department, a government department, and concentrates on the social development of clients with disabilities, primarily in adult training centres, day centres and disability living centres. The general aim is to promote integration into the community and to encourage effective use of the community-based services. This model focuses on employment as one of many possible goals the client may wish to work towards. The adult training centre is part of the regional council's social work department and as such is funded by the local authority, and governed by its procedural guidelines relating to day-care services. This provision is targeted towards clients with learning disability. Most centres operate a key-worker system of client care whereby needs and abilities are assessed and individual goals set through programmed daily activities. The evaluations of these activities is ongoing, with annual reviews for each client as a focus for considering effectiveness, progress and future goals. Whilst historically the adult training centres have seen considerable change and the services now concentrate more on developing social and domestic skills, the general aim of this approach is to enhance the individual's potential for integrating freely in the community. Many clients who attend the centres also attend college-based support-for-learning services. Whilst staff are not directly involved in providing formal education, supported employment or independent living, the philosophy encourages clients to make informed choices about options for themselves. Social work departments also provide social support for clients with specific needs, an example of this is the services for the hearing and visually impaired. These services are not specifically involved in providing vocational training, but offer support in relation to this. The main remit of specialist services is to provide social rehabilitation and to maximize independent-living skills. For clients interested in pursuing further education or employment, the skills gained in social rehabilitation scenarios may enhance employment prospects.

Rehabilitative model

Rehabilitation focuses on the collaborative development of skills and abilities integrating social, medical, vocational and educational factors. This model adopts a holistic perspective, recognizing the diverse needs of the job seeker, attempting to concentrate on the redevelopment of functional, personal and vocational skills that need to be redeveloped in order to return to the job market. Hagedorn (1992) summarized the rehabilitation model as: 'nominally holistic, and the importance of taking a broadly based view of the patient and her needs, and of considering ability as well as disability, is often stressed.'

Occupational therapy model

Occupational therapists encompass the rehabilitation model into their practice, and traditionally they have provided their service within the structure of the National Health Service and local authority. Hospital-based occupational therapists worked in light and heavy workshops and clients were referred by medical consultants. Many patients needed to undergo a period of rehabilitation of skills and function before returning to work after illness or injury, in many cases patients still remained in employment and intended to return within due course, vocational competence was a major factor influencing treatment. In more recent years, unemployment has become a major problem in the UK and many patients are unemployed or there is less prospect of returning to work after injury. As a result, patients have to consider career changes and alternatives to employment as a more realistic scenario. In the past industrial therapy units flourished and assisted in returning clients directly back to work, offering training in traditional work skills and process skills. More recently this service has been viewed as outdated and inappropriate to today's employment demands. In more recent years there have been dynamic developments in the area of work practice in the UK. The Department of Education and Employment has rationalized and developed its function. European funding and other enterprise grants have been made available to develop services for adult returners to work. Occupational therapists must develop roles within the new structures, and this is slowly becoming apparent. Occupational therapists are employed within educational environments, as vocational guidance counsellors and training managers, they are also integrating into voluntary and training organizations. The opportunities for the profession are endless, and practitioners are increasingly working within and as part of the Employment Service. Recent changes in health and social-care initiatives, e.g. care in the community legislation, have promoted increased community intervention and a shift in funding responsibility from statutory health-care providers to contracting with community-based services. New areas of practice are abundant with potential for therapists to engage in many new areas. Occupational therapists are becoming independent care providers and working in private practice, functioning in a wide range of new and innovative areas including extended learning and special needs support in education facilities, industrial consultation within occupational-health services, employee assistance programmes, health promotion, ergonomic consultation, offering on-site work adaptation and return-to-work programmes.

References

Employment Department Group (1990). *Consultative Document. Employment and Training for People with Disabilities*. Employment Department, London.

Employment Service (1992). *PACT – A New Service for People with Disabilities*. Employment Department Group, London.

Employment Service (1992a). *Ability Development Centres Scotland*. Employment Department Group, London.

Employment Service (1992b). *Information on Disability and Employment*. Employment Department Group, London.

Employment Service (1994a). *Access to Work*. Employment Department Group, London.

Employment Service (1994b). *Jobs in Supported Placements, Jobs in Supported Employment*. Employment Department Group, London.

Employment Service (1994c). *Job Introduction Scheme Information for Employers*. Employment Department Group, London.

Hagedorn, R. (1992). *Occupational Therapy: Foundations for Practice*. London: Churchill Livingstone.

Pratt, J. (1995). *Employment Services for People with Disabilities in Scotland Work: A journal of prevention, assessment and rehabilitation*, **5**, 11–16.

Royal Association for Disability and Rehabilitation (1994). *Training for Disabled People Factsheet 4*.

Section II

Performance Contexts

4

Environment

Barbara Cooper, Mary Law, Susan Strong and Debra Stewart

Learning objectives

At the end of this chapter, the reader should be able to:

1 Identify and describe key theoretical ideas about the relationship between people and environment.
2 Identify five characteristics of the environment that act as barriers to satisfactory work and five characteristics that promote this.
3 Identify five ways in which he or she might adapt the work environment to facilitate work performance.
4 Develop a complete treatment plan that considers suitable adaptations to the environment, occupational performance and behaviour.

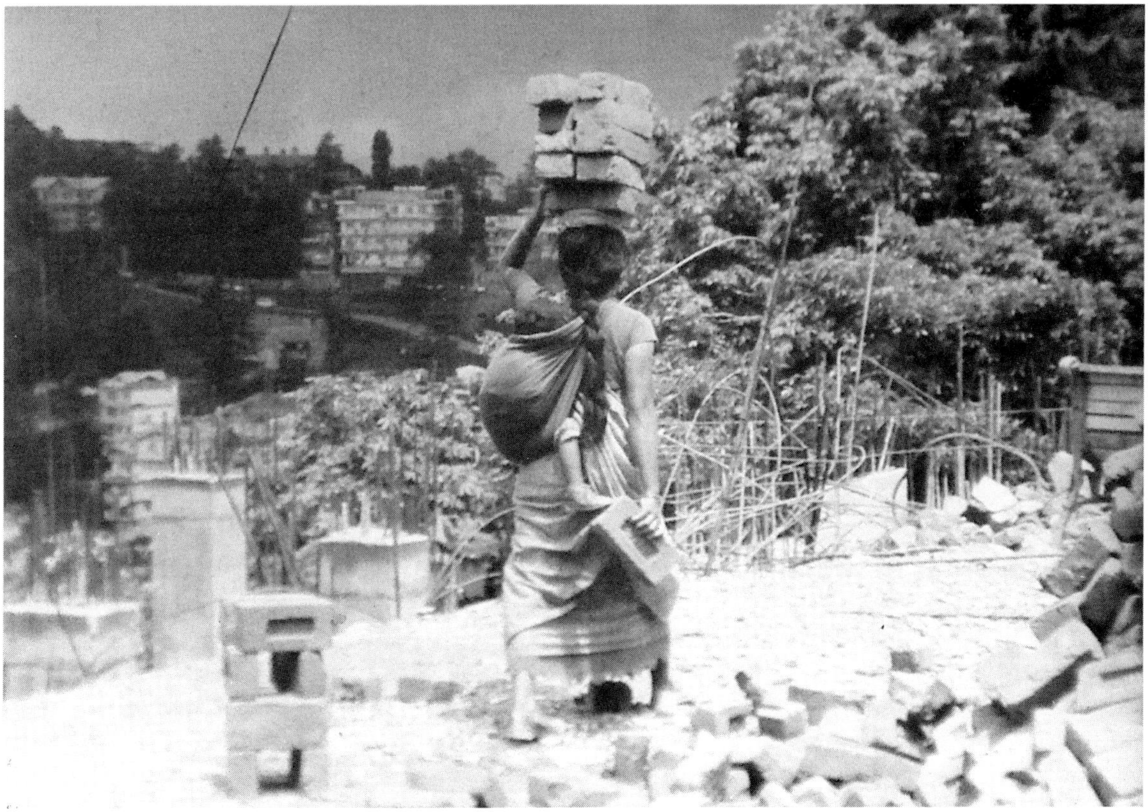

Keywords and definitions used in this chapter

Theoretical models: describe, explain and predict observed phenomena
Transactive interactions: in person–environment theoretical models are those where the relationships being explored are so interwoven and interdependent that they cannot be teased apart easily for examination
Person–environment fit: is a term describing the degree of congruence that exists between an individual and his or her surroundings
Client-centred: refers to services that are focused upon and organized around the self-perceived needs of the individual(s) receiving the professional interventions
Occupational performance: is a general term that describes the functional tasks of self-care, work and leisure, conducted by individuals during the course of a day in the area of work; for children this usually means play and for adults this encompasses both paid and voluntary employment.

Abstract

In this chapter, major theories of person–environment fit, used to describe, explain and predict the relationship between a person and his environment, are presented. A variation of these, the Person–Environment Model of Occupational Performance, has been developed for the use of professions addressing work dysfunction. This suggests that optimal work performance results when the person, his environment and his occupation fit harmoniously with each other. The model demonstrates how strategies enabling work performance can be developed for all component domains, and in particular, in the previously neglected area of the environment. A case history illustrating this approach is given.

Introduction

People view the world in different ways. These variations are expressed by differences in the way human beings observe, explore and relate to the environment in which they live and work. Variations in personal experiences and beliefs also colour these differences; cultural and professional outlooks distinguish them further.

The generally accepted view is considered the current *paradigm* (Guba, 1991). When changes disturb this set of beliefs and practices and a new view is adopted, a *paradigm shift* is said to have occurred. The changes seen over the past generation in patterns of employment for women represents an example of a paradigm shift for society. This paradigm shift in normative work patterns varies among countries and within subsets of each country, but nonetheless, demonstrates shared convictions.

In health and vocational services, the present paradigm of practice requires service providers to make or facilitate adjustments in clients' behaviours and their environment in order to allow these individuals to carry out necessary functions to their satisfaction. In the past, input from all professions has focused primarily on assisting clients to make the essential behavioural changes. However, a paradigm shift is evident in the current emphasis being placed on environmental concerns. These are now considered equally important when considering ways to facilitate clients' ability to work (Law, Cooper, Stewart *et al.*, 1994).

Theoretical models of person–environment relations

Theoretical models provide a vehicle for organizing related ideas on particular topics. Such a structure allows us to describe, explain and predict the observations made about these issues. Theoretical models are also used to guide clinical practice. Outcomes consistent with the theory and related research studies provide a way of confirming, developing and refining the body of knowledge represented by the model being applied (Cooper and Saarinen, 1985).

Theoretical models of person–environment interaction have been proposed by many different professions, in particular, environmental psychology, sociology, anthropology, architecture and occupational therapy. Although the theoreticians come from diverse backgrounds, and the purposes for which their models have been developed vary, nonetheless, the basic building blocks or concepts and principles underlying these models are similar. Fundamental to all models is a particular conceptualization of the person and the environment, and common themes, such as the individuality of people, the important influence of environmental characteristics, and the interdependence of persons and the environments in which they live and work.

Basic concepts

The person

The person is pivotal to all theoretical considerations of person–environment (P–E) models influencing work-related issues. However, the concept of person is often emphasized differently by each. For example, the model may conceptualize the person as an individual or as part of a group (Law, Cooper, Stewart *et al.*, 1994); the functional activities carried out by the person can also be considered specifically or broadly (Lawton, 1986). Nonetheless, in keeping with this emphasis, most theoretical P–E models consider the person as the main unit or focus of interest and measurement.

The person is sometimes conceptualized as possessing a set of competencies that are observable and can be measured (Lawton, 1986). The internal attributes of the person, such as beliefs, values, knowledge and needs, are also recognized as important to assess (Lawton, 1986). These too can be measured using self-report or by using reliable, valid psychometric measures. Both types of assessment are often used to determine a person's ability to work.

The environment

The context in which people live and work is described as their environment. There is no agreement on how the environment should be defined, but most authors acknowledge that the definition should be broad and include physical, psychological, social, organizational and cultural considerations (Law, Cooper, Stewart *et al.*, 1994). This too represents a paradigm shift from a previous focus that tended to limit our considerations of the environment to just the physical concerns, and in particular, to barrier-free design environments.

Similarly, there is no agreement on how to organize environments. Some authors believe this should be by attribute (e.g. privacy, safety); others, that the classification should be by function (e.g. school, farm, office, home); still others order the environment by scale (e.g. room, home, factory, community, country) (Weisman, 1981). In health care, professionals often classify environments by their enabling or disabling qualities (Law, 1991). Clearly no one method is more correct than any other, and the importance lies in applying the most appropriate categorization for the occasion and in being aware of these differences when discussing such issues interprofessionally or assembling information on the subject.

Most authors agree that it is often easier to modify the environment than to change behaviour (Lawton, 1986). In keeping with the broad definition of environment, modifications to promote work and function can be made to any of the component areas. These strategies can include everything from physical considerations, such as barrier-free design and good ergonomic planning, to the implementation of flexible working hours and job sharing. Similarly, the presence of barriers impeding work or function can be addressed in each area.

Person–environment relations

Person–environment theorists consider that the relationship between users and the milieux in which they live and work is complex and inseparable rather than linear.

They believe that the environment influences the person's behaviour and that, equally, the person shapes the environment. This view also emphasizes the dynamic temporal aspects of the person–environment relationship. This interwoven interaction is difficult if not impossible to tease apart and is referred to as a *transactive process.*

Environments that support human behaviour in an optimal manner are referred to as *enabling* (Law, 1991; Swain, Finkelstein, French and Oliver, 1993). Theorists use different expressions to describe the degree to which this occurs, most commonly: *fit* (Baker and Intagliata, 1982), *adaptation* (Lawton, 1986), *congruence* (Kahana, 1982), *compatibility* (Kaplan, 1983), and *accommodation* (Bronfenbrenner, 1977). Regardless of which expression is used, the concept of enabling environments is central to rehabilitation and to positive work experiences.

Measurement

Given the complexity of the transactive interaction, measuring the fit of the person and environment becomes challenging. It calls for the ability to assess many variables consistently and accurately across time, for example: the status of the person and the environment; all personal and other user needs; and, the results of interventions. Instruments of measure that allow us to meet these demands are not yet well developed nor are common methods of investigating such concerns.

Letts and colleagues (1994) have addressed this issue through a review and categorization of instruments of measure that consider both the person and the environment. Many of these instruments are not sufficiently sensitive to measure transactive relationships across time, and still take a linear, discrete, cross-sectional approach to measurement. However, it is worth noting that, for practical reasons, therapists and other health-care professionals usually need to employ these measures. Nonetheless, it is likely that this area will receive considerable attention in the future as clinicians and academics wrestle with the dilemmas of transactive measurement in research.

Key theoretical models influencing the field

There are several environmental models that have influenced our thinking about the relationship between people and the work environment. In this section, the theoretical work of Baker and Intagliata, Kaplan, Bronfenbrenner, Weisman and the Healthy Communities Approach will be discussed.

The origins of the ideas expressed in these models have roots in the works completed by Lewin (1935) on environmental press theory and by Murray (1938) on need–press theory of human behaviour. Kaplan (1983), an environmental psychologist, developed the Model of Person-Environmental Compatibility, to conceptualize the relationship between the internal environment of the individual and the opportunities and choices offered by the external environment. Baker and Intagliata (1982) were more concerned with quality-of-life issues for chronic psychiatric patients, but acknowledge the importance of both the individual's perception of the environment and the 'real' characteristics of the environment as contributing factors. The models by Kaplan (1983) and Baker and Intagliata (1982) focus upon the internal environment of the individual and how this influences the relationship between the individual and the external environment. Bronfenbrenner (1980) studied human development and, as a consequence, his Ecological Systems Model centres on the social development of the individual over his or her life span. Weisman (1981) has a background in architecture and psychology. These influences have directed him towards examining how the physical environment of an organization can be designed to influence the behaviours of employees towards meeting organizational goals and objectives. Uniquely, the Healthy Communities conceptual model (Hancock, 1993) emerged from a public health planning initiative which attempted to renew grass-roots links between community and health.

Baker and Intagliata

Baker and Intagliata (1982) conceptualized the individual as a broad bio-psycho system,

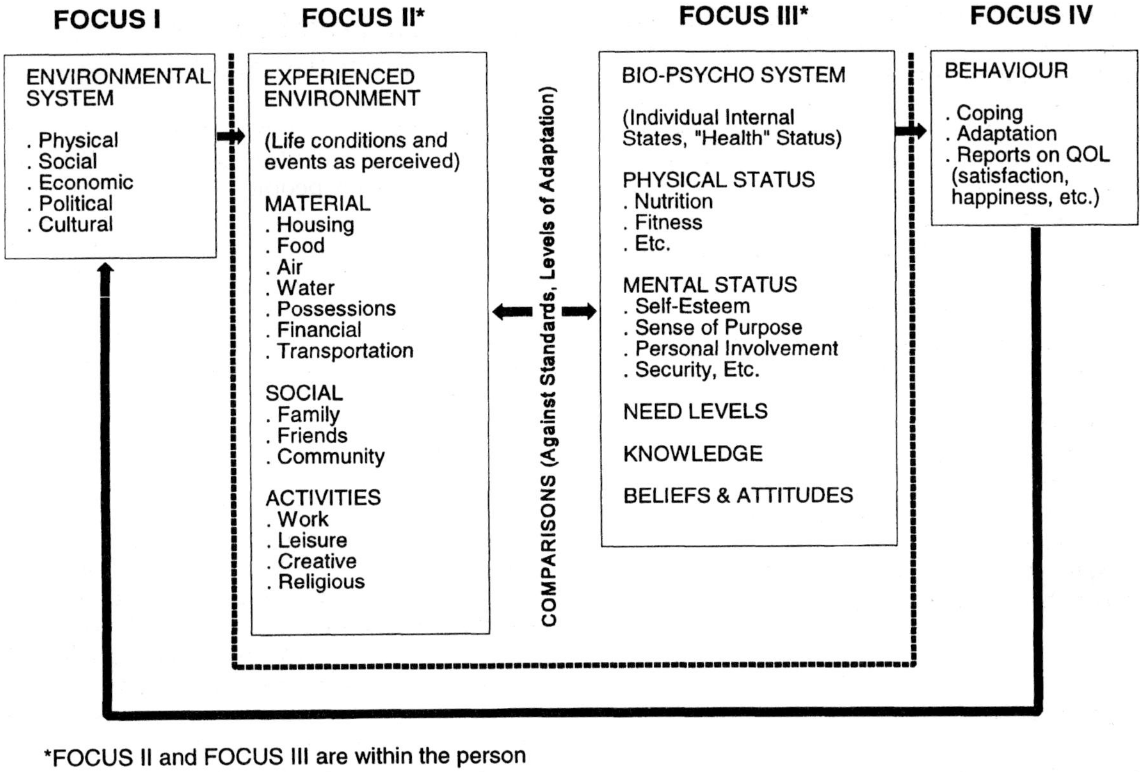

Figure 4.1 Baker and Intagliata's Model. Reprinted with permission from Baker and Intagliata (1982).

which is delineated as: internal states of needs, desires, knowledge, beliefs, values and attitudes. The model provides an explanation of the relationships between the external environmental system, the individual's experienced environment, the individual's health status and the individual's behaviour (Fig. 4.1).

While Baker and Intagliata believe that it is important to identify how the individual perceives the environment, they also note that the actual environment should be defined in terms of its physical, social, economic, political and cultural characteristics. An individual's knowledge, beliefs and attitudes affect how he will relate to the environment. Thus the individual may respond to environmental situations at work with active participation, seeking to increase skills and competence, or with instinctive avoidance, to cope with memories of unpleasant experiences.

Kaplan

Kaplan (1983) also focuses on how the individual perceives the external environment. He describes the internal organization of informational processes (e.g. perception, attention and planning processes) which mediate all functions within an individual, emphasizing the opportunities and choices offered to the individual by the work environment. Kaplan describes the individual's internal environment in terms of 'temporal flexibility'. This means that the individual brings memories of past experiences to each work experience. These in turn influence current and future perceptions and anticipation. A poor environmental relationship occurs when the external environment is not seen as supportive to the individual. A supportive work environment is viewed as an environment which makes it possible for an individual to strive towards goals by

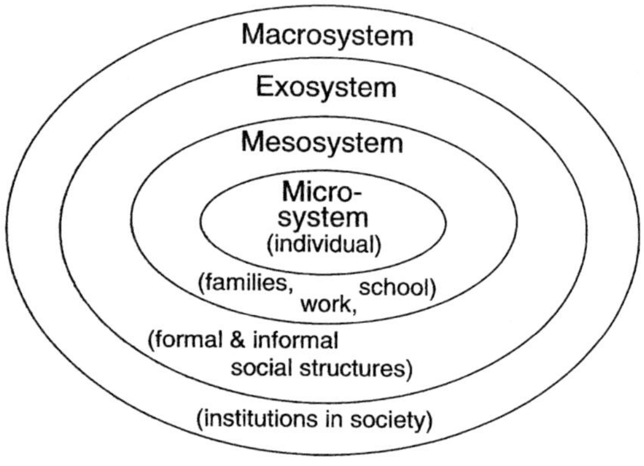

Figure 4.2 Bronfenbrenner's Ecological Systems Model. Reprinted with permission from Bronfenbrenner (1980).

providing information and opportunites for choices and reflection.

Bronfenbrenner

Bronfenbrenner's model centres on the individual acting as a social agent to seek and create meaning in the social environment. However, while Bronfenbrenner places most emphasis on the social environment, he does so without excluding the consideration of other environmental components. Bronfenbrenner (1980) stresses the interdependence of the social environmental systems within which each individual interacts (Fig. 4.2). He proposes that the environment is structured as four inter-related systems: the microsystem involving the immediate environmental setting (time, place, physical features, activity and participants); the mesosystem, involving interacting microsystems; the exosystem, consisting of formal and informal social structures; and the macrosystem, consisting of institutional patterns (economic, social, legal, educational).

Social relationships create formal and informal social groups. Bronfenbrenner proposes that change in one domain of the social environment will effect change in interacting domains. For example, workplace decisions about environmental hazards and resource management are influenced by all systems, including personal concerns, societal interpretation of environmental events and worksite response (Duncan, 1985).

Weisman

Weisman (1981) is the one theorist whose major focus is on work environments. His ideas centre on the organization and its policy and objectives. He is also the only theorist to emphasize the physical environment more than the other components of the environment. Weisman describes how the other parts of the environment are conceived through a filter of the physical environment (Fig. 4.3). His perspective is somewhat more linear than those of the other theorists, but provides a targeted approach to work-related concerns.

Weisman takes an interventionist approach to describe, explain and predict behavioural outcomes of work situations. He suggests that the behaviours of employees of an institution can be shaped by the physical properties of the environmental setting, for example, to improve work performance. The physical setting is described as having two levels: the actual components of the setting (structure, materials, equipment, etc); and the sensory and spatial properties of the setting (temperature, illumination, shape, etc.). The structure of the physical environment affects patterns of behaviour. For example, walls and barriers reduce interaction and create a more formal atmosphere in a workplace, while an open-concept design creates informality and encourages interaction (e.g. a lawyer's office versus a newsroom).

Healthy communities model

The Healthy Communities Model focuses on social policy and the distinctive needs of the community (Hancock, 1993). It depicts the environment in very broad terms to include biological, physical, cultural and economic components (Fig. 4.4). The beginnings of these ideas can be traced to work by Han-

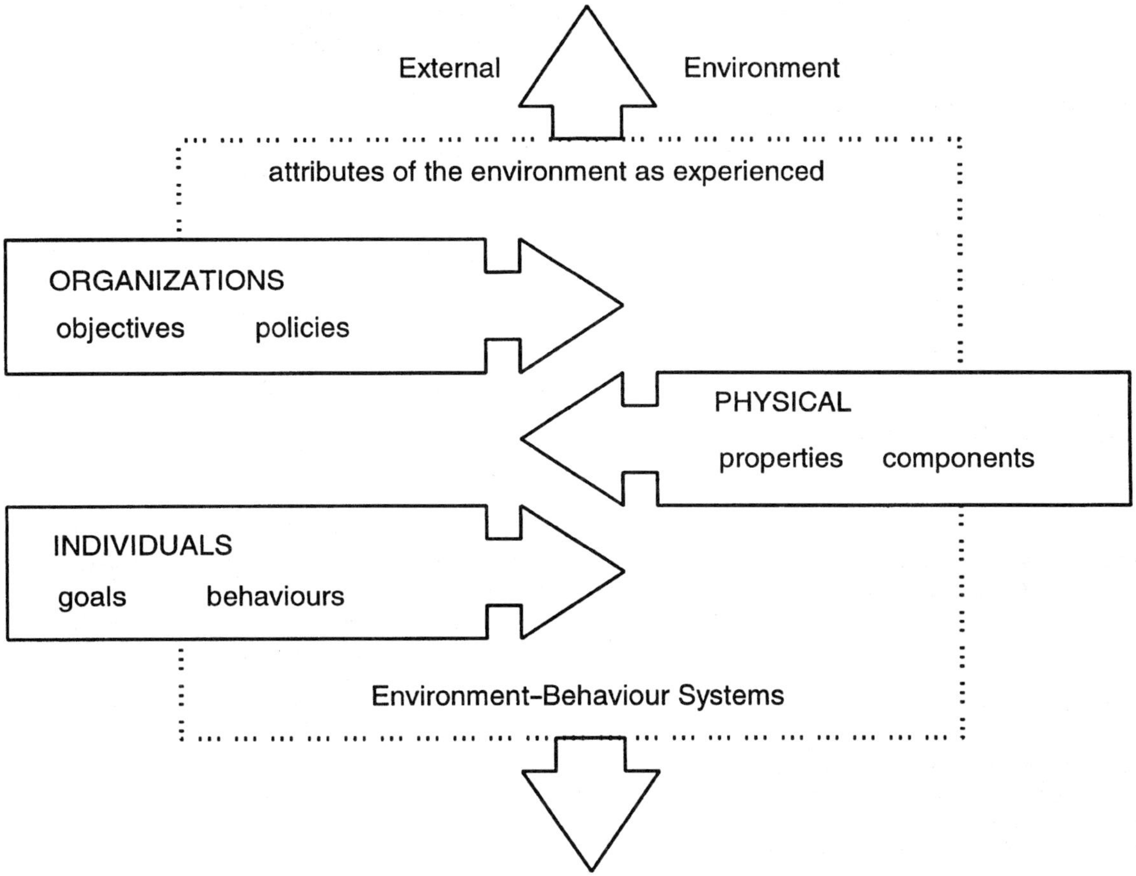

Figure 4.3 Weisman's Model. Reprinted with permission from Weisman (1981).

cock (1993), who discussed the need for communities to promote healthy work and living environments for their citizens. In this model, parameters for a healthy city such as a clean, safe environment, participation, economic diversity and high health status are outlined.

The central behavioural concept found in the Health Communities Model is the need to change environments to fit community needs rather than trying to change individuals to fit environments. There is recognition of the social and political barriers to the achievement of a healthy environment. These include: inertia; fragmentation in the political/bureaucratic process; vested interest; and the philosophical belief that an element of misery is part of the human condition. This model provides perhaps the broadest base for conceptualizing work environments.

Person–environment fit

Environmental theorists use the term person–environment fit to describe the degree of adaptation that exists between a person and his environment. The models described have developed over the past two decades and reflect a theoretical process that has evolved over time to help us understand the relationship of persons in their environment. All recognize the complexity of the relationship. It is important to stress that changes in *any* component of this relationship will influence the balance of the system as a *whole*, often making it difficult to achieve an acceptable fit between a person and the work environment. When this occurs, it becomes the responsibility of the health-care worker to help facilitate the re-establishment of congruence between the two.

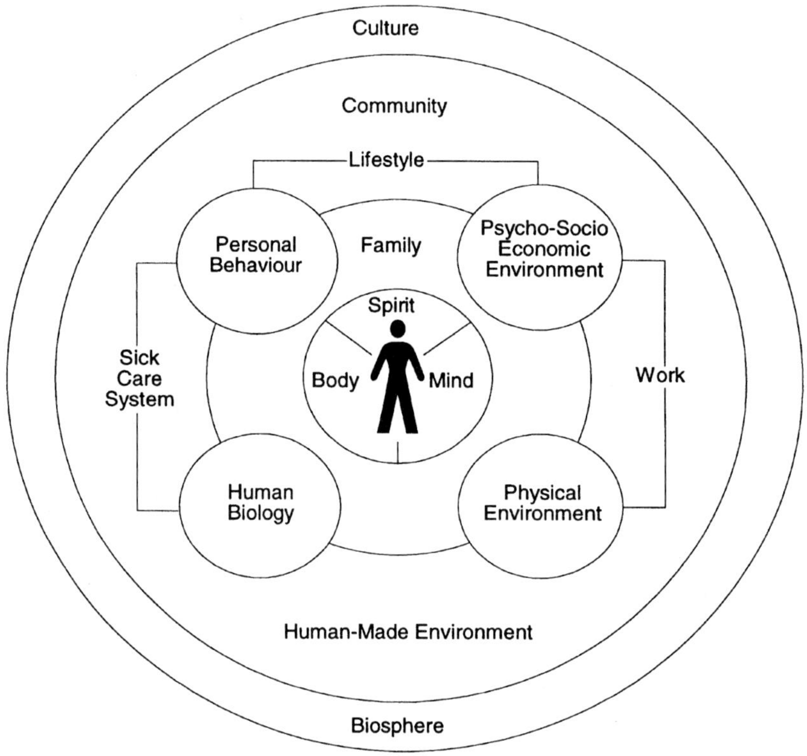

Figure 4.4 Healthy Communities Model. Reprinted with permission from Handcock (1993).

Person–environment fit and work

Work is highly valued in our society and provides several different functions: the means for practical survival, improved feelings of self-worth and a sense of belonging and contributing to the community (Clutterbuck and McKay, 1984; Liebermann, 1988; Campbell, 1989). A job also links people to reality (Olshansky, 1962), provides structure to one's life, and increases social connections (Bellamy, Rhodes, Mark and Albin, 1988). The value and meaning of work will vary for different groups and individuals, particularly between clients and professionals (Tebes and Kramer, 1991). Consequently, there is increased awareness that what constitutes meaningful work should be defined by the client involved (Strong, Law, Willus, Eyles, 1995).

Ochocka and colleagues (1994) found that the quality of the fit between the person and the culture of the workplace is the prime determinant for successful employment. There is not one factor most responsible for determining a good fit, however, allowing clients to perceive control over facets of their employment situation appears to be an important variable in increasing job satisfaction and reducing stress (Karasek and Theorell, 1990).

A move towards proactive strategies

Today's health-care professional will be asked to address person–environment fit and work-related issues from both a reactive (rehabilitation) and proactive (health promotion) perspective. This too represents a paradigm shift, for the proactive stance is relatively new. Recent legislation, such as the Americans with Disabilities Act of 1990 (Public Law 101–336) and parallel moves in other countries (United Nations, 1989), is primarily responsible for these views. They reflect the concerns and lobbying of the large numbers of people with disabilities now living in the community who have indicated their desire to lead productive lives, as well as changes in societal views. In addition, employers have come to the realization that it is ultimately less expensive, if not a better course of action, to anticipate work-related problems than to deal with them after the fact. However, there is no doubt that legislation is the driving force, and that this is beginning to have a major impact on the demands made on health-care professionals to maintain and improve the health of employees. Creative solutions will be required to meet the challenges of developing enabling environments for all workers in a manner that strives to prevent the occurrence of disability.

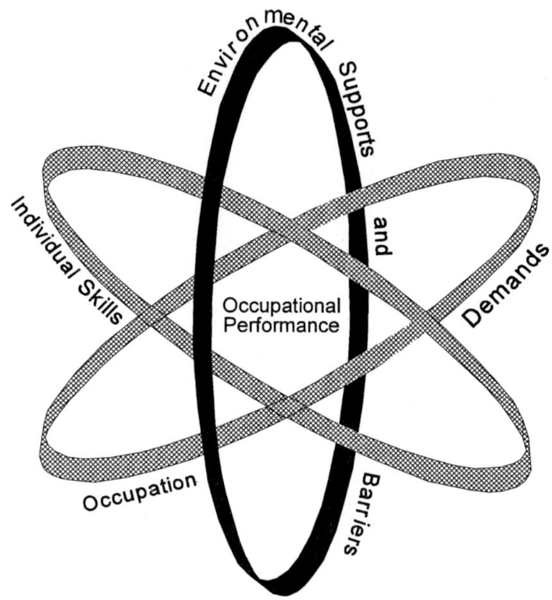

Figure 4.5 Person–Environment Model of Occupational Performance. Reprinted from Law *et al.* (in press).

The person–environment model of occupational performance

Law and colleagues (in press) have proposed a person–environment model that specifically addresses the occupational performance of the individual. This builds upon the multiprofessional models described above and other relevant sources. While developed primarily for occupational therapy practitioners, it nonetheless is sufficiently generic to provide a useful model for any profession addressing client issues of work–performance dysfunction.

Sources of influence

The occupational therapy literature of the 1980s and early 1990s reflects the growing importance of the environment as a treatment modality for that profession. Examples of these trends are found in publications by Kiernat (1982), the Guidelines for Client-Centred Practice of Occupational Therapy (CAOT, 1991), Dunn, Brown and McGuigan (1994) and Christiansen and Baum (1991). The last of these authors developed a person–environment–performance framework that focuses in particular on the influence of the environment on *roles and tasks*. Dunn and colleagues emphasize the importance of *context* in assessing a person's functional performance.

Parallel work by other scholars also influenced the development of the Person–Environment Model of Occupational Performance, most importantly, the ideas presented by Csikszentmihalyi and Csikszentmihalyi (1988) and Lawton (1982). The former described the challenges of the relationship between an activity and individual skills. They suggested that satisfaction with the experience is greater when environmental attributes and resources are in harmony with the individual's level of skills. Lawton developed a theoretical model, the Ecological Theory of Aging, that matched demands made by the environment (press) with the person's competence, in order to estimate the degree of healthy adaptation possible. Lawton makes the important point that when competence is dimished, press can have a greater negative impact on behavioural outcomes than when competence is high. Conversely, small positive changes to the environment of a person functioning with a disability can have a major beneficial impact on performance. This final point is critical for practitioners responsible for making environmental adaptations that enhance clients' ability to work.

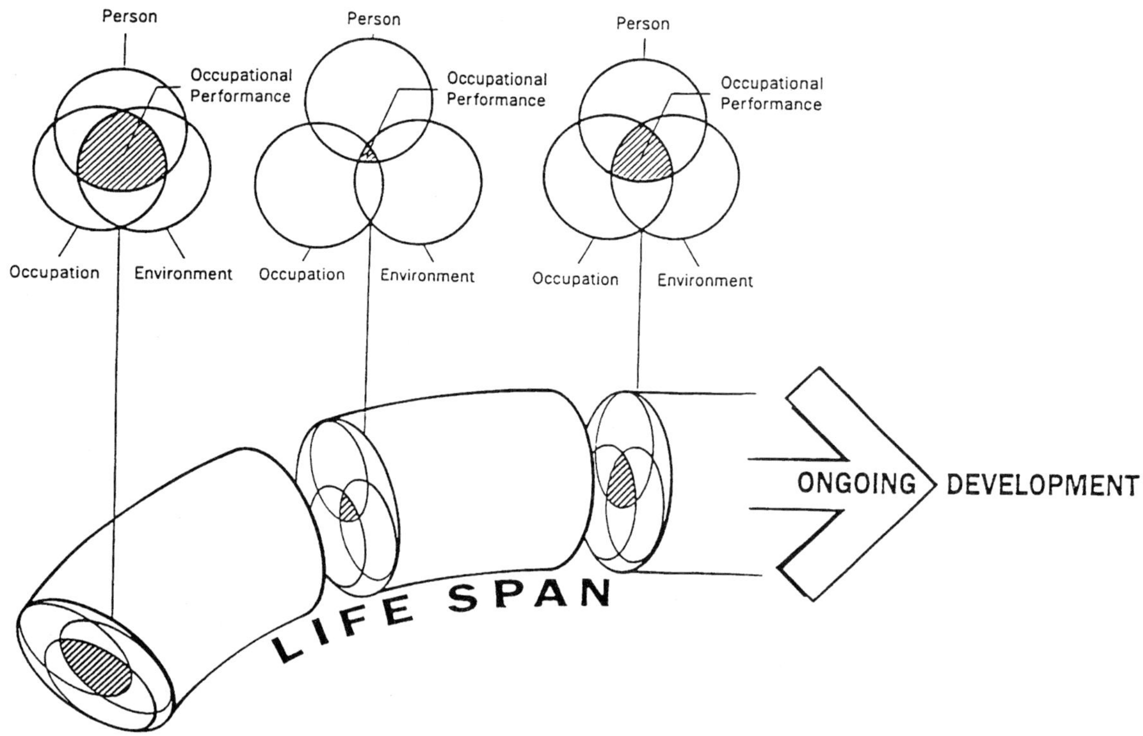

Figure 4.6 Depiction of the Person–Environment model of Occupational Performance across the life span illustrating hypothetical changes in occupational performance at three different points in time. Reprinted from Law *et al.* (in press).

These ideas have been incorporated into the Person–Environment Model of Occupational Performance. Law and colleagues defined *occupational performance* as the overlap produced by the person, environment and occupation (see Fig. 4.5). The closer the overlap or fit, the greater the area of good occupational performance. Fit reduces or increases according to the degree that the three contributing components complement each other. The temporal aspects of this transactive process are addressed by conceptualizing the overlap as dynamic and changing throughout the life span (see Fig. 4.6).

The following example illustrates the application of the model broadly and from a pragmatic perspective. If an individual sustains injuries that cannot be modified, then interventions that allow the person to return to work can only focus on the two remaining components: the environment and the person's occupation. On the contrary, if some aspects of the environment cannot reasonably be changed, then clearly the only recourse is to develop interventions that include some personal adaptation, the amenable factors of the environment and the occupation in which he is involved. Evaluation allows further refinements to be made across time as the relationship among these components changes dynamically. The case study below applies these ideas further, concentrating in particular on the effects of modifying different aspects of the environment.

Case study

Fred is a man in his late thirties who sustained a closed head injury as a child. His residual impairments include a right hemiparesis and problems with speech articulation, short-term memory and perseverance. Fred received rehabilitation services when he was a child and adolescent. During his teenage years, he worked in several summer jobs, including gas bar attendant, cleaner and filing clerk.

Fred grew up in a small town and, when he was 20 years old, moved to a large city where he currently resides. He began experiencing mental-health problems soon after his move, when he found himself unable to cope with the stress of his job. Fred experienced delusional thoughts, and was hospitalized several times for this. For the past two years, Fred has been living in a boarding house with eight other residents. This provides supervised living services for people with persistent mental illness. He shares a room there with one other person.

During past hospitalizations, Fred was enrolled in an industrial therapy programme. His most recent vocational assessment suggested that he was ready for work in a 'transitional' setting, and his counsellor referred him to a new cooperative business where he was employed in production-line work requiring a moderate amount of manual dexterity and bilateral hand coordination.

After six months, Fred indicated that he was not satisfied with his employment, and staff reported that he was not adjusting well. He was therefore referred for assessment and consultation. The therapist interviewed Fred and staff members; observed his work performance, and used two standardized assessments, the Canadian Occupational Performance Measure (COPM) (Law, Baptiste, Carswell *et al.*, 1994) and the Work Environment Scale (Moos, 1980) to identify and evaluate target areas. The assessment pointed out personal, environmental and occupational elements influencing Fred's current occupational performance.

Fred's personal assessment

Through the COPM, Fred identified that he considered work an important activity in his life, but that he was not satisfied with his current performance. Observations and staff reports showed that Fred was experiencing difficulty with responsibilities involving short-term memory, manual dexterity and the simultaneous management of tasks. He stated that the work did not suit his interests, values, or lifestyle of working and that he never saw any results for his efforts. Fred had developed a friendship with one other person, but otherwise, felt no connection with his coworkers. He identified living on his own as an important goal.

Environment

Several environmental supports and constraints to occupational performance were identified by the assessment. The physical environment was fully accessible for Fred, but the linear arrangement of the tables in the production line did not facilitate interaction among the workers.

Occupational performance

Although the staff at work were supportive of Fred and had provided a flexible work schedule, it was clear that they did not fully understand the implications of his closed-head injury. Fred's work required a moderate amount of manual dexterity and bilateral hand coordination. Accommodations had also been made for Fred's slower pace, with unit production organized around this. However, the production-line work was very segmented, which resulted in Fred feeling further isolated from his coworkers and unable to understand how his efforts contributed to the final production goal.

Improving person–environment–occupation fit

Based on this assessment, the therapist identified areas where the fit between Fred, the environment and his occupation were of concern. Overall, a lack of partnership between Fred and the staff existed. Because staff did not fully understand the limitations caused by Fred's head injury, their expectations for his occupational performance were not always in line with his abilities. Additionally, the poor fit between Fred's work interests and needs and the requirements of his current job caused him to feel frustrated and increased his inability to complete work tasks successfully. Although the work setting supported his need to be around others, the type of tasks and physical layout of the production line did not encourage social interaction nor foster emotional support from coworkers.

In summary, Fred was not enjoying his current work experience because of problems with person–environment–occupation fit. He did not feel a sense of belonging or commitment to the group, and was frustrated with himself and with the staff's efforts to help him.

Interventions

Direct and indirect strategies aimed at improving the fit between Fred and his work environment were implemented by the therapist. His work tasks were modified to be more in line with his abilities and interests by reducing the time he spent on the production line to a half day, and by assigning responsibilities that required less manual dexterity. The other half day, Fred did cleaning tasks and helped in the store, which proved to be more satisfying for him. To encourage social interaction, but not interfere with productivity, the tables in the production line were changed to circular ones. Fred was also encouraged to join the social committee. The therapist conducted a staff in-service on head injury, and consulted with fellow workers on ways to assist Fred when he experienced difficulty with specific tasks. At an organizational level, recommendations were made to orient and train all new employees to help them feel more at ease in the work setting and familiarize them with relevant work issues. The therapist met with Fred to discuss his current living arrangements, and subsequently referred him to a community therapist for independent-living skills training. Several months later, Fred was able to move into his own apartment.

As a consequence of these varied interventions, Fred now reports increased satisfaction with his life and employment situation. He states that his occupational environment seems more responsive to his greater sense of purpose and accomplishment.

Summary

Person–environment models augment and expand the number and types of strategies available to health-care personnel responsible for helping people with disabilities to work more productively. Most P–E models propose that changes or modifications to the person or to the environment will promote work outcomes and worker satisfaction. More recent thinking, exemplified by the Person–Environment Model of Occupational Performance, suggests that a triad of components exists: this considers the person's occupation as well as the person and environment. Optimal fit of all three areas furthers productive work or occupational performance outcomes. Time introduces a dynamic dimension to this last approach, and the choice of intervention for a given moment will fluctuate according to component responsiveness. In particular, all these theoretical models suggest that the environment provides a rich resource that can be adjusted to fit the needs of individuals with disabilities better and thereby enable more productive work to take place.

Multiple choice questions

1 Theories are used in service roles to:
   (a) predict outcomes
   (b) explain observations
   (c) guide practice
   (d) determine treatment.

2 A person–environment theory which focuses on social policy is work by:
   (a) Baker and Intagliata
   (b) Weisman
   (c) Healthy Communities Movement
   (d) Bronfenbrenner.

3 Occupational performance can be enhanced by:
   (a) enhancing the enabling qualities of the environment
   (b) reducing the complexity of the task
   (c) introducing barrier-free design
   (d) developing good economic strategies.

4 Intervention strategies to facilitate satisfactory work performance focus on:
   (a) removal of environmental barriers
   (b) development of environmental supports
   (c) reduction of enablers to occupational performance
   (d) a and b.

5 An individual's work performance is determined by:
   (a) the person's skills
   (b) the work environment
   (c) the work task
   (d) all of the above.

For answers to multiple choice questions see p. 309.

References

Americans with Disabilities Act. (1990). Public Law 101–336, 42 USC 12101.

Baker, F. and Intagliata, J. (1982). Quality of life in the evaluation of community support systems. *Evaluation and Program Planning*, **5**, 69–79.

Bellamy, G. T., Rhodes, L. E., Mamk, D. M. and Albin, J. M. (eds) (1988). *Supported Employment: A Community Implementation Guide*. Paul H. Brookes.

Bronfenbrenner, U. (1977). Towards an experimental ecology of human development. *American Psuchologist*, 513–531.

Bronfenbrenner, U. (1980). Ecology of childhood. *School Psychology Review*, **9**(4), 294–7.

Campbell, J. F. (1989). Employment programs for people with a psychiatric disability: An overview. *Community Support Network News*, **6**(2), 1–11.

Canadian Association of Occupational Therapists (1991). *Occupational Therapy Guidelines for Client-centred Practice*. COAT Publications.

Christiansen, C. and Baum, C. (1991). *Occupational Therapy: Overcoming Human Performance Deficits*. Slack Incorporated.

Clutterbuck, P. and McKay, S. (1984). *Work and Well-being, the Changing Realities of Employment*. Canadian Mental Health Association.

Cooper, B. and Saarinen, H. (1985). The interrelationship of theory and clinical practice. *Physiotherapy Canada*

Csikszentmihalyi, M. and Csikszentmihalyi, I. S. (1988). *Optimal Experience: Psychological Studies in Flow in Consciousness*. Cambridge University Press.

Duncan, J. (1985). Individual action and political power: A structuration perspective. In *The Future of Geography, 342*. Methuen.

Dunn. W., Brown, C. and McGuigan, A. (1994). The ecology of human performance: A framework for considering the effect of context. *American Journal of Occupational Therapy*, **48**, 595–607.

Guba, E. (1991). *The Paradigm Dialogue*. Sage Publications.

Hancock, T. (1993). Health, human development and the community ecosystem: three ecological models. *Health Promotion International*, **8**(1), 41–7.

Kahana, E. (1982). A congruence model of person–environment interaction. In *Aging and the Environment: Theoretical Approaches* (M. P. Lawton, P. G. Windley and T. O. Byerts, eds) pp. 97–121, Springer.

Kaplan, S. (1983). A model of person–environment compatibility. *Environment and Behaviour*, **15**, 311–32.

Karasek, R. and Theorell, T. (1990). *Healthy Work, Stress, Productivity, and the Reconstruction of Working Life*. Basic Books.

Kiernat, J. M. (1982). Environment: the hidden modality. *Physical and Occupational Therapy in Geriatrics*, **2**(1), 3–12.

Law, M. (1991). The environment: A focus of occupational therapy. *Canadian Journal of Occupational Therapy*, **58**(4), 171–9.

Law, M., Baptiste, S., Carswell *et al.* (1994). *Canadian Occupational Performance Measure Manual* (2nd edn). CAOT Publications ACE.

Law, M., Cooper, B. A., Stewart *et al.* (1994). Person–environment relations. *Work*, **4**(4), 228–38.

Lawton, M. P. (1982). Competence, environmental press, and the adaptation of older people. In *Aging and the Environment: Theoretical Approaches* (M. P. Lawton, P. G. Windley and T. O. Byerts, eds) pp. 33–59, Springer.

Lawton, M. P. (1986). *Environment and Aging* (2nd edn). Plenum.

Letts, L., Law, M., Rigby, P. *et al.* (1994). Person–environment assessment in occupational therapy. *American Journal of Occupational Therapy*, **48**(7), 608–18.

Lewin, K. (1935). *Dynamic Theory of Personality*. McGraw Hill.

Liebermann, R. P. (1988). *The Psychiatric Rehabilitation of Chronic Mental Health Patients*. American Psychiatric Press Inc.

Moos, R. H. (1980). *Work Environment Scale Manual*. Consulting Psychologists Press.

Murray, H. (1938). *Explorations in Personality*. Oxford.

Ochocka, J., Roth, D., Lord, J. and Mac Gillivary, H. (1994). *Workplaces that Work*. Centre for Research and Education.

Olshansky, S. (1962). Preventing relapse of ex-mental patients. *Journal of Rehabilitation*, **28**, 34–5.

Olshansky, S. and Unterberger, H. (1963). The meaning of work and its implications for the ex-mental hospital patient. *Mental Hygiene*, **47**, 137–49.

Report on national legislation for the equalization of opportunities for people with disabilities: examples from 22 countries and areas (United Nations, 1989). United Nations.

Strong, S., Law, M., Willus, D. and Eyles, J. (1995). Listening and learning from the clients perspective. *Canadian Journal of Occupational Therapy*, **62**.

Swain, J., Finkelstein, V., French, S. and Oliver, M. (1993). *Disabling Barriers: Enabling Environments*. Sage Publications.

Tebes, J. K. and Kramer, D. J. (1991). Quantitative and qualitative knowing in Mutual Support Research: Some lessons from the recent history of psychology. *American Journal of Community Psychology*, **19**(5), 739–56.

Weisman, G. D. (1981). Modelling environment–behaviour systems: A brief note. *Journal of Man–Environment Relations*, **1**, 32–41.

5

Legislation

Mildrette Hill, Robina McDonald and Karen Jacobs

Learning objectives

At the end of this chapter the reader should be able to:

1 Describe the nature of legislation which shapes work practice in three developed countries.
2 Discuss the opportunities and constraints which this legislative framework provides.

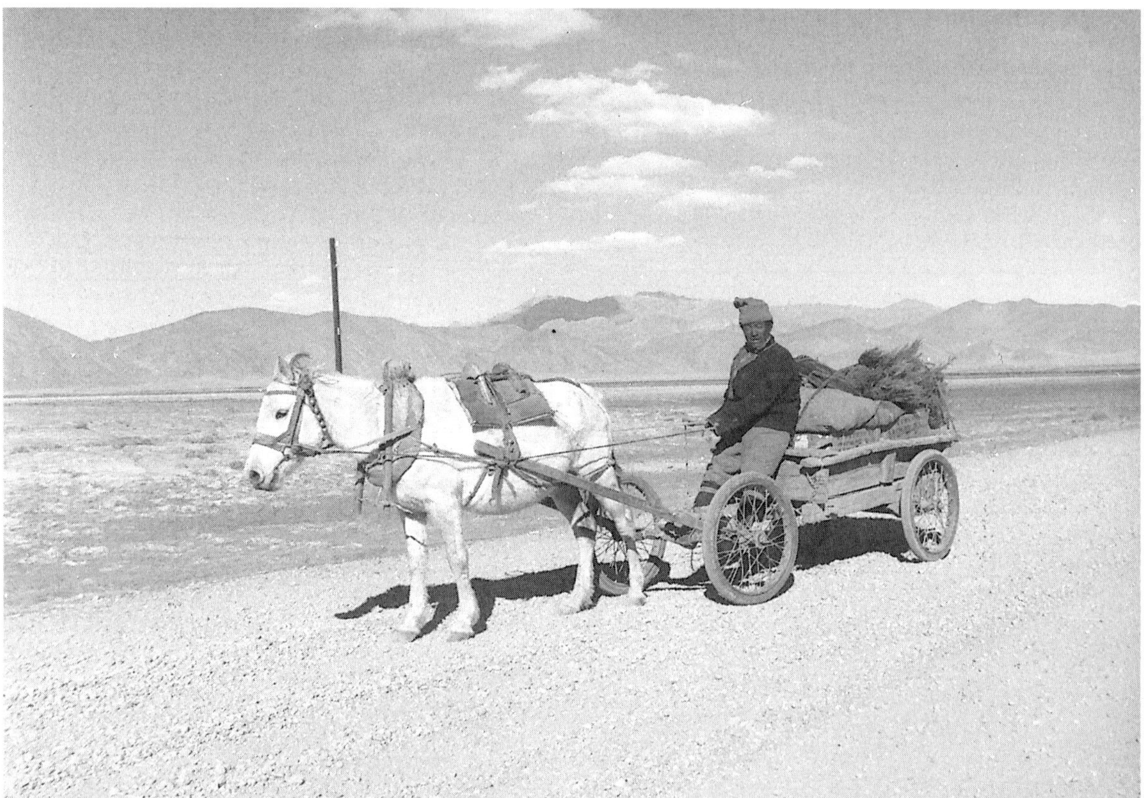

Introduction

Robert Owen, a philanthropist and social reformer, made the following observations on the effects of manufacturing in 1815:

> The employer regard the employed as mere instruments of gain while these acquire a gross ferocity of character which, if legislative measures shall not be judiciously devised to prevent its increase and ameliorate the conditions of this class will sooner or later plunge the country into a miserable and perhaps inextricable state of danger.

He supported his observations by building a woollen mill in New Lanark, Scotland which in its day was considered a model of good working practice by many of its international visitors. Workers lived on site in the housing provided by Owen, while their children were schooled in the nearby Institute for the Formation of Character. Everyone had Sundays off from work, and Owen encouraged the development of a cooperative food store and savings scheme, again on site. While many of Owen's views are considered normal today in most developed countries it is also still true that the framework provided by legislation and regulation is as necessary as it was in 1815.

Occupational therapy practice is framed within a legislative context. This drives both current service provisions as well as the development of new areas of practice. Additionally for our clients it enables access to work and support services, as needed. A knowledge of this legislative framework allows practitioners to direct their practice within the ever-changing political environment. Brief descriptions of the legislation which frames work practice in several countries follows.

Key words and definitions used in this chapter

Disabled person (person with a disability): any person who has a physical, sensory, learning, multiple impairments or disability, who experiences mental health difficulties or who is HIV + or who has AIDS.
Disablism: the discrimination and exclusion that disabled people experience because of their impairments. This can be institutional or individual discrimination and is based on the belief that to be non-disabled is to be superior.
Registered disabled person: (UK) any person whose name is on the register of disabled persons maintained under s. 6 of the Disabled Persons (Employment) Act 1944 shall be deemed to be a disabled person for the purposes of the application of any provisions of the Act in which the term appears.

An Australian perspective

In Australia, there are several major legislative instruments that aim to protect the rights of employees, including disabled employees. These rights are enshrined in law both at the Federal (Commonwealth) level and that of its jurisdictions (states and territories).

States and territories

At the level of the jurisdictions there exist historical reasons for their autonomy pertaining to the interpretation and administration of legislation. This is particularly evident in occupational health and safety legislation, regulations and codes of practice designed to assist employers to reduce the risk of injury to employees. The jurisdictions have their own compensation schemes and legislation for injured workers; for example, in the State of Victoria this is known as Workcover. Under this scheme employers pay premiums to insurance companies who administer arrangements to support injured workers such as rehabilitation or income payments. Similarly, jurisdictions have their own system of insurance for transport-accident victims. In Victoria this is called the Transport Accident Commission. It covers people injured on the way to or from work and during recess periods. This is a 'no fault' system which provides, as appropriate, hospitalization costs, rehabilitation, a percentage of earnings, in some cases a lump-sum benefit, or in the case of death, a lump-sum benefit to dependants.

Federal legislation

Federal legislation may promulgate a particular law, for example, the Disability Discrimination Act 1992 (DDA). This Act supplements and protects anti-discrimination legislation at the level of the states and territories where it is found in equal opportunity legislation. Through the DDA, anti-discrimination legislation broadly covers discrimination in work, education, access to public places, associations and accommodation. Given the large volume of legislation in Australia which deals with disability, disability discrimination and occupational health and safety, it is not within the scope of this chapter to describe such capacious information. Therefore an overview of the essential Federal legislation is outlined. Where necessary, reference is made to non-legislative material. Thus the Acts described here are:

The Disability Discrimination Act 1992 (DDA)
The Disability Services Act 1986 (DSA)
The Occupational Health and Safety (Commonwealth Employment) Act 1991.

The Disability Discrimination Act 1992 (DDA)

The DDA describes and defines disability in broad terms. Disability may involve total or partial loss of function which may be physical, psychological, originate from disease-causing organisms, illness, deformity and learning disorders. It is unlawful to discriminate where circumstances lead a person to suspect: the presence of a disability; a disability that may have existed in the past and is now terminated; or a disability which may currently exist or perhaps may develop in the future.

Part Two, Division One of this Act deals with discrimination in employment. It protects all persons who have a disability and who are seeking employment, are employed, or who have been unlawfully dismissed from employment because of disability or when a disability has been ascribed to an individual. Conditions of service, pay, access to training, transfers and promotions are also protected under the Act.

This does not mean that an employer is obliged to employ a person who has a disability. The individual's experience, training, qualifications and, if employed, his or her performance must be appropriate to the requirements of the position. If, by employing a person who has a disability the employer is likely to suffer unreasonable hardship, then the employer is not obliged to offer or to maintain employment. However, if necessary, the employer needs to be able to justify that alterations to the work environment might cause unreasonable hardship to the employer.

It is also unlawful to discriminate against those who care for, or are related to, a person who has a disability. This also extends to discrimination against those who may associate with persons who have a disability in business, recreation or other settings. An important issue in this Act is that persons who have disabilities are not disadvantaged in employment when compared with individuals without a disability matched for qualifications, training and experience. The Act also preserves the rights of the person who has a disability and his or her associates to protection from harassment in employment.

If discrimination is believed to have occurred then several processes are in place to handle complaints either at the level of the jurisdictions, or the Commonwealth. For example, in the State of Victoria complaints are referred to the Equal Opportunity Commission who determine whether the complaint falls under state or Commonwealth anti-discrimination legislation. A process of investigation commences in which both sides present their point of view. The Commission will decide whether or not further investigation is required. If a complaint proceeds, a conciliator is appointed to assist the parties through a conciliation process. Where conciliation is unsuccessful, the matter may be referred to the Human Rights and Equal Opportunity Commission who have the power to instigate a public hearing. The Commission has the power to order that the employee is reinstated, that an apology is made by the discriminator, or that damages are paid to the employee.

The Disability Services Act 1986 (DSA)

The purpose of the DSA is to enable people with a disability to obtain services which assist them towards greater participation in the community, for example integration, independence and employment. Services provided under this Act are intended to complement existing services in the community. The Act relates to areas as diverse as accommodation, advocacy, respite care, independent living, print disability services, recreation services, and specialized rehabilitation and employment services. It provides access to Competitive Employment Training and Placement (CETP) agencies, whose purpose is to assist persons who have a disability to find and to retain paid employment. This type of service also helps them to integrate into a workplace setting by provision of suitable work preparation strategies. A service is also rendered to persons who have accessed special education, or who wish to make the transition from a supported work environment into the open employment market. Supported employment services are available to those who are unable because of disability to participate in open competitive employment, or who require significant support to find and to keep employment. Part Three of the Act describes the provision of rehabilitation programmes funded by the Commonwealth government (through the Commonwealth Rehabilitation Service). In order to access rehabilitation services, people with a disability should be aged between 14 and 65 years, and be able to make significant progress towards employment which is supported or unsupported. There are four main categories of disability: psychiatric, physical, intellectual and sensory impairments. In some cases, persons accessing rehabilitation have multiple and complex disabilities. Rehabilitation programmes are restricted to Australian citizens or to persons who have the status of permanent residents of Australia. The costs of programmes are borne by the Commonwealth government where the individual is a beneficiary or a pensioner. The exception to this is where the costs are recoverable through a compensation scheme.

Under Section Five, guidelines pertaining to the Act, rehabilitation personnel who have delegation under the Act to assess persons who have a disability need to be mindful of the costs of a programme, the stability of the medical condition, and that rehabilitation will greatly enhance the person's chances of employment and remaining in employment. The guidelines outline the general processes for consideration when deciding if the individual is eligible for rehabilitation services. All rehabilitation programmes include a plan developed with the individual (client) and the rehabilitation case manager. Such plans include goals, strategies to achieve goals, programme costs, a timetable for reviewing and achieving goals, who is responsible for implementing strategies, and how and when the programme is likely to end. The case manager regularly reviews and updates the programme plan with the client. In order for the programme to commence or to continue, the case manager must be satisfied that the client is making reasonable progress towards attaining a vocational outcome, either supported or unsupported. The client has the right of appeal if the decision is made not to offer a programme or to close an existing programme.

The Occupational Health and Safety (Commonwealth Employment) Act 1991

This Act covers only employees of the Australian Federal Government and is similar to legislation in the states and territories. It incorporates Robens' (1972) enabling legislation.

Part Two, Division One of the Act deals with general information regarding occupational health and safety. Commonwealth employers are expected to ensure that all judicious steps are taken to protect the health and safety of their employees. They must adhere to the specific regulations, standards and codes of practice which are relevant to their workplace. The workplace should not pose risks to the health of employees, and suitable facilities to protect their welfare must be available. It is the responsibility of the employer to preserve the work environment including plant, access to, and exit from the workplace. Additional safeguards are the maintenance of safe storage and transportation of substances, as well as the use of correct handling techniques by employees when using substances. In conjunction with the appropriate unions the employer must develop occupational health-and-safety policies for the workplace and promulgate strategies for the protection of employees. Satisfactory review processes are necessary to evaluate such policies. Instruction, training and supervision are essential to reduce the risks of harm to employees. Information needs to be provided in languages congruent with employees' needs. The Act also refers to the provision of first-aid facilities and to the monitoring of the health and safety of employees. Persons who are at or near the workplace and who are not employed by the employer are also protected under the Act. This is because they are deemed to be under the control of the employer for the purposes of occupational health and safety. Manufacturers of plant also have a duty to ensure that plant is properly designed, assembled, researched and tested for faults. Proper instructions and conditions for use must be made available to the employer. Suppliers are not exempt from conditions imposed by the Act and must ensure that plant or substance will not be injurious to the health and safety of employees.

Responsibilities under the Act also lie with employees to maintain a safe working environment, not only for themselves but also for their coworkers. Unnecessary actions should not be taken which might create a risk or exacerbate a current risk. The employee has an obligation to use equipment consistent with proper instructions relating to health and safety as directed by the employer. This duty also extends to others who may be in the vicinity of the employee's workplace.

In accordance with the Act, specific regulations also exist in regard to the health and safety of employees or contractors. Regulations cover a broad number of areas and cannot be described in detail here. However, some examples of those areas covered by regulations include manual handling, labelling substances, testing plant, transporting plant, protective clothing or equipment, granting, renewal or cancellation of licences, and the qualifications and training deemed necessary to do the job.

There is provision within the Act for industrial democracy through health-and-safety representation in the workplace. Where work groups are concerned, the employer needs to consult with employees and appropriate unions. A health-and-safety representative may be chosen from designated work groups where such groups perform similar tasks. Only employees are eligible to represent the group and must be chosen by election or the unanimous agreement of their fellow employees. All employees must be notified by their employer regarding the selection of occupational health-and-safety representatives. Representatives must undergo relevant training in occupational health and safety. It is unlawful for employers to penalize representatives in the execution of their duties, or by loss of entitlements or pay during training periods.

Health and safety representatives have the power to inspect the workplace if an accident has occurred. They also have a role to play in the prevention of accidents, for example if there exists the threat of an accident or harmful incident. These representatives may accompany any investigator inspecting or conducting an investigation of the workplace. Representatives may also investigate complaints by employees and access information held by the employer relating to health-and-safety issues. Access to medical information is not available to representatives without the express authority of the person concerned. An exception to this is when it is impossible to identify the employee in any way. Where it is believed that there has been contravention of the Act, occupational health-and-safety representatives must enter into consultation with the employer or the supervisor to improve the situation. If agreement cannot be reached following due process, the representative has the power to issue what is known as a 'provisional improvement notice'. This outlines the regulations or how the Act has been contravened. The representative must justify the purpose of the notice, including what is happening, or may happen, in contravention of the Act; state a period of time (not less than 7 days) in which the employer must rectify the situation or request that an investigation is conducted. Provisional notices become ineffective when cancelled by the occupational health-and-safety representative, the investigator, or the employer complies with the notice.

Employers, when requested to do so, must consult with occupational health-and-safety representatives regarding any proposed changes to the workplace which may potentially affect the health and safety of employees. Health and safety committees are required by law where an employer has fifty or more employees. Such committees meet every three months and maintain minutes of their meetings which they are obliged to keep for up to three years. The employer has a duty to assist the committee regarding information relating to occupational health-and-safety matters. The employer cannot penalize employees who are committee members in the execution of their role in participating in the functions of the committee.

Further considerations of the Industry Commission

The three Acts described here have briefly outlined Federal legislation in relation to disability and discrimination, disability services and occupational health and safety. An inquiry by the Industry Commission into work, health and safety in Australia produced a draft report in April 1995. This report highlighted a number of problems pertaining to the regulation, enforcement and practice of occupational health and safety. The Commission's authors (Rae and Easson, 1995) proposed a number of recommendations to improve work and safety in industry and thus reduce work injury and disease. It appears that every year in Australia, work related injury or disease is estimated to affect 650,000 people. Around 2700 workers die annually from health problems originating at work. Many of these deaths are due to hazardous substances. The authors report that there is a case for serious reform in respect of occupational health and safety at the Federal level and that of the jurisdictions.

Jurisdictions in Australia have incorporated elements of the Robens (1972) report (UK Committee on Safety and Health at Work) into their occupational health legislation. The National Occupational Health and Safety Commission (NOHSC) have through Worksafe Australia strived to achieve national uniformity through creation of 'national standards'. Worksafe Australia was specifically initiated in 1988 to assist this process of uniformity. The effect of incorporating these standards into legislation has shown that confusion and inconsistencies regarding regulatory approaches still exist. The Commission also reports that there is widespread apathy amongst governments, employers and unions. When workplace accidents occur, fault is often attributed to the worker involved. Many employers and employees fail to perceive that better work practices including suitable design of workplaces and work tasks will serve to reduce injury and disease.

The Commission has recommended modifying regulations to ensure clarification of individual employer and employee responsibilities and to increase state enforcement when employers fail to meet their legal obligations. Other proposals include improvement of safety by financial incentives through workers compensation; greater cooperation between national and state government agencies; and a change of role by governments. They suggest that employers and employees are the best managers of a safer workplace, and the government's role is to: set enforceable standards of occupational health and safety; reduce impediments to employers and employees managing safety in the workplace; to provide employers with incentives; and both employers and employees with greater assistance towards meeting responsibilities for safety in the workplace.

Conclusion

Good occupational health and safety practices are essential to reduce the cost of personal injury to employees and their families. Occupational therapists are involved in prevention of work injury; rehabilitation of injured workers; and training and advocacy for clients who have disabilities. Therefore it is important that they have an understanding of aspects of the law pertaining to these areas. This chapter has given a brief overview of the legislation pertaining to disability, disability discrimination and occupational health-and-safety legislation in Australia and its relevance to persons who have a disability.

References

Disability Discrimination Act 1992. Canberra, ACT: Australian Government Publishing Service.

Disability Services Act 1986. Canberra, ACT: Australian Government Publishing Service.

Disability Services Act 1986: Section 5 Guidelines. Canberra, ACT: Commonwealth Rehabilitation Service.

Equal Opportunity Guidelines: Disability Discrimination Act 1992. Melbourne, Victoria: Office of the Commissioner for Equal Opportunity.

Occupational Health and Safety (Commonwealth Employment) Act 1991. Canberra, ACT: Australian Government Publishing Service.

Racial Discrimination Act, Sex Discrimination Act, and Disability Discrimination Act: Complaints Procedure. Melbourne, Victoria: Equal Opportunity Commission.

Rae and Easson, M. (1995). Work, health and safety: inquiry into occupational health and safety (draft report). Melbourne, Victoria: Australian Government Bookshop.

The USA perspective

Significant legislation related to work

1916 National Defense Act: Improved military efficiency and enabled soldiers to become more competitive in civilian life. The focus was educational, but no agency was established to carry out the directives.

1917 PL 64–347 Smith-Hughes Act (Vocational Education Act): Created the Federal Board for Vocational Education (FBVE).

1918 PL 65–178, Smith-Sears Act (Soldiers Rehabilitation Act): Enlarged the role of the FBVE to provide programmes for disabled veterans who were unable to succeed at gainful employment.

1920 PL 66–236, Smith-Fess Act (Civilian Rehabilitation Act): Initiated rehabilitation for the general public. Provided funds for vocational guidance and training, occupational adjustment, prostheses, and placement services. Occupational therapy was reimbursed if it was part of medical treatment. No reimbursement for psychiatric or developmentally disabled people.

1921 PL 67–47, Veterans Bureau Act: Established the Veterans Bureau as an independent agency with a director responsible to the President.

1933 PL 73–2, Veterans Administration Act: Recognized the Veterans Bureau and designated this federal agency as the Veterans Administration.

1935 PL 74–271, Social Security Act: Established unemployment compensation, old-age insurance, child health and welfare services, crippled children services, and public assistance for the aged, blind and dependent children.

1943 PL 78–16, Welsh-Clark Act (World War II Disabled Veterans Rehabilitation Act): Provided vocational rehabilitation for disabled veterans of the Second World War.

1943 PL 78–113, Barden-LaFollette Act (Vocational Rehabilitation Act): Changed the original provision of PL 66–236. Physically disabled, blind, developmentally delayed, and psychiatrically disabled were added to those served. Office of Vocational Rehabilitation (OVR) established. New emphasis on activities of daily living (ADL) and adaptation. Removed ceiling on appropriation.

1944 PL 78–346, Servicemen's Readjustment Act (GI Bill): Provided for the education and training (tuition and subsistence) of individuals whose education or career had been interrupted by military service.

1945 PL 79–176, Joint Congressional Resolution for a National Employ the Physically Handicapped (NEPH) Week: Established an annually observed NEPH week. In 1954, Truman changed it to President's Committee on Employment of the Physically Handicapped; in 1962, Kennedy changed it to President's Committee on Employment of the Handicapped.

1954 PL 83–565, Hill-Burton Act (Vocational Rehabilitation Act Amendments): Greater financial support, research and demonstration grants, professional preparation grants, state agency expansion and improvement grants, and grants to expand rehabilitation facilities. Many occupational therapists received this money for training and education.

1965 Vocational Rehabilitation Act Amendments of 1965: Increased services for several types of disabled and socially handicapped people. Construction money made available for rehabilitation centres and workshops.

1968 PL 90–480, Architectural Barriers Act: Led the way to changes in access for disabled people.

1970 PL 91–517, Developmental Disabilities Services and Facilities Construction Act: States were given broad responsibility for planning and implementing a comprehensive programme of services to developmentally delayed, epileptic, cerebral palsied, and other neurologically impaired people.

1973 PL 93–112, Rehabilitation Act: Expanded services to the more severely disabled. Also provided for affirmative action in employment (Section 503) and non-discrimination in facilities (Section 504) by federal contractors and grantees.

1975 PL 94–142, Education for all Handicapped Children Act: Provided educational assistance to all handicapped children in the 'least restrictive environment'. Occupational therapists included as 'related personnel'.

1978 PL 95–602, Amendments to the Rehabilitation Act of 1973: Expansion of rehabilitation to include independent living. Established the National Institute of Handicapped Research. Provided employer incentives for training and hiring disabled people.

1983 PL 98–199, Education of the Handicapped Act Amendments of 1983: Established better transition from school to work.

1984 PL 88–210, Carl D. Perkins Vocational Act: Authorized federal grants to states to assist them in (1) extending, improving and maintaining existing programmes of vocational education; (2) developing new programmes; (3) providing part-time employment for youths who need earnings to continue their vocational training on a full-time basis; and (4) assisting people of all ages (secondary, postsecondary, and adult levels) to enter the labour market, upgrade their skills, or learn new ones. Provides funding for the following grant programmes: Adult training and Retraining, Career Guidance and Counselling, High Technology Training, Title II Basic Grants, Consumer and Homemaking Education, and Community-Based Organizations (CBO) programmes.

1986 PL 99–357, Carl D. Perkins Vocational Education Act Amendment: A technical amendment to rectify a problem with state allocation of funds, particularly for the Consumer and Homemaking Education programme.

1986 PL 99–457, Education of the Handicapped Act Amendments: Provides a significant increase in federal funds to encourage states to provide special education and related services to preschoolers aged 3 through 5 years. Federal funds for this age group will be terminated if this is not initiated by school year 1990–91. Also included is a mandate for a new, comprehensive, interagency programme to provide early intervention to infants and toddlers with handicaps, aged birth through 2 years.

1990 PL 101–336, Americans with Disabilities Act: Provides comprehensive civil rights protection from discrimination in employment, transportation, public accommodations, telecommunications, and the activities of state and local government for people with disabilities.

Extract from Hopkins H, Smith H, 1993, Willard and Spackman's Occupational Therapy, 8th edition, p. 229. Reprinted with the kind permission of the author Karen Jacobs and the publisher Lippincott-Raven, East Washington Square, Philadelphia, PA 19105.

A British perspective
Disabled people and disability legislation: The legislative framework of work practice

Introduction

There are approximately 6.5 million people with physical, mental or sensory impairment in Britain (OPCS, 1991). In November 1995 the Disability (Discrimination) Act will be enacted. It will make unlawful discrimination against disabled people in connection with employment, the provision of goods, facilities and services or the disposal or management of premises. It will also establish a National Disability Council to oversee the implementation and enforcement of the Act. However, the DDA 1995 will not make it totally unlawful to discriminate against disabled people. It is limited in scope and the 'get out' clauses within the Act mean that disabled people may still receive lesser services, education, jobs and other opportunities compared to non-disabled people. Determined outright discrimination of disabled people can also still take place in many areas of mainstream life not included within the Act. They will continue to occupy an inferior status to most other citizens and will still be some of the most severely disadvantaged members of society. Thus, despite DDA 1995 disabled people will continue to experience some form of discrimination in many areas of their lives.

In the following section the present situation will be briefly outlined with reference to education and employment and the changes that the DDA 1995 will make to them. I also examine the DDA 1995 in relation to the provision of goods and services and highlight the main provisions of welfare rights and community-care legislation. I also explain some of the reasons why disabled people and their organizations continue to argue for full comprehensive civil rights legislation despite the enactment of DDA 1995.

Education rights

After the establishment of mass education a corresponding system of mainly segregated 'special' schools education for disabled pupils and young people was developed. The Education Act 1944 laid the foundation for the education systems in England and Wales though it has been much amended by later Acts. This Act expressed a commitment to the equality of opportunity in education for all pupils. This, however, did not extend to disabled children as local education authorities (LEAs) were instructed to make special provisions for pupils who had so-called 'special educational needs' (SEN).

Present educational provisions

The most recent legislation that governs the education of disabled children is the Education Act 1993. It consolidated or amended much of the previous legislation and included revision of the law on special educational needs.

Part 111 S.(1) of the Act states that a child has 'special educational needs' if he has a learning difficulty which calls for special educational provision to be made for him. Special educational provision is provision for children of two years or more which is above or different from the educational provision made for other children of his age in schools maintained by the local educational authority or grant-maintained schools in their area.

Around 93 per cent of all children attend state maintained schools. Although moves are being made in certain quarters to further the inclusion of disabled children in mainstream schooling, it is still the case that the majority of learning disabled children still attend special schools (ACE, 1995).

Presently, physically disabled children may be refused entry to mainstream education simply because of a lack of ramps, lifts and other facilities that would enable them to use the school fully. As a result many physically disabled children are also obliged to attend segregated special schools (ACE, 1995). Though several attempts have been made to introduce adequate legislation to outlaw such discrimination, the practice is still common. It is more a matter of luck or discretion whether a physically disabled pupil will be allowed entry to a mainstream school.

The DDA 1995 and education

The DDA 1995 amends section 161(5) of the Education Act 1993 which relates to the publishing of schools' annual reports. This will make no immediate practical changes for disabled pupils. Simply, the DDA 1995 will require the annual report for each country, voluntary or grant-maintained school to include a report containing information as to:

- the arrangements for the admission of disabled pupils;
- the steps to be taken to prevent disabled pupils from being treated less favourably than other pupils; and
- the facilities provided to assist access to the school by disabled pupils.

Conclusions

Even after more than a century of largely state-sponsored education, disabled children are still not legally entitled to the same type of schooling as non-disabled children. The introduction of the DDA 1995 will make little difference to the present situation for at least another decade. The overwhelming majority of British schools and colleges cannot accommodate disabled students within a mainstream setting. As a consequence, many children with physical or learning impairments have no option but to continue to accept segregated, so-called 'special' school education (Barnes, 1991).

Employment rights

Until the provisions of the DDA 1995 are fully implemented, the only law specifically protecting disabled workers is the Disabled Persons (Employment) Act 1944. The Act was brought into force initially to cater to the employment needs of ex-service men who returned from the war injured or disabled.

The main provisions of the 1944 Act:

- establishes a register of disabled people;
- imposes a quota of 3 per cent registered disabled employees in companies with twenty or more staff;
- prohibits the recruitment of non-registered disabled staff if employers are below quota, unless they have a permit from the Employment Department; and
- prohibits the dismissal of registered employees without reasonable cause if this reduces staff below quota level.

The quota was set at 3 per cent as at the time it was thought that that was the percentage of the population who had some form of disability or impairment. In the 1981 OPCS report it was stated that 10 per cent of the population were disabled while some disabled people's associations estimate the figure to be around 12 per cent.

The Disability (Discrimination) Act 1995 and employment

When the DDA 1995 comes fully into force, it will be unlawful for an employer of more than twenty people to discriminate against a disabled person. According to the Act a person has a disability if he has a physical or mental impairment which has a substantial and long-term adverse effect on his ability to carry out normal day-to-day activities.

The main employment provisions of the 1995 Act

Prohibits an employer from discriminating against a disabled person:

- in the arrangements which he makes for the purpose of determining to whom he should offer employment;
- in the terms on which he offers that person employment; or
- by refusing to offer, or deliberately not offering, him employment.

In addition, it will be unlawful for an employer to discriminate against a disabled person whom he employs:

- in the terms of employment which he gives him;
- in the opportunities which he offers him for promotion, a transfer, training or receiving any other benefit;
- by refusing to afford him, or deliberately not affording him, any such opportunity; or
- by dismissing him, or subjecting him to any other detriment.

A complaint that a disabled person has been discriminated against can be presented to an industrial tribunal. If the industrial tribunal considers the complaint well founded, it will:

- make a declaration as to the rights of the person complaining and the person responding to the complaint on issues relating to the complaint;
- order the person responding to the complaint to pay compensation to the person complaining;
- recommend that the person responding take action within a specified period of appearing before the tribunal to rectify the issues to which the complaint relates.

Conclusions

It is generally accepted that work is crucial to an individual's social and economic well-being. Yet many of the environmental barriers, discriminatory attitudes and practices that stop disabled people's gainful employment will not be overcome with the DDA 1995. The new law will give some employment protection to disabled people. However, the test of whether it is reasonable for an employer to take steps to comply with the Act will make it possible for them not to adhere to it. Therefore, for some considerable time, disabled people will continue to occupy an inferior employment status.

Welfare rights

The present welfare benefits system for disabled people has its origins in the period immediately preceding the First World War. Until the 1970s, state-funded welfare payments were focused mainly on people who had acquired impairments due to war or industrial accident and who had a qualifying record of National Insurance contributions.

In the 1970s there was a sea-change in the provision of social security benefits which saw the introduction of a series of non-means-tested entitlements. Until that time disabled people who were not eligible for any form of compensatory benefit had to rely entirely on means-tested assistance. In 1971 the Invalidity Benefit (IVB), a long-term benefit to replace earnings, was introduced.

In an effort to cover some of the impairment-related expenses incurred by disabled people the higher and lower rates of Attendance Allowance (AA) were introduced in 1970. AA was ostensibly intended to provide funds to cover the extra expenses incurred by disabled people with high levels of care needs.

In 1975 Mobility Allowance (MA) was introduced and was paid to those individuals who are unable or virtually unable to walk. In April 1992 the AA and MA were combined when the provisions of the Disability Living Allowance (DLA) Act came into force. DLA therefore has two parts, the care component and the mobility component.

In 1975, the Severe Disablement Allowance (SDA), formally known as the Non Contributory Invalidity Pension, was introduced for people who have not paid enough National Insurance contributions to qualify for IVB. 1975 also saw the introduction of the Invalid Care Allowance (ICA), a benefit paid to people of working age who act as personal assistants (PAs) to disabled people in receipt of AA. It was not however available to married women, who are the vast majority of PAs, until 1986 and is not available to those people who act as PAs to disabled people who are not in receipt of AA. This allowance is significantly lower than the wages of full-time workers. The means-tested Disability Working Allowance (DWA) was introduced in April 1992 to encourage disabled people on benefit to take up employment. Basically, it tops up the wages of disabled people in full-time employment. Unfortunately, many disabled people derive little benefit from DWA, while others actually lose out financially in as much as they must give up other benefits when claiming it.

Other impairment-related benefits to which disabled people are entitled include Statutory Sick Pay while those with long- and short-term disability or impairment are entitled to Incapacity Benefit. Invalid Care Allowance (ICA) may be paid to PAs who are caring for a disabled person (DSS, 1995).

Disabled people are also entitled to other benefits which are not impairment related, such as income support, supplementary benefit, housing rebate, and so forth.

Conclusion

The bureaucratic regulation of disability benefits carries with it unmistakable assumptions of social incompetence which might prove unacceptable to other sectors of the community. Moreover, the language used in relation to them often emphasizes and reinforces difference and dependence (Barnes, 1991). This serves only to perpetuate and reinforce the myth that disabled people are incapable of taking control of their own lives and allows the state to intrude into their lives in ways and to an extent which would be unacceptable to others.

Besides emphasizing differences between disabled people and non-disabled people, the organization of the benefits system also creates significant economic and social divisions within the disabled population as a whole. Most disability benefits have a different set of eligibility criteria. As a result disabled people with similar impairments can be entitled to vastly differing sums of money (Barnes, 1991).

Community care legislation

The National Health Service and Community Care Act 1990 established the guidelines by which local authorities are required to provide care services for adults who may require some extra help and support at some stage in their lives. This includes those people who may have a continuing need for care such as disabled and elderly people and those with mental ill health or dementia. People with drug and alcohol related disorders and those with HIV and AIDS also come within the regulations for community care services.

The intention of the community care legislation was to enable local authorities 'to provide the right level of intervention and support to enable people to achieve maximum independence and control over their own lives.' It sought to enable people to live as independent a life as possible out in the community. The provision of the right amount of care and support to maximize independence was the cornerstone of the Act.

The main provisions of the Act are:

- to promote the development of domiciliary, day and respite services to enable people to live in their own homes wherever feasible and sensible.
- to ensure that service providers make practical support for carers a high priority.
- to make proper assessment of need and good case management the cornerstone of high quality care.

- to promote the development of a flourishing independent sector alongside good quality public services.
- to clarify the responsibilities of agencies and so to make it easier to hold them to account for their performance.
- to secure better value for taxpayers' money by introducing a new funding structure for social care.

The primary focus of the Act is the reform and reorganization of social care funding. The legislation sought to foster the development of a wide range of services provided in a variety of settings. These services were to form 'a spectrum of care' for people in need, ranging from home care support strengthened by respite and day care through to sheltered housing, group homes and hostels, depending on the levels of care required. Provisions were also made for residential, nursing homes and long-stay hospital care for those for whom other forms of care are considered no longer enough.

Community services for disabled children

Guidelines for the provision of similar services for disabled children are outlined in the Children Act 1991. The Children's Act was designed to be consistent with and complementary to the Community Care Act and together the two pieces of legislation were heralded as setting a 'fresh agenda and new challenges for social services authorities for the next decade.'

According to the Children's Act, every local authority shall open and maintain a register of disabled children within their area. Disabled children are automatically considered children in need. However, the Act ascribes no protective function to the register of disabled children thereby distinguishing it from the child protection register. Thus, although disabled children are considered to be in need, this does not necessarily mean that they are in need of protection.

The overall intention of the legislation appears to be to assist with the planning of future services of disabled children into adulthood. It recognizes that disabled children may have specific needs and seeks to provide a framework in which local authorities can begin to incorporate them within mainstream service provision.

By bringing together relevant sources of finance, improving accountability and providing the right incentives, the legislation sought to establish the right financial and managerial framework which would help to secure the delivery of good-quality local services in line with national policy objectives. Many recent reports have concluded that progress toward achieving these objectives has been somewhat slow. Only time will tell whether the provisions of these acts will be implemented to the best advantage of disabled people.

The DDA 1995 provision of goods, facilities and services

The provision of more general services to disabled people is now covered by the DDA 1995. According to the Act it is unlawful for a provider of services to discriminate against a disabled person:

- in refusing to provide, or deliberately not providing, to the disabled person any services which he provides, or is prepared to provide, to members of the public;
- or making it impossible or unreasonably difficult for the disabled person to make use of any such service;
- in the standard of service which he provides to the disabled person or the manner in which he provides it to him; or in the terms on which he provides a service to the disabled person.

Provisions for people in employment

The main statutory provisions for people at work are enacted through the Health and Safety at Work Act (HSW). This Act provides the legislative framework to promote, stimulate and encourage high standards of health and safety at work. All 'persons at work', whether employers, employees, or self-employed, are covered with the exception of domestic servants in a private household. This legislation is designed to protect not only people at work, but also the general public whose health and safety may be affected by work activities. Statutory arrangements are underpinned by regulations, which in turn can be supported by codes of practice. The latter are not statutory requirements, but they may be used in criminal proceedings, as evidence that statutory requirements have been contravened.

Administration of the Act

The Health and Safety Commission consists of representatives of local authorities and both sides of industry. It has the remit to develop policies in the field of health and safety and to propose new regulations to the government minister when appropriate. The Health and Safety Executive works under the direction of the Commission. It enforces legal requirements and advises both sides of industry. It also houses the major inspectorates in the health and safety field.

Duties of employers

Employers have a statutory responsibility to safeguard so far as is reasonably practical, the health, safety and welfare of the people who work for them. Some examples of the matters which need to be considered by employers are highlighted below.

- Is all the plant up to the necessary standards with respect to safety and risk to health?
- When new hardware/plant is installed, is the latest god practice taken into account?
- Are systems of work safe? Thorough checks of all operations, especially those operations carried out infrequently, will ensure that danger of injury or to health is minimised. This may require several special safety systems, such as 'permits to work'.
- Where known toxic contaminants are present, do protection measures conform to current hygiene standards?
- Is safety equipment regularly inspected?
- Risks to health from the use, storage, or transport of articles or substances must be minimised.

Taken from: *The Act Outlined*, 1992, Health and Safety Commission

Duties of employees

- Employees have a duty under the Act to take reasonable care to avoid injury to themselves or to others by their work activities, and to co-operate with employers and others in meeting statutory requirements. The Act also requires employees not to interfere with or misuse anything provided to protect their health, safety or welfare in compliance with the Act.
- No charge may be levied on any employee for anything done or provided to meet any specific requirement for health and safety at work.

Taken from: *The Act Outlined*, 1992, Health and Safety Commission

References

ACE (1995). Advisory Centre for Education: *Special Education Handbook*. London.

Barnes, Colin (1991). *Disabled People in Britain and Discrimination: A Case for Anti-Discrimination Legislation*. Hurst & Company, London.

Barnes, Colin (1994). *Discrimination Against Disabled People in Britain*. Hurst & Company, London.

Bingley, William and Hurst, Rachel (1987). *Getting In On The Act*. Thames Television, London.

Cash for Care (1992). RADAR & DIG, London.

Community Care and the Benefits Research Unit (1990). *The New Poor*, London.

CSIE (1989). *The National Curriculum and Integration*. Centre for Studies on Integration in Education, London.

DA (1990). *Social Security Bill: Government Proposals for Changes in Benefits for People with Disabilities*. Disability Alliance, London.

Disability and Discrimination in Employment (1993). RADAR, London.

Disability – on the Agenda: Summary of a Consultation on Government Measures to Tackle Discrimination Against Disabled People (1994). Bristol.

Disabled People Have Rights (1994). RADAR, London.

DSS (1995). *Benefits for Disabled People*. Department of Social Security, Makerfield.

Employment Rights: A Guide for Disabled People (1992). RADAR, London.

Evers, H., Badgers, F., Cameron, E., Atkin, K. (1989). *Community care project working papers*. Department of Social Medicine, University of Birmingham.

Finklestien, Vic (1992). Being disabled. *The Open University, K665 The Disabling Society*, Milton Keynes.

Gooding, Caroline (1994). *Disabling Laws, Enabling Acts – Disability Rights in Britain and America*. Pluto Press, London.

Hansard (1990). 16 January.

Hansard (1991). 25 March.

Hansard (1994). 11 March.

Hansard (1995). 9 February.

Hansard (1995). 10 February.

Hansard (1995). 27 April.

Hansard (1995). 28 April.

Health and Safety Commission (1992). *The Act Outlined*.

HMSO (1944). *Disabled People (Employment) Act 1944*. London.

HMSO (1970). *The Chronically Sick and Disabled Persons Act 1970*. London.

HMSO (1981). *The Education Act(s) 1981, 1991, 1993*. London.

HMSO (1981). *Disabled Persons Act 1981*. London.

HMSO (1986). *The Disabled Persons (Services, Consultation and Representation) Act 1986*. London.

HMSO (1989). *Caring for People: Community Care in the Next Decade and Beyond*, London.

HMSO (1989a). *The Children's Act 1991*. London.

HMSO (1989b). *The National Health Service and Community Care Act 1989*. London.

HMSO (1995). *Disability Discrimination Bill 1995*. London.

HMSO (1995a). *The Civil Rights (Disabled Persons) Bill 1995*. London.

Macdonald, Sheila (1991). *All Equal Under The Act*. Race Equality Unit (REU), London.

Oliver, Michael (1990). *The Politics of Disablement*. Macmillan Education Ltd., Hampshire.

OPCS (1991) OPCS monitor, Government Statistical Services, London.

Putting Teeth in the Act (1981). RADAR, London.

The Legal Rights of People with Disabilities (1991). The Castlemilk Law Centre & The Scottish Society for the Mentally Handicapped, Scotland.

Section III

Performance Components

6

Work Assessments

Joanne Pratt

Learning objectives

At the end of this chapter, the reader should be able to:

1 Describe methods and contexts for assessment which can be used to identify environment- or person-focused issues which have an impact on work performance.
2 Describe the features of standardized assessments.
3 Understand the ethical issues related to assessment.
4 Offer examples of tools which assess occupational performance enablers and specific components of performance.

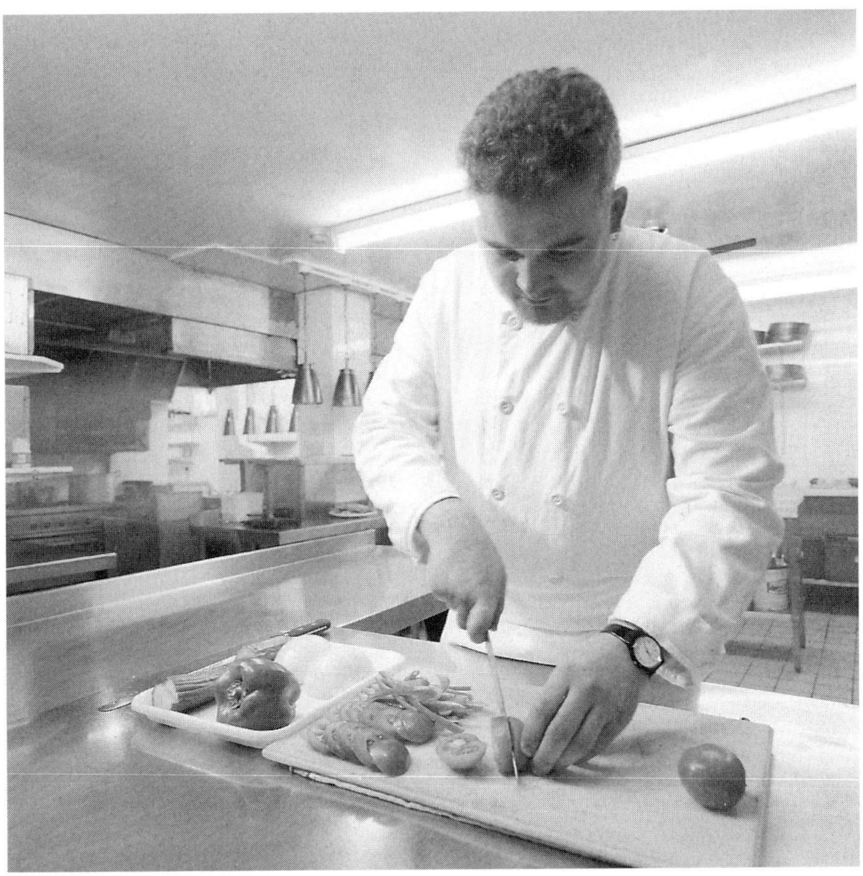

Introduction

Assessment takes many forms in the practice of occupational therapy. The methods used have arisen from a number of potential and diverse sources. These include, but are not limited to: professional philosophy and values; the varied theoretical perspectives which underpin these values; the frames of reference used to bridge theory into practice; the culture of the organization delivering service(s) to the client; the nature of the referral to the service as well as the practitioners' interpretation of client needs. Each of these sources will have an impact, to a greater or lesser extent, on the methodology the practitioner uses. The diversity of methodologies available for use in this process has paralleled the development of the profession's knowledge base and consequent research activity.

The need for objectivity in the assessment process is a challenge continually being addressed by researchers, academics and clinicians, most of whom will agree with Dunn (1993) who asked 'how do we capture the essence of life as a human being, the meaningful nature of a person's choices, and the functional integrity of performance?' The answer to this relies on the use of both quantitative information on an individual's occupational behaviour and the subjective and qualitative information which is needed to describe the context and meaning of that behaviour to the individual. In considering the former of these, objectivity can be increased with the use of tests which standardize administration, scoring and interpretation procedures. The latter issue is addressed in many ways, through interviews with the client, his or her employer, family members, and direct observation of performance in simulated and real situations. In discussing work performance, however, it is necessary to distinguish work skills, work behaviours and work tolerance (Northern Ireland Committee of the College of Occupational Therapists, 1992):

- *Work skills* are those psychomotor and social skills related to the demands of employment. These include.
  - (i) the *physical demands* required by the environmental conditions in which the employment takes place, and by the nature of the employment activities
  - (ii) *worker functions in relation to data, people and things*, components of which range from compiling, analysing, computing, comparing data; advising, supervising, persuading, serving people, through to precision working, driving or operating, manipulation or handling equipment or things;
  - (iii) *temporal demands* which is comprised of the number of working hours and whether these are required in a full-, part- or shift-time mode.
- *Work behaviours* are those expected of a person in an employment situation. They consist of:
  - (i) *work attitudes* which are the expression of an individual's feelings towards his or her work. These are naturally related to that person's values, work ethic, motivators, ambitions, attitude to authority and perception of the self as a worker;
  - (ii) *work habits* which are the individual's patterns of behaviour in the workplace including attendance, punctuality, concentration etc;
  - (iii) *work traits* which are defined as the personal qualities of the person required to perform a job. These could include reliability, adaptability, initiative, speed and perseverance.
- *Work tolerance* is defined by the individual's ability to endure the requirements of a job in a timely and appropriate manner.

Dunn has described assessment as the

> planned process of obtaining, interpreting and documenting the functional status of the individual. The purpose of the assessment is to identify the individual's abilities and limitations, including deficits, delays or maladaptive behaviour that can be assessed in occupational therapy intervention. Data can be gathered through a review of records, observation, interview and the administration of test procedures. Such procedures include, but are not limited to, the use of checklists, activities, and tasks designed to evaluate specific performance abilities. (Dunn, 1993)

This chapter provides an introduction and describes current methods which can be employed in practice to measure the diverse factors which impact on work performance.

Person–environment models

Person–environment models have been used in diverse scientific and applied professional practice areas such as occupational and environmental psychology, engineering, applied ergonomics, anthropology and organizational behaviour. Increasingly in health and social care, person–environment models are being used to both describe and frame clinical reasoning processes and the resultant services that are delivered. The development of clinical and social applications of this model has been propelled by the increasing number of community-based services. The assessment process can therefore be viewed as the key element in the person–environment interface. Assessment tools used in occupational therapy have arisen from a perspective in which humans are seen as having an innate occupational nature which is being compromised by a medical condition and/or overwhelming environmental demand(s). A recent review of assessments used in practice which consider environmental influences on performance revealed a range of 42. However only two of these focus on work performance (Letts *et al.*, 1994). Hence, it is true to say that, at present,

Community profile in occupational therapy

Aims

- to increase awareness of local provision
- to identify gaps or duplication in service provision
- to audit existing local services

Stages

1. **Define the community** Identify and describe the geographical boundary and the sociological features of the environment which make up the population to be profiled.
2. **Collect data** A variety of sources should be used to collect information on the health, social and environmental needs of the defined community. Government, statutory, voluntary and private agencies can all contribute relevant data.
3. **Analyse data** An analysis of the data is essential in order that an interpretation of local need can be made. A statistician may provide valuable support if complex analysis proves necessary.
4. **Compile the profile** The information requires to be recorded and presented in a single file, which can be either a paper or computer document.
5. **Disseminate the findings** The value of the profile is dependent on widespread dissemination so that gaps or duplication in OT provision may be clearly identified. Information could be disseminated through, for example, marketing brochures, client information leaflets or oral presentation and publication.

Limitations

- Data Protection Act and client confidentiality MUST be observed
- The profile requires regular updating
- The profile is specific to the defined community and cannot be generalized

Whyte L. and Ferguson D. 1996, Adapted from a paper 'Community Profile in the Occupational Setting' presented at the annual conference of the Royal College of Nursing Occupational Health Nurses Forum, Scotland, 1995, Edinburgh. Reprinted with permission.

assessment in this domain of practice is either environment-focused or person-focused. Each of these two broad categories will be considered in turn.

Environment focused assessments

Community profile

Community profile is a method of assessing the resources and needs within the specific community in which the practitioner's service is based. One model proposed by Whyte and Ferguson (1995) suggests that community profiling can be applied to the occupational health setting, although it could equally be applied to rehabilitation, social and employment services for those working with clients, who for diverse reasons are unable to access, adapt or maintain their work performance. This focus on the wider community context of a service serves several purposes: it increases awareness of local provision for particular client groups; it can serve as a means of identifying a potential network for communication between service providers; it can also assist in identifying gaps or duplication in service provision; it is one method of auditing local needs to compare with existing services and as an impetus for change in these services.

Workplace assessment

The effects of the work environment on performance, productivity level, efficiency and the health of employees are well recognized. The technical, medical and social elements of the workplace ultimately combine in ways which will give a particular workplace a unique identity. When problems arise or when change is planned or needed in a workplace a multidisciplinary assessment process can be employed to find solutions, to recommend adaptations or to plan goals. Health and rehabilitation practitioners may become involved in this assessment process, either as consultants, service providers or on behalf of injured workers. Any workplace assessment can involve a range of personnel, such as environmental hygienists, toxicologists, health and safety inspectors, ergonomists, medical personnel and external consultants. In addition, the assessment will take place within cultural, organizational and legislative contexts which have been described in earlier chapters. Simmons and Oland (1992) have proposed a framework for workplace assessment which is a useful means of organizing and conducting this process in employment environments which are focused in a physical plant. The core elements of their framework are:

1 *the manufacturing process* which consists of technical systems, people, raw materials, organizational and management systems.
2 *work environment factors* which they delineate as consisting of physical, toxic, physiological, biological and psychological factors. The emissions from these factors most frequently considered in the workplace include air, solid waste, waste water, soil, noise and vibration.
3 *work environment consequences* which include occupational disease, occupational discomfort, hazards and accidents. The consequences for the environment include ecological damage, nuisance, environmental health effects, and environmental contamination.

The authors describe two models – problem orientated or planning – as well as two types of assessment – strategic or thematic – which can be applied to this framework. The *problem orientated model* is familiar to many disciplines and includes the components of problem identification, problem analysis, identification and appraisal of options, decision, implementation and operation of the solution. Feedback on the outcome of this process links the final and initial components, effectively forming a loop or system which is used to focus on existing problems and their resolution. The *planning model* is used when changes are planned or already occurring in the workplace. Examples could include the introduction of new working practices, policies, the introduction of new equipment or alterations to the physical plant. Planners are challenged to integrate health, safety and environmental issues into the planning process. The five basic stages in this model are *briefing*, whereby performance criteria will be devised against which various options can be

Ergonomic chair assessment

Manufacturer: ______________________________ Model: ______________

Yes or No responses

_____ Does the seat height adjust easily while you are seated?
_____ Does the seat height allow you to rest your feet on the floor?
_____ Does the seat pan tilt forward and back easily while you are seated?
_____ Does the backrest adjust easily up and down while you are seated?
_____ Does the backrest move forward and backward easily for adjustment while you are seated?
_____ Does the backrest provide firm support to the lower part of your back?
_____ Can you make adjustments easily without assuming awkward positions?
_____ Are the seat and back contoured and comfortable to adjust to your movements and body shape?
_____ Have you been instructed in how to adjust this chair to fit you properly?
_____ Does the seat support your thighs to just behind the back of the knee?
_____ Do you experience a shock when you touch the seat in cold weather?
_____ Do you seat and back dissipate body heat?
_____ Do you feel supported and comfortable in this chair? If not, why?
_____ Do you like the overall appearance of the chair?

If arms are featured on this chair,

_____ Are you able to get in close to your desk?
_____ Do the armrests allow your elbows to remain comfortably by your side with your shoulders relaxed?
_____ Are the armrests contoured and comfortable?
_____ Are the armrests adjustable in height and distance from your body?
_____ Can the armrests be removed easily without affecting the appearance of the chair?

Manager or purchaser

_____ Does this chair come in a variety of models to accommodate variations in size of people, yet give a uniform look?

By Diane Hermenau in K. Jacobs and C. M. Bettencourt (eds) (1995). *Ergonomics for Therapists*. Reprinted with the kind permission of the publishers Butterworth-Heinemann, 313 Washington Street, Newton, MA 02158, USA.

tested. Examples derive from legislative guidelines, environmental constraints, users' needs and demands, among others; *proposals*, which involve the identification of potential options; *finalization*, where the technical, costing and practical aspects of the selected option are determined, tenders are invited and a contract awarded; *implementation*, where the project is monitored to ensure health, safety and environmental protection issues are addressed; and *application*, at which point the project becomes operational, evaluation against the initial criteria is undertaken and the experience gained during the process is documented for future reference.

While many types of assessment are needed and undertaken in the workplace, Simmons and Øland (1992) contend that they can be divided into two broad categories of strategic and thematic assessments. *Strategic assessments* occur when all areas of a company's activities are subjected to systematic and critical examination with the aim of reducing risk and/or increasing performance in health and safety and environmental management. The main tool used for this purpose is *audit* which the authors report is widely used throughout the European Community with respect to health and safety issues. The findings of these audits are ultimately useful in forming or adapting company strategies. *Thematic assessments* are used to identify and 'evaluate health, safety and environmental problems associated with particular aspects of

FACTORS	QUESTIONS
1 The task	Does it involve: – holding load at distance from trunk? – unsatisfactory bodily movement or posture especially: twisting at the trunk? stooping? – excessive movement of the load? – risk of sudden movement of the load? – frequent or prolonged physical effort? – insufficient rest or recovery periods?
2 The load	Is it: – heavy? – bulky or unwieldly? – difficult to grasp? – sharp, hot or otherwise potentially damaging? – unstable, or with contents likely to shift?
3 The working environment	Are there: – space constraints preventing good posture? – uneven, slippery or unstable floors? – variations in level of floors or work surfaces? – extremes of temperature, humidity or air movement? – poor lighting conditions?
4 Individual capability	Does the job: – require unusual strength, height, etc? – create a hazard to those who are pregnant or have a health problem? – require special knowledge or training for its safe performance?

Reprinted with the kind permission of the Health and Safety Executive, 1996 IND (G) 143L.

an operation.' These include environmental impact assessments; health and safety assessments; risk assessments with regard to air, noise, vibration, lighting, thermal, physiological, psychological, waste or discharge; machinery hazards; hazardous substances. Both strategic and thematic assessment methods need to identify those factors involved in a problem, as well as their causes and consequences, to be effective.

Ergonomic assessments

The introduction of computers has caused rapid and significant changes in the work environment. The ever increasing number of person–machine interfaces has resulted in an increased susceptibility to constrained postures, visual strain as well as mental and physical stresses (Grandjean, 1988). A number of tools have been developed to assess the *fit* between a worker and his or her workstation. These tools mainly focus on the design features of equipment, postural support devices or manual operations a worker is expected to use or perform while carrying out his or her duties. For example, many types of work can require the employee to sit for prolonged periods of time in what is considered sedentary work. Workplace seating then becomes a critical feature as well as a capital expenditure for most companies. Hermenau (1995) argues that the most important feature of good chair design for the workplace is adjustability. This can encompass adjustable seat height and tilt, which should be independent of backrest height adjustment. A good backrest should be able to support the lumbar spine in both vertical and horizontal directions. There should be adequate buttock space, the seat edge should not cause pressure under the legs and the base of support should have five points or a 'star' design for safety purposes. Similarly, computer keyboard design and work heights have received increased attention with the increase in musculoskeletal conditions which can be linked to repetitive patterns of movement required by work tasks. These good design features can then be used to construct an observational checklist which can be used to ensure a workstation is individualized to a worker's postural needs. One example of a self-administered ergonomic chair assessment is presented in the box on p. 105.

Another example of ergonomic assessment for the workplace can be found in manual handling operation guidelines. Many countries will have government agencies to regulate and monitor health and safety practices in the workplace. In the UK this body is the Health and Safety Executive, which issues directives on the standards to be implemented by industry as well as guidelines on good practice. One example of this occurs with regard to the manual handling of goods. Proposals for regulation and guidance in this area include the duties of employers and employees as well as a self-administered checklist of factors an employer must attend to when making an assessment of manual handling operations. The box on p. 106 highlights the main considerations.

Work-related stress

Stress has become a major workplace issue with 48 per cent of European workers sharing the belief that their health is affected by work-related stress (European Foundation for the Improvement of Living and Working Conditions, 1995). The Occupational Stress Indicator was authored by Cooper, Sloan and Williams (1988) who acknowledged the wide range of meaning inherent in the term 'occupational stress'. For the purposes of test construction it has been broadly regarded as 'a response to

Occupational Stress Indicator questionnaires and subscales

1 Biographical

2 Job satisfaction
- (i) satisfaction with achievement, value and growth
- (ii) satisfaction with the job itself
- (iii) satisfaction with organizational design and structure
- (iv) satisfaction with organization processes
- (v) satisfaction with personal relationships

3 Mental and physical ill health
- (i) how you feel/behave
- (ii) physical symptoms of stress

4 Type A Syndrome*
- (i) attitude to living
- (ii) style of behaviour
- (iii) ambition

5 Individual's interpretation of events around them
- (i) organizational forces
- (ii) management processes
- (iii) individual influence

6 Sources of job pressure
- (i) factors intrinsic to the job
- (ii) managerial role
- (iii) relationships with other people
- (iv) career and achievement
- (v) organizational structure and climate
- (vi) home/work interface

7 Coping with stress
- (i) social support
- (ii) task strategies
- (iii) logic
- (iv) home and work relationship
- (v) time
- (vi) involvement

*Type A Syndrome: a set of behavioural characteristics which have been established as an independent predictor of coronary heart disease

Occupational Stress Indicator (OSI) sample items

How you feel about your job

1	Communication and the way information flows around your organization	6 5 4 3 2 1
9	The style of supervision that your superiors use	6 5 4 3 2 1
11	The kind of work or task you are required to perform	6 5 4 3 2 1
22	The degree to which you feel extended in your job	6 5 4 3 2 1

How you assess your current state of health

Part A How you feel or behave

7	As you do your job have you noticed yourself questioning your own ability and judgement and a decrease in the overall confidence you have in yourself?	6 5 4 3 2 1
16	When you think about your past events do you feel regretful about what has happened, the way *you* have acted, decisions *you* have taken, etc?	6 5 4 3 2 1

Part B Your physical health

1	Inability to get to sleep or stay asleep	6 5 4 3 2 1
11	Feeling as though you do not want to get up in the morning	6 5 4 3 2 1

The way you behave generally

5	When I am doing something, I concentrate on only one activity at a time and am fully committed in giving it 100% of my effort	6 5 4 3 2 1
12	I am a fairly easy going individual, who takes life as it comes and who is not especially 'action oriented'	6 5 4 3 2 1

How you interpret events around you

4	It is not possible to draw up plans too far ahead because so many things can occur that make the plans unworkable	6 5 4 3 2 1
9	Being an effective leader is more often a function of personal skills than it is of taking advantage of every available opportunity	6 5 4 3 2 1

Sources of pressure in your job

13	Not being able to 'switch off' at home	6 5 4 3 2 1
19	My spouse's attitude towards my job and career	6 5 4 3 2 1
27	A lack of encouragement from superiors	6 5 4 3 2 1

How you cope with the stress you experience

3	'Buy time' and stall the issue	6 5 4 3 2 1
13	Deliberately separate 'home' and 'work'	6 5 4 3 2 1
20	Use distractions (to take your mind off things)	6 5 4 3 2 1

situations and circumstances that place special demands on an individual with negative results'. This tool was designed to be used within organizations for the purposes of creating a 'group profile', its use is generally precipitated by management's perception of issues like an increased sickness rate, absenteeism or staff turnover. Conversely, a decrease in performance rates may also warrant the use of this measure in an attempt to identify causes of these changes. It is stressed that the OSI is not intended for individual diagnostic purposes, but to provide a picture of the overall situation. The OSI is based on a model of stress which has four main elements: sources of stress; the individual who may be experiencing stress; coping strategies; and the effects of stress on the individual and the organization. The measure is comprised of seven pen-and-paper questionnaires, designed to be administered to groups of respondents, which takes 45 minutes to complete. The titles of these seven questionaires and their subscales are presented below. The data collected from individuals is scored with a scoring key and a total obtained for each subscale. Two scoring methods are possible, the first provides 25 subscale sores which can provide a detailed view of the situation while the second produces 17 subscale scores to offer a broad view of a situation. A group profile is then constructed with these scores which are interpreted qualitatively and in the light of precipitating factors noted above. Profiles can be created, for example, between groups within one office or section of an organization, or if needed, between units or plants of a parent organization.

Person-focused assessments

The Jacobs Prevocational Skills Assessment was developed by Karen Jacobs in 1979 and revised in 1988 as a screening tool for school-aged children with learning difficulties. It has three categories – physical capacities, work behaviours and work aptitudes – which are assessed through observation of a client's performance on fifteen standard tasks which are designed to simulate real work skills as closely as possible. It is intended for use as a tool to assist therapists to plan goals for intervention programmes.

Psychometric tests

Objective testing can be thought of as the sampling of an individual's (or group's) behaviour and represents another aspect of the

<table>
<tr><th colspan="2">The Jacobs Prevocational Skills Assessment</th><th>Work skills</th></tr>
<tr><td>Physical capacities</td><td>Fine motor coordination
Eye-hand coordination
Motor planning
Use of tools</td><td rowspan="3">1 Quality control
2 Filing
3 Carpentry assembly
4 Classification
5 Office work
6 Telephone directory
7 Factory work

8 Environmental mobility

9 Money concepts
10 Functional banking
11 Time concept
12 Work attitudes
13 Assembly
14 Leather assembly
15 Food preparation</td></tr>
<tr><td>Work behaviours</td><td>Task focus
Ability to follow directions:
visual
written
verbal
Organizational skills
Decision making</td></tr>
<tr><td>Work aptitudes</td><td>Sorting
Attention to detail
Classification sequencing
Problem solving
ADL knowledge</td></tr>
</table>

Ethical responsibilities in OT evaluation

- Recognize the value of standardized tests
- Distinguish standardized from non-standardized tests
- Distinguish objective from subjective data
- Know that using standardized tests incorrectly invalidates them
- Recognize one's own abilities and limitations

assessment process. A number of standardized tests, used to translate behaviours into numbers or quantitative information, are used in the practice of occupational therapy to make inferences or predictions about a person's occupational performance. Standardized tests can vary in the complexity of their administration, scoring and interpretation. The term 'psychometric test' is used to describe those measures used to collect quantitative information or data on the psychological attribute(s) of a person. Psychometric tests are distinguished from others by their reliability, validity and the standardization process. These qualities, and their principles of measurement theory, are increasingly being used as the benchmarks against which new tools are developed in areas of practice outside psychology, including occupational therapy (Benson and Clark, 1982). Occupational therapists are increasingly using the information provided by such measures when assessing or planning intervention for a client, particularly in an area like work practice. There are well-established tools developed for the field of occupational psychology, and practitioners may well work in teams where this information is collected and interpreted by a psychologist or vocational rehabilitation specialist. Additionally, occupational therapists may, following additional training, qualify to administer and interpret tests themselves.

Psychometric testing considers the reliability and validity of assessments. *Validity* is most simply defined as the quality of a test to measure what it claims to measure. Evidence

1 **Tests of attainment** These usually reflect a client's level of general educational attainment and come in two main forms:

(a) standardized or 'critierion-referenced' tests that produce a single score, and
(b) batteries, modules or banked materials that produce a number of subtest scores or profiles.

2 **Measures of attributes or dispositions** These cover typical behaviour patterns, aptitudes, interests and cognitive abilities. The different types of tests which comprise this category include:

(a) pencil and paper tests for groups or individuals which produce quantitative scores,
(b) those which involve the use of apparatus or complex materials for use with individuals and designed on the same principles as those above,
(c) computer-based versions of the above tests which may include provisions in their design which allow them to be tailored for individuals through item choice selection,
(d) *projective* tests which produce qualitative information largely and
(e) *idiographic* procedures which are those which measure patterns or profiles of the attributes of interest *within* an individual. There is therefore no reference to membership of specified groups.

3 **Procedures that assess 'dysfunction' or occupational performance deficits** This category is comprised of those tests used as diagnostic measurements, including:

(a) observer rating scales made in structured or real-world situations and
(b) those which assess an individual's level of performance, quantitative information may or may not be produced.

From: British Psychological Society (1992) Psychological Testing: a guide. Steering Committee on Test Standards, Leicester.

of validity can be obtained in various ways: through satisfactory statistical correlations with other tests of the same ability or skill, or with practitioners' estimates of their clients' abilities, or with clients' subsequent achievements. *Reliability* is a quality whereby a test is considered capable of producing consistent results. The reliability coefficient, a statistical calculation, indicates the extent to which an instrument is 'stable'. The validity and reliability of assessments is usually enhanced when the test is administered, scored and interpreted using standardized methods. In this way, the data obtained from the test are more likely to yield objective information. Psychometric tests can be divided into three broad categories. These are tests: (1) of attainment, (2) which measure attributes or dispostions, or (3) which assess 'dysfunction' or psychological deficits (British Psychological Society, 1992).

This categorization is equally useful when considering the range of standardized tools available to measure work performance from occupational or functional perspectives. For organizational purposes, the next section of this chapter will utilize these categories to provide readers with descriptions of tools used in the varied aspects of work practice.

Tests of attainment

Assessment for Training and Employment

This psychometric battery of 25 tests was first published in 1988 and again in 1991 and is designed for use in occupational consultancy. Use of all 25 tests leads to the creation of four separate client profiles:

1. *Foundation skills* This set of tests produces adult measures of attainment in numeracy and literacy. A short simple screening test is administered first to determine which of the three levels of the main test is appropriate to administer to a client. A single scaling system runs through all three levels. Raw scores can be converted into percentiles, norm tables are available for US, Canadian and UK adult samples.
2. *Vocational interests* Clients are presented with 253 different job activities which they rate on how much they would like to perform each task on a full-time basis using a five-point scale. A Vocational Interest Exploration profile can then be created. Clients' preferences are assessed on the dimensions of data/people/things which are related to these same three dimensions in occupations rated by job holders. Twenty-three separate job clusters have been identified which can then be used as a basis for discussion or counselling with the client for goal planning.
3. *Aptitudes* Culturally appropriate versions of the Differential Aptitude Test by Bennett, Seashore and Wesman (1947) (cited in The Psychological Corporation Ltd, 1991) which focuses on aptitudes in the distinct areas of: verbal reasoning, numerical ability, abstract reasoning, clerical speed and accuracy, mechanical reasoning, space relations, spelling, language use. Raw scores can be converted to percentiles with norm tables available for male, female and combined samples.
4. *Personal qualities* A Personal Qualities Inventory highlights those styles of behaviour and attitudes which can be important in accessing and maintaining employment. The publishers stress that this is not a formal objective test or a personality measure. Five dimensions important to employers are assessed, these are sociability, work orientation, adaptability, self-presentation and self-directedness.

General Clerical Test – Revised

First published by the Psychological Corporation in 1936, this test is widely used to provide estimates of clerical ability. It focuses on three areas of competence: perceptual accuracy, verbal ability and numerical ability. These divide into ten subtests which include: checking, filing, calculation, error location, estimation, problem solving, spelling, vocabulary, language use and comprehension. The battery consists of 265 items which are administered in timed sections. Raw scores can be converted with thirteen norm tables which use various educational and occupational populations to provide a percentage score; T-score, stanine or sten scores. The publishers provide extensive validity and reliability information including test-retest reliability, standard error of measurement, content validity and subtest intercorrelations. The test has also been adapted for use in North America and the United

Problem Solving

4 Susan repairs appliances. She made two service calls. She spent 3 1/2 hours on the first one and 1 1/2 hours on the other. Also, she spent 1 hour in driving time. How many hours did she spend all together?

A 5 hours
B 6 hours
C 7 hours
D Not Given

SALE!
5 tins for
£1.50

5 This week you can buy 5 tins of soup for £1.50. At this rate, how much does each tin cost?

A £0.25
B £0.30
C £0.35
D Not Given

£200 cash now
or £25 for each month
for 10 months

6 A new sewing machine costs £200. How much will you save if you pay for it in cash, instead of paying 10 monthly payments of £25?

A £5
B £25
C £50
D Not Given

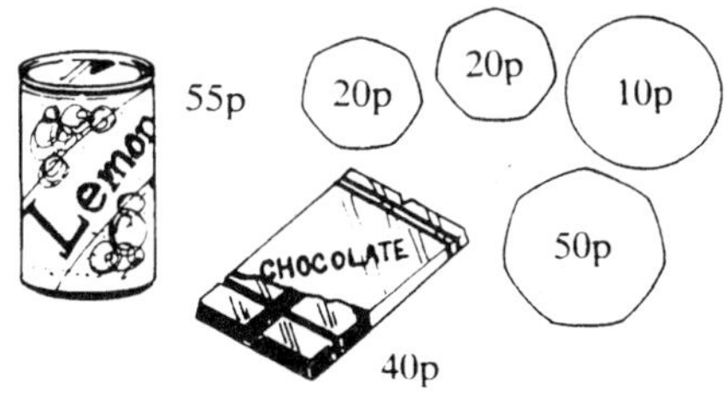

7 Anne bought a 40p bar of chocolate and a 55p can of lemonade. She gave the shop assistant a 50p piece, two 20p pieces, and a 10p piece. How much change should she get back?

A 5p
B 10p
C 15p
D Not Given

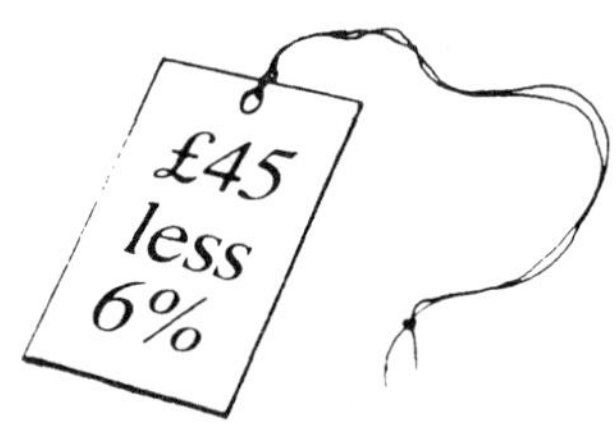

8 Frances works in a shop. She has just sold a coat that was reduced from £45.00 in a sale. If the reduction was 6%, what is the saving?

A £0.27
B £2.70
C £27.00
D Not Given

GO ON TO NEXT PAGE ➤

Figure 6.1 Extract from Assessment for Training and Employment (ATE). Reproduced with kind permission by The Psychological Corporation. Copyright The Psychological Corporation Ltd, 24–28 Oval Rd, London, NW1 7DX, UK.

Kingdom. Assessors are asked to note when a candidate's first language is not English as this can obviously influence and possibly limit interpretation of the results.

Valpar work samples

The Valpar International Corporation produces a range of tools which are used to measure work-related task performance. They were first introduced to the field of vocational rehabilitation but have since been applied in a number of related practice areas, including occupational therapy. A series of 'work samples' which simulate various aspects of job performance have been manufactured to assess performance using criteria which have been derived from Methods–Time Measurement (MTM) which is defined as a job analysis system using systematic, motion–time methods' (Hertfelder and Gwin, 1989) and from the Worker Qualifications (Trait) Profile of the Dictionary of Occupational Titles. The work samples which have most commonly been used in occupational therapy to date are described further.

VCWS 1 small tools (mechanical)

This work sample measures a client's ability to understand and work with small tools, such as screwdrivers, pilers and wrenches. Through observation of task performance the occupational therapist will also be able to assess several components of neuromotor performance, including motor coordination, manual dexterity and finger dexterity. In addition, the cognitive components of perseverance, tolerance of frustration and performance on long, repetitive tasks can also be observed. The work sample is divided into six timed exercises, five of which comprise assembly tasks and one disassembly. It is appropriate for use with disabled and non-disabled clients, including people with visual impairments or blindness.

VCWS 4 Upper extremity range of motion

This work sample measures a client's range of movement and work tolerance in tasks that involve all the upper limb joints in a range of bilateral manual activities. There are two timed sections involving the assembly and disassembly of nuts onto bolts. Components of performance which can be assessed through observation include reaching, handling, fingering, feeling, seeing, motor coordination and manual dexterity. A series of questions designed to identify positions of fatigue and possible pain are also used with this sample in conjunction with an Upper Extremity Body Position chart.

VCWS 8 Simulated assembly

This work sample is designed to be characteristic of conveyor assembly using a three-step task. The client places a pin on the assembly wheel, followed by a plastic spacer and then a cap as the wheel rotates at a constant speed. The score for the VCWS 8 is derived from the number of correct units assembled in a 20-minute time period on an automatic counter built into the hardware. This task measures a client's ability to work at an assembly task requiring repetitive physical manipulation, bilateral use of the upper limbs, finger dexterity and motor coordination. The assessor may also choose to determine endurance for work hardening by extending the 20-minute time limit, or choose to observe the client's ability to adapt their pace of work by increasing or decreasing the speed of the wheel.

VCWS 9 Whole body range of motion

This work sample measures a client's ability to work at four different heights: overhead, shoulder height, waist height and crouching. The task involves transferring three forms and screwing them into place at each of these heights. The components of performance which can be observed through this task include: transitional movements between each of these body positions, reaching, handling, feeling, seeing, coordination and dexterity. This work sample is also used in some work hardening programmes to build work tolerances in common working positions.

VCWS 11 Eye-hand-foot coordination

A maze, mounted on a standing frame is used to measure a client's ability to use hands, eyes and feet simultaneously in a coordinated manner. Scores are awarded based on which of thirteen holes in the maze small steel balls fall through as they traverse the maze. Three timed trials are made to determine the score.

VCWS 19 Dynamic physical capacities

The main hardware used with this work sample includes a shelving unit and small table, scale, three-step ladder, cartons of varying weights, and twelve shaped parts. The tasks involve having a client read an invoice, locate a shipping carton, remove a carton from a shelf, climbing one step up the ladder, weighing the carton and putting it in its proper place for shipping. In this way the physical demand factors at sedentary, light, medium, heavy and very heavy levels can be measured. The components of performance which can be observed include: climbing and balancing, fingering, reaching and pulling, kneeling, stooping, seeing and handling. There are 28 individual exercises in the work sample which are used to establish whether a client can lift the required weight and perform physical tasks required at each strength level.

Measures of attributes or dispositions

The Coping Responses Inventory (CRI)

This test, authored by Moos in 1990, can be administered as a questionnaire or structured interview. The client is asked to make an appraisal of a stressful situation they have experienced during the past year. The 48 coping items are then answered in relation to the identified stressor and are rated on a four-point frequency scale. Eight subscales are used to classify answers: approach coping vs avoidance coping responses; and cognitive coping vs behavioural coping strategies. In order that a coping profile can be constructed raw scores are converted to standard scores, where a standard score of 50 represents the average and one standard deviation is ten points. The CRI is considered to be of particular use in identifying adaptive changes in client's coping and in measuring change over time, i.e. before and after intervention.

Raven's progressive matrices and the Mill-Hill Vocabulary scales

The aim of the MHV is to record a person's 'present recall of acquired information and ability for verbal communication'. There are supposedly no demands on a person's present capacity for intellectual activity or rational judgement, it is purely an estimate of a person's recall of verbal information. The MHV consists of 88 words which are divided into two sets of Definitions and Synonyms. The test is published at three levels: junior, standard and senior. Scoring involves comparing the respondant's raw score with his or her chronological age to obtain a percentile score. The Standard Progressive Matrices consist of 60 problems divided into five sets of twelve. The problems become progressively more difficult and training is inherent in the progressive method of working through the test. The five tests provide five opportunities for grasping the method and five progressive assessments of a person's capacity for intellectual activity. The test was designed to be used across the widest possible range of mental ability and with people of all ages. It can be administered either timed or untimed, depending on the reason for assessment, i.e. for clinical purposes an untimed 'capacity' test is recommended by the authors. For vocational guidance and occupational selection a 'speed or efficiency' test is more useful. In the latter case the authors recommend using the senior version of the test. Considerable research attention was paid to the test's standardization from its first publication in 1936 until the 1970s. Scoring is done with an answer key provided in the manual, this raw score is then compared to a norm table constructed with chronological age categories to obtain a percentile score. These percentile scores can then be assigned a Grade 1 'intellectually superior' through to a Grade V 'intellectually impaired'.

The authors state that there are advantages to the combined use of the SPM and MHV together in place of a single test of general intelligence. For instance, the vocabulary test indicates where a person must begin any course of training he wishes to pursue or work he will have to undertake while the SPM indicates the rate at which he might be expected to progress.

Valpar Prevocational readiness battery (VCWS 17)

This group of work samples is produced by Valpar International Corporation to assess a client's 'ability to function in a vocational, educational, sheltered or independent living setting.' It is divided into four subtests each of which is independent of language and reading skills, i.e. clients are able to respond non-verbally, if appropriate.

1 Development assessment which has four parts: patterning/colour discrimination/manipulation; manual coordination; range of motion/dynamic strength/walking; matching/vocational knowledge/measurement
2 Workshop evaluation: three of four workstations have a three-step assembly process. At the fourth station, completed assemblies are sorted into pass or reject bins. This task allows observation of interpersonal skills and teamwork in a workshop setting. Problem solving, adjustment to the working pace of others and behaviour during testing can also be observed.
3 Interpersonal/social skills: there are four parts to this subtest, practical skills; socialization skills; aggravating behaviours; and work-related skills. Behaviours are observed and assigned a point value on a Critical Barriers Inventory. This subtest is designed to identify a client's ability to make appropriate social judgements as well as to highlight any social behaviours which could act as barriers to employment or independent living. It involves practical evaluation of skills independently of an interview.
4 Money handling skills: this subtest involves a series of progressive tasks which measure a client's understanding of money concepts from addition and subtraction through to saving and working for money.

Procedures that assess 'dysfunction', functional or occupational performance deficits

Perceived Stress Scale (PSS)

Authored by Cohen, Karmack and Mermelstein (1995), this test attempts to measure the degree to which individuals appraise situations in their own life as 'stressful'. While the term 'stress' is used widely in everyday language its use in health psychology can be related (1) to the behaviour or responses individuals make, (2) to the identification of stressors or (3) to the transactions that an individual uses to meet the demands of his or her environment (Johnston, Wright and Weinman, 1995). The 14 items on the PSS-14 can be administered by self or through interview and are designed to elicit subjective appraisals of events occurring within a one month time period. The test comes in three versions PSS-14, PSS-10 and PSS-4. Items are scored from 0 to 4 in both directions and then totalled to achieve an overall score within the range of 0–56. Higher scores then are indicative of more perceived stress. Cohen *et al.* found the internal consistency of the PSS-14 to be 0.75, 0.78 for the PSS-10 and 0.60 for the PSS-4 using Cronbach's alpha when they administered the test to 2387 people in a stratified random sample. Evidence of concurrent validity has been found in studies of college students where there was some correlation found with number of life events and impact of life events. Additionally, the PSS has been found to correlate with indices of depressive symptomology. The PSS-10 is recommended for use over the PSS-14 and PSS-4 because of 'its good internal reliability, tighter factor structure and equivalent value in predicting outcomes' (Johnston, Wright and Weinman, 1995).

McGill Pain Questionnaire

This first appeared in 1975 and has since become one one of the most widely used tools in the assessment of a patient's subjective experience of his or her pain. Melzack authored this questionnaire when it became evident that there were no measures available at that time which addressed this subjective experience of pain adequately, if at all. Currently, at least five versions of the test are published. While Melzack recommends that the test is administered verbally it has also been used as a self-administered tool. A respondant is asked to select a word from a presented list, which has been organized into 20 categories, which best describes his or her pain. On the standard form a single pain

Client's name: . . . . **Age:** . . . .

File no.: . . . . **Date:** . . . .

Clinical category (e.g. cardiac, neurological, etc.): . . . .

Diagnosis: . . . .
. . . .
. . . .

Analgesic (if already administered):

1. Type . . . .
2. Dosage . . . .
3. Time given in relation to this test . . . .

- -

This questionnaire has been designed to tell us more about your pain. Four major questions we ask are:

1. Where is your pain?
2. What does it feel like?
3. How does it change with time?
4. How strong is it?

It is important that you tell us how your pain feels now. Please follow the instructions at the beginning of each part.

Part 1. Where is your pain?

Please mark, on the drawing below, the areas where you feel pain. Put E if external, or I if internal, near the areas which you mark. Put EI if both external and internal.

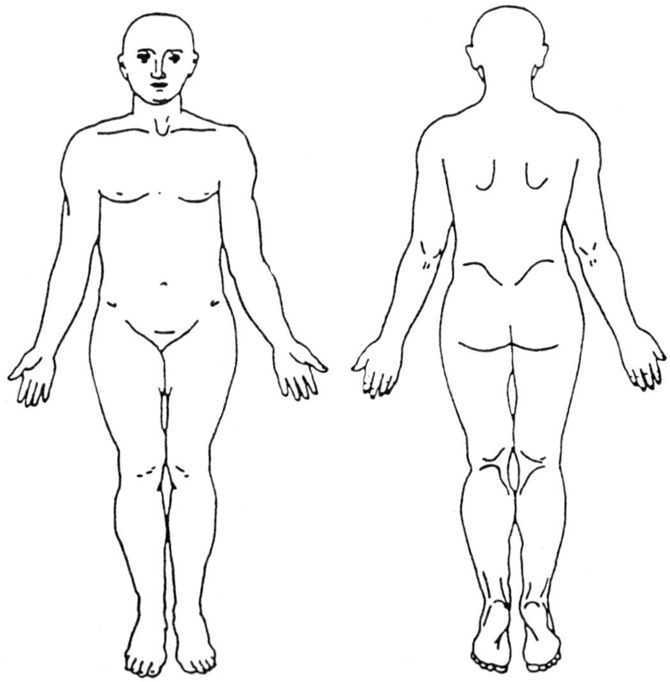

Figure 6.2 Extract from The McGill Pain Questionnaire, copyright Melzack 1975 from 'The McGill Pain Questionnaire: major properties and scoring methods, *Pain* **1**, 277–99. Available in *Assessment: A Mental Health Portfolio*, published by NFER-Nelson, Darville House, 2 Oxford Road East, Windsor, SL4 1DF, UK. Reprinted with kind permission of the author and publisher.

intensity score is calculated along with six pain quality scores. Ranks or a weighted rank score can be calculated. Reliability evidence is available as well as that which supports concurrent, predictive and construct validity (Wilkin, Hallam and Doggett, 1993). The MPQ has been used with clients with a range of medical conditions, and as one of the best available measures it is used extensively in clinical practice and research.

Pain Coping Strategies Questionnaire (CSQ)

This is a 44-item, self-administered questionnaire authored by Rosentstiel and Keefe (1983) which assesses the type and effectiveness of coping strategies used by clients when experiencing pain. Six different cognitive and one behavioural strategy are identified through the items on the test which then form subscales. These include: diverting attention, reinterpreting the pain sensation, catastrophizing, ignoring sensations, praying or hoping, coping self-statements and increased behavioural activities. Scores for each subscale range from 0–36 after clients have rated each item on a 7-point scale ranging from 0 or 'never do' to 6 or 'always do that'. A higher score indicates a greater use of the strategy identified by a particular subscale. Clients are also assessed by two items on their perceived ability to control or reduce their pain. It is also possible to generate three total scores on cognitive coping and suppression; helplessness and diverting attention and praying/hoping by adding specified subscale scores. While there is currently no normative data for this measure, there is some evidence that the internal consistency of the tool is satisfactory (Johnston, Wright and Weinman, 1995).

The Functional Assessment Inventory

This was created by Crewe and Athelstan and developed for clinical use to describe a client's potential for vocational rehabilitation. It is intended to be used with all types of disability by summarizing the functional limitations as well as the personal and environmental resources that a client can use to help cope with problems. The FAI identifies a person's strengths and limitations that predict ability to return to work, and those which should be taken into account when planning a programme of intervention. Thirty items describing functional limitations are rated on a four-point scale representing current levels of impairment. A ten-item checklist of assets or unusual strengths is also incorporated into this measure, which are marked present or absent by the respondant. The FAI is completed by an observer using a range of data sources, i.e. interview records, direct observation etc. Reliability and validity studies have been conducted with some reported success (McDowell and Newell, 1987), however work is ongoing to determine and strengthen the predictive validity of this measure.

Functional Capacity Assessments

Occupational therapists are skilled in identifying the determinants of role performance, task breakdown and activity analysis. Functional Capacity Assessments (FCAs) are increasingly being used to determine an individual's overall physical capacities for work-related tasks which mainly involve use of the hands in bimanual activities, lifting and bending. Many of the components of these assessments can be linked to the US Dictionary of Occupational Titles (Department of Labor, 1977) and later the Revised Handbook for Analysing Jobs (1991), while in the UK the three volumes of the Standard Occupational Classification (Office of Population Censuses and Surveys, 1990) will act as increasingly useful references for practitioners. Currently there are standardized and non-standardized versions of FCAs being used in clinical practice. The results are used in a number of ways, i.e., to determine if an individual can return to work; compensation entitlements; to support claims or benefits applications; to explore alternative career options; and as a basis for recommending modifications to the individual's workstation or workplace. FCAs can be used to delineate the individual's physical abilities from subjective issues which may also impact on performance. The basis of FCA lies in neuromuscular performance. Analysis of muscular effort, torque patterns, heart rate, pain behaviours, physiological consistencies, provide an assessment of the person's functional ability, not a diagnostic analysis of a specific injury or illness. Figure 6.2 is an example of a Physical Capacities Evaluation, developed for clinical use with clients. Assessment takes

Injured WORKERS program

SACRED HEART GENERAL HOSPITAL
1255 HILYARD STREET POST OFFICE 10905 EUGENE, OREGON 97440 (503) 686-7331

PHYSICAL CAPACITIES EVALUATION

DATE:
Name:
MRUN, Hosp#:
CC:

Treating MD:
DI/DX:
Insurer:

POSTURAL ENDURANCE

	Hours at a Time					Duration of Postural Change (After ____ Mins, then resume position)	Total Hours in 8 Hour Day								
SIT	.5	1	2	3	4	____	.5	1	2	3	4	5	6	7	8
STAND	.5	1	2	3	4	____	.5	1	2	3	4	5	6	7	8
WALK	.5	1	2	3	4	____	.5	1	2	3	4	5	6	7	8

PHYSICAL DEMAND CATEGORY

Estimated functional capacity level as defined by US Department of Labor:

_____SEDENTARY	Lift, carry, push, and/or pull 10# maximum, walk occasionally, mostly sit.
_____LIGHT	Lift, carry, push, and/or pull 20# maximum, frequently lift and/or carry up to 10#. Can include walk and/or stand frequently.
_____MEDIUM	Lift, carry, push, and/or pull 50# maximum, frequently lift and/or carry up to 25#.
_____HEAVY	Lift, carry, push, and/or pull 100# maximum, frequently lift and/or carry up to 50#.
_____VERY HEAVY	Lift, carry, push, and/or pull over 100#, frequently lift and/or carry 50 + #.

MAXIMUM LIFT__________ MAXIMUM CARRY__________

COMMENTS__________

HAND/FOOT USE

Worker can use hands for repetitive:	RIGHT YES	RIGHT NO	LEFT YES	LEFT NO
Fine Manipulation	___	___	___	___
Simple Grasping	___	___	___	___
Pushing and Pulling	___	___	___	___
Dominant Hand	___		___	

Can worker use feet for repetitive raising and push (as in operating foot controls)? ___YES ___NO

RANGE OF MOTION

_____ No significant limitations observed	COMMENTS:__________
_____ See DIF Spinal ROM form	__________
_____ See attached	

6/13/94. ot\pce.new

Figure 6.3a Physical Capacities Evaluation, Sacred Heart General Hospital, Eugene, Oregon. Reprinted with permission.

CLIENT NAME / MRUN:
DATE:

POSTURAL ACTIVITIES

	Continuously 67-100% of day	Frequently 34-66% of day	Occasionally 6-33% of day	Intermittently 1-5% of day	Not At All
Bend	____	____	____	____	____
Twist	____	____	____	____	____
Crawl	____	____	____	____	____
Hands/Knees	____	____	____	____	____
Kneel	____	____	____	____	____
Squat	____	____	____	____	____
Climb	____	____	____	____	____
Balance	____	____	____	____	____
Reach above shoulder level	____	____	____	____	____

STRENGTH

____ No significant limitations observed	COMMENTS: ____________________

ENDURANCE

		Limiting Factor: Pain	Fatigue	COMMENTS:
Bicycle Ergometer	____mins @ ____kgm	____	____	____________
Upper Body Ergometer	____mins @ ____kgm	____	____	
Treadmill	____mins @ ____mph	____	____	____________

Maximum achieved heart rate ____ BPM
Calculated Target Zone ____________ BPM
Estimated MET level ____

RELIABILITY OF TEST RESULTS

Maximum Effort Tests	Not Tested	Normal	Abnormal
Static Lift Strength	____	____	____
Hand Grip Dynamometer			
Coefficient of Variation: (Consistent Effort)	____	____	____
Bell Curve: (Maximal Effort)	____	____	____

	Not Tested	Normal	Abnormal	SCORE
Perceived Exertion	____	____	____	____
Pain Diagram	____	____	____	____
Pain Rating Scale	____	____	____	____
Waddell's Signs	____	____	____	____

ADDITIONAL COMMENTS ______________________________

Estimations are based on client report, available medical records, and observations of performance.

EVALUATORS/DATE: ______________________________

FOR TREATING PHYSICIAN USE AND COMMENT (OPTIONAL)

____ I agree with the above findings and release the patient to work at this physical level. Effective Date: ________

PHYSICIAN COMMENTS ______________________________

Treating Physician   Date

6/13/94. ot\pce.new

Figure 6.3b (continued): Physical Capacities Evaluation, Sacred Heart General Hospital, Eugene, Oregon. Reprinted with permission.

place through observation of an individual's performance on a number of tasks which generally simulate real work.

The development of standardized methods of determining the individual's functional ability have largely taken place in the USA, although different versions are used in Canada, Australia and the Netherlands. Two tools, the Ergos and KEY methods have been introduced to the UK and are based at the Rehabilitation Resource Centre at City University, London. Both these methods of assessment are designed for use by experienced and trained clinicians and take approximately four hours to administer.

Ergos Work Simulator is a computer-based assessment which incorporates bar-code technology. These codes are used as a basis for comparison with US standards for job requirements, work speed and manual lifting. It is comprised of five work-simulation panels, each of which is linked to an on-line computer. These can be used for assessment or intervention purposes. The box *below* shows the layout of activities on the unit.

KEY Method is designed to assess injured workers to determine their safe capabilities and tolerances for the work environment using data gathered from physical, medical, behavioural and ergonomic perspectives. The KEY Method is comprised of a series of 22 protocols which are administered in a defined progression by a therapist specifically trained in the method. The client is free to terminate each test when they wish. The main focus is on whole body function along with specific upper-body

Panel 1
Strength measurement

static/isometric and dynamic strength lifting, pushing, pulling, trunk rotation, safe lifting limits, average lifting frequency, action limits, lift origin and destination

Panel 2
Whole body range of motion

reaching, standing, stooping, bending, crouching, seeing, trunk rotation, balancing, kneeling

ERGOS

- **Standardized procedures & reporting**
- **Computer-generated charts, scores, reports**
- **Relates performance to job-spectic activities**

Panel 5
Seated work tolerance

reaching, handling, fingering, feeling, sitting, range of motion, wrist flexion/extension, grip strength, finger flexion, pinch, forearm/wrist supination and pronation, vision, hearing

Panel 3
Standing work tolerance

walking, climbing (ascending/descending), balancing, pushing, pulling, lifting, carrying, stooping, seeing, work endurance

Panel 4
Work endurance

handling, reaching, feeling, stooping, standing, walking, seeing

KEY protocols

Lifting	Head and neck mobility
Pushing	Work height levels
Sitting	Grip tolerance
Bending	Walking tolerances
Kneeling	Climbing stairs
Crouching	Keyboard tolerances
Crawling	Small tool manipulation
Squatting	Normal tool manipulation
Balancing	Pinch capacity
Carrying	Torque capacity
Pulling	Fine hand movements
Standing	Hand movements
Stooping	Repetitive foot movements
	Hand and body position tolerances

capabilities. An individual's results can be compared to data of injured and uninjured worker's functional capacities, which is available in the databank provided. The box *above* lists the protocols used with this apparatus.

The publishers state that testing can discriminate performance at four levels, these are defined as: *valid* – the numbers generated can be used as safe capabilities; *conditionally valid* – although the numbers are safe and can be used they are usually lower than actual capabilities. The client has not intentionally manipulated the results, but has demonstrated an 'early' termination point; *invalid* – the numbers do not represent safe capabilities as the client may have intentionally manipulated the results of the assessment; *conditionally invalid* – the numbers are not true representations of the client's capabilities. The client did not demonstrate an awareness of his or her safe capabilities and worked beyond them.

In the UK, the introduction of the Disability Discrimination Act will make it advantageous for employers to have an understanding of the fundamental physical tasks of any job they advertise. The Ergos and KEY Method FCAs could be used for both job analysis and job description purposes. Once the employer is cognizant of the essential physical requirements of a job, they must then be satisfied that an applicant can meet the physical and intellectual demands of the post, and if not, the ways in which a job may reasonably be modified can then be explored.

Outcome measures in occupational therapy

Outcome measures used for work hardening programmes appear to have largely been devised for two of the three levels of occupational performance. At the lowest level, components of task performance, commonly used outcome measures focus on the client's push, pull, lift and carry capacities. At the level of occupational role performance, the outcome measures shown in the box *below* have been applied.

A 50–80 per cent return-to-work success rate with work hardening programmes has been reported (King, 1993). However, the need for uniform standards in outcome data collection as a basis for comparison has also been documented (Neimeyer *et al.*, 1994). These measures of the outcomes of intervention programmes contrast with the Canadian Occupational Performance Measure (COPM), which has been designed for use with individuals.

The Canadian Occupational Performance Measure, by Law *et al.* (1994), is one tool which was developed following the recommendations of a task force on guidelines for client-centred practice in Canada which advised that a tool or tools should be developed to measure

Outcome measures used in work hardening
Same job, same employer
Same job, different employer
Different job, same employer
Different job, different employer
Retired
Medical absence

occupational therapy outcomes with a primary focus on the three areas of occupational performance – self-care, productivity and leisure. Performance in these three areas is grounded in the interaction of an individual's mental, physical, sociocultural and spirtual performance components (Reed and Sanderson, 1980). Outcome measures describe and/or quantify the impacts of a programme of intervention which contrasts with other assessment tools, which are generally used earlier on in the therapeutic process for screening or diagnosing performance deficits, establishing performance baselines, planning purposes and for measuring change. However, increasingly the management of health and social care services requires quality assessment of these services. The COPM is one such individualized measure which tracks a client's self-perceived change in his or her occupational performance problems over time. As such, it can offer a valuable contribution to the overall evaluation of the package of care the client has received. The COPM is used to document the results of a face-to-face interview between the client and therapist during which the therapist asks the client to identify occupational performance problems and concerns or issues through consideration of a typical day. This could include the vocational activities undertaken by the client in the occupational performance area of productivity. The five most important problems are confirmed and recorded. The client is then asked to score their perceived level of current *performance* and *satisfaction* for each of these problems on a scale of one to ten. The averaged performance and satisfaction scores are then calculated. Reassessment involves revisting these problems during a second interview following intervention(s) and having the client score their performance and satisfaction levels again. The initial interview can assist the therapist to gain an understanding of a client's perceived needs and insight into their problems. The results can act as indicators for interventions which are likely to have the most meaning for the client, including counselling in work-related issues where appropriate. Although the COPM was designed to fit the Canadian cultural environment, it has recently been introduced in a number of clinical situations in the UK, with reports of its utility starting to appear in the professional literature.

Acknowledgements

The author wishes to thank: Lesley Whyte and Dorothy Ferguson, lecturers in the Department of Nursing and Community Health, Glasgow Caledonian University, for the use of their information on Community Profiling; Diana Landymore, for contributing the information on the Ergos and KEY Method functional capacity.

References

Benson, J. and Clark, F. (1982). A guide for instrument development and validation. *Am. J. of Occup. Ther.*, **36**(12), 789–800.

Bonder, B. (1985). Standardized assessments: ethical principles for use. *Am. J. of Occup. Ther.*, **39**, 473–4.

British Psychological Society (1992). *Psychological testing: a guide*. Steering Committee on Test Standards, Leicester.

Christiansen, C. and Baum, C. (1991). *Occupational Therapy Overcoming Human Performance Deficits*. New Jersey. Slack, pp. 395–404.

Cohen, S., Kamrack, T. and Mermelstein, R. (1995). Perceived Stress Scale. In *Measures in Health Psychology Stress, Emotion and Life Events* (J. Weinman, S. Wright and M. Johnston, eds) pp. 23–6, NFER-Nelson.

Cooper, Sloan and Williams (1988). *Occupational Stress Indicator Management Guide*. ASE, a Division of NFER-Nelson, Berkshire, UK.

Dunn, W. (1993). Measurement of function: actions for the future. *Am. J. of Occup. Ther.*, **47**(4), 357–9.

European Foundation for the Improvement of Living and Working Conditions (1995). *Stress at Work: Causes, Effects and Prevention: A guide for small and medium sized enterprises*. London: HMSO.

Grandjean, E. (1988). *Fitting the Task to the Man*, 4th edn. New York: Taylor and Francis.

Health and Safety Executive (1996). Getting to grips with manual handling, HSE IND(G) 143L.

Hermenau, D. C. (1995). In *Ergonomics for Therapists* (K. Jacobs and C. M. Bettencourt eds) pp. 137–55. Oxford: Butterworth-Heinemann.

Hertfelder, S. and Gwin, C. (eds) (1989). *Work in Progress*. Rockville MD: American Occupational Therapy Association, pp. 132.

Hopkins, H. L. and Smith, H. D. (1988). *Willard and Spackman's Occupational Therapy*, 7th edn pp. 272–307.Philadelphia: JB Lippincott Company.

Jacobs, K. (1991). *Occupational Therapy Work Related Programs and Assessments*, 2nd edn pp. 23–114. London: Little Brown and Company.

Johnston, M., Wright, S. and Weinmann, J. (1995). *Measures in Health Psychology*. Berkshire: NFER-Nelson.

Kanawaty, G. (ed.) (1992). *Introduction to Work Study*, 4th edn. International Labour Office, Geneva.

King, P. M. (1993). Outcome analysis of work-hardening programs. *Am. J. of Occup. Ther.*, **47**(7), 595–603.

Kopec, J. A. and Esdaile, J. M. (1995). Functional disability scales for back pain. *Spine*, **20**(17), 1943–9.

Law, M., Baptiste, S. Carswell, A. *et al.* (1994) *Canadian Occupational Performance Measure*, Canadian Association of Occupational Therapists, ACE Publishers.

Letts, L., Law, M., Rigby, P., Cooper, B., Stewart, D. and Strong, S. (1994). Person–environment assessments in occupational therapy. *Am. J. of Occup. Ther.*, **48**(7), 608–18.

McDowel, I. and Newell, C. (1987). *Measuring Health: A guide to rating scales and questionnaires*. Oxford: Oxford University Press.

Maure, P., Barris, R., Bonder, B. and Gillette, N. (1984). Hierarchy of competencies relating to the use of standardised instruments and evaluation of techniques by occupational Therapists. *Am. J. of Occup. Ther.* **38**(12), 803–4.

Mayer, T. G., Gatche, R. J., Kishino, N., Keeley, J., Capra, P., Mayer, H., Barnett, J. and Mooney, V. (1985). Objective assessment of spine function following industrial injury. *Spine*, **10**(6), 482–93.

Melzack, R. (1992). In *Assessment: A Mental Health Portfolio Psychological Adjustment to Illness* (D. Milne, ed.) pp. 4–9. Berkshire: NFER-Nelson.

Northern Ireland Committee of College of Occupational Therapists (1992). *Employment assessment and preparation in occupational therapy.* College of Occupational Therapists.

The Psychological Corporation Ltd (1991). *Assessment for training and employment: project manua*. Kent.

Reed, K. L. and Sanderson, S. R. (1980), cited in Canadian Association of Occupational Therapists and the Health Services Directorate, Health Services and Promotion Branch, Health and Welfare, Canada, *Occupational therapy guidelines for client-centred practice* (1991). CAOT/ L'ACE Publications

Rosenstiel, A. and Keefe, F. J. (1995). In *Measures in Health Psychology Pain and Pain Behaviours* (J. Weinman, S. Wright, M. Johnston, eds) pp. 31–40, NFER-Nelson.

Simmons, S., Stampe Øland J. (1992). *Workplace assessment*. European Foundation for the Improvement of Living and Working Conditions, Luxembourg.

Trickey, G. (ed.) (1993). *General Clerical Test: Revised manual*. Kent: The Psychological Corporation.

US Department of Labor (1991). *The Revised Handbook for Analysing Jobs*. Indianapolis: JIST Works Inc.

US Department of Labor, Employment and Training Administration (1977). *Dictionary of Occupational Titles*, 4th edn.

Whitmore, D. A. (1975). *Work Measurement: Institute of Practitioners in Work Study, Organisation and Methods*. London: Heinemann.

Whyte, L., Ferguson, D. (April 1995). Community profile in the occupational setting. Paper presentation, Occupational Health Nurses Forum Scotland, Edinburgh.

Wilkin, D., Hallam, L., Doggett, M. (1993). *Measures of Need and Outcome for Primary Health Care*. Oxford: Oxford Medical Publications.

Appendix

Assessment tools used in work practice

Name	Description and/or publisher and/or supplier
Assessment for Training and Employment	See text. Published by The Psychological Corporation.
BTE Work Simulator	Baltimore Therapeutic Equipment (BTE) work simulator allows job activities to be replicated in the clinical area through use of a number of optional handle attachments which can be adjusted for work height and resistance offered to client. Used for intervention and observation of performance. Supplier: BTE Ltd.
Canadian Occupational Performance Measure	See text. Published by Canadian Assoc. of Occupational Therapy.
Coping Responses Inventory	See text. Published by NFER-Nelson.

Name	Description and/or publisher and/or supplier
EPIC Functional Capacity Evaluation	Employment Potential Improvement Corp (EPIC) developed a set of test protocols designed to perform a comprehensive functional capacity evaluation (FCE). Measures lift capacity; motor coordination; finger and hand dexterity; standing whole body range of motion; balance while walking, carrying and climbing; industrial pushing and pulling. See text. Supplier: Work Evaluation Systems Technology (WEST).
ERGOS Work Simulator	A computerized Functional Capacity Assessment which utilizes bar code technology. Compares client's performance with US standards for job requirements, work speed and manual lifting. See text. Supplier: Work Recovery Inc.
Functional Assessment Screening Questionnaire	The FASQ: application for evaluating pain-related disability Millard RW (1989), *Arch. Phys. Med. Rehabil.* **70**, 303–7.
(GCET) General Clerical Test – Revised	See text. Published by The Psychological Corporation.
Grip strength dynamometers	A range of devices are available which measure grip strength in lbs, kPa or kgs. Normative data also widely published. Supplier: Smith & Nephew Roylan Ltd.
Goniometer	Measures joint range of movement in degrees. Supplier: Smith & Nephew Ltd.
Hassles and Uplifts Scales	Kanner, Coyne, Schaefer and Lazarus (1981) from: Comparison of two modes of stress management: daily hassles and uplifts versus major life events. *J. of Behavioural Medicine* **4**, 1–39 Published: NFER-Nelson.
Inventory of Interpersonal Problems	Horowitz, Rosenberg, Baer, Ureno and Vellasnor (1988) from: 'Invertory of interpersonal problems: psychometric properties and clinical applications,' *J. of Counselling and Clinical Psychology* **56**(6), 885–92. Pub. NFER-Nelson.
Life Experiences Checklist	Ager (1990) Publisher: NFER-Nelson.
McCarron–Dial Work Evaluation System	Norm referenced set of tests which assess neuropsychological components i.e. emotional, motor, verbal–spatial–cognitive, sensory and integrative coping ability. Supplier: McCarron-Dial Systems.
McGill Pain Questionnaire	Melzack, R. (1975). The MPQ: Major properties and scoring methods. *Pain*, **1**, 277–99, and pub. by NFER-Nelson. See text.
MOS 36-Item Short Form Health Survey	Ware, J. E. and Sherbourne C. D. (1992). The MOS (Medical Outcomes Study) 36-item short form health survey. *Med. Care*, **30**, 473–83.

Name	Description and/or publisher and/or supplier
Occupational Stress Indicator	See text. Published by ASE, a division of NFER-Nelson.
Oswestry Low Back Pain Questionnaire	Fairbank, J. C. T., Couper, J., Davies, J. B. and O'Brian, J. P. (1980). *Physiotherapy*, **66**, 271–3.
Prevocational Assessment	Etheridge, D. A. (1968). Prevocational assessment of rehabilitation potential of psychiatric patients. *Am. J. of Occup. Ther.* **22**, 161.
Purdue Pegboard Test	A test of UE dexterity with child and adult norms available. Supplier: Science Research Association.
Raven's Progressive Matrices and Mill-Hill Vocabulary Scales	See text. Supplier: NFER-Nelson.
System 2000	A computer-based, modular package which assesses aptitudes and general educational attainment. Supplier: Valpar Corp.
Valpar Work Samples	A series of work samples with varied activities which measure work-related motor and cognitive abilities. Criterion referenced scoring based on US industrial standards. See text. Supplier: Valpar Corp.
WEST Tool Sort	West Evaluation Systems Technology (WEST) measures can be used for screening and intervention purposes. Focuses on assessment of: whole body flexibility; dynamic lifting ability, UE strength and fatigue tolerance; tool handling ability. Norms and motion-time measurement (MTM) standards are provided. Supplier: WEST.
Work Cube	A frame with optional activities which can be adjusted to work heights to allow simulation of job tasks. Used in intervention and for observation of client's performance. Supplier: Advanced Therapy Products.
Work Environment Scale	Moos RH, Published by Consulting Psychologists Press.

Address of suppliers and publishers

Advanced Therapy Products, Baltimore Therapeutic Equipment Ltd., Consulting Psychologist Press and McCarron–Dial Systems: PO Box 45628, Dallas TX 75245, USA.

NFER-Nelson, Darville House, 2 Oxford Rd East, Windsor, SL4 1DF, UK.

Science Research Association, 155 Wacker Drive, Chicago, Illinois 60606, USA.

Smith and Nephew Roylan Inc., Main Office, One Quality Drive, PO Box 1005, Germantown, WI 53002, USA.

The Psychological Corporation Ltd, A Division of Harcourt Brace & Company Ltd, 24–28 Oval Road, London, NW1 7DX, UK.

Valpar International Corporation, PO Box 5767, Tuscon, Arizona 85703–5767, USA.

Work Evaluation Systems Technology (WEST), 22741 N Highway 1, PO Box 2477, Ft. Bragg, CA 95437, USA.

Work Recovery Inc. 2341 S Friebus, Suite 14, Tuscon, Arizona 85713, USA

7

Work Programmes to Enhance Psychosocial Performance Components

Rosie Hallam and Jonathan Leach

Learning objectives

At the end of this chapter the reader should be able to:

1. Describe the value of psychosocial work programmes for clients with mental health problems.
2. Describe a range of different psychosocial work programmes.
3. Identify the core skills needed to devise a psychosocial work programme in practice.
4. Discuss how psychosocial programmes can contribute to the normalization of the client's life and their integration in the community.

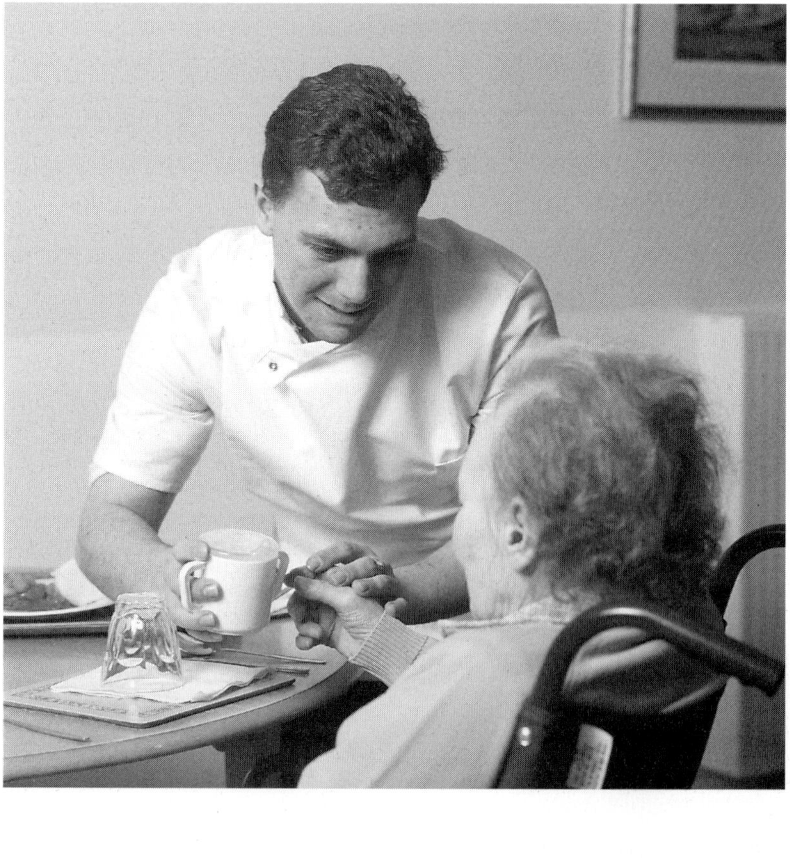

Introduction

Psychosocial work rehabilitation – current and future perspectives

Over the last twenty years, there have been significant changes in the development of vocational rehabilitation services for people with mental health problems. Increasingly this has involved moving away from the traditional sheltered workshops (often hospital-based) where people performed low-skilled industrial tasks and clients had few or no social contacts beyond the workshop setting. Often, a place in the workshop became a 'job for life' with neither rehabilitation staff nor clients having much expectation of the clients achieving any degree of economic independence or social integration into the community.

Research shows that the ability to handle social relationships is more crucial than the possession of task skills in successfully resettling people with mental health problems. Watts (1983: 219) found that poor social relationships with other workers and with supervisors coupled with low levels of motivation and initiative were more often responsible for a person's inability to secure and maintain employment than their poor task performance. These views have been supported by several other researchers in the field including (Anthony and Jansen, 1984). Indeed work is a social activity – with there being few occupations where people work single-handedly or where communication with others bears no relevance or importance to an individual's or a business's success. Furthermore, communication in the workplace has become a complex process with employees expected to cope with the numerous forms of communication which are now available. Phones, faxes, computers, e-mail and videos, while helping to speed processes and increase efficiency, also add considerably to the pressures of work and the need to be able to communicate effectively.

The developments in technology have also made unnecessary many of the manual jobs to which people with mental health problems often returned. Even where lower skilled jobs still exist they often place much greater demands upon the employee. One only has to see how fast people have to work in a fast food outlet, or watch the concentration needed to input data at speed into a computer, to realize that a world of work where the demand is for consistently high-speed, efficient, high-quality work can be demanding even for a healthy person. For those with mental health problems (especially severe and enduring), it can be very threatening and if people feel inadequate to cope with these demands this will make the whole idea of returning to work more formidable. Yet, at the same time 'there is a growing national consensus – among consumers of mental health services and their families, mental health professionals and vocational rehabilitation providers – that individuals with psychiatric disabilities can indeed work' (Baron, 1994: 1–2).

Furthermore, work is also becoming an increasingly skilful activity. Over the last two decades, the workplace has undergone a fundamental change. Technology has changed both our lives and our working environments; and the increasingly competitive marketplace means that the workplace is becoming more demanding. Employers are looking for more highly skilled, flexible and adaptable employees to cope with a competitive and fast moving world. For those people with mental health problems who seek to return to employment, this means that the 'requirements are more stringent' than in the past particularly for 'key technical and social skills' (Seyfried, 1992: 9–11).

Indeed, occupational stress has become a major factor in the UK workplace and is fast becoming the primary cause of absenteeism and reduced work performance. The Health and Safety Executive estimates that 80 million working days are lost every year due to stress-related illnesses compared with 250,000 days lost due to strikes, and this figure is increasing by the year. Britons work longer hours than their European counterparts and according to the pressure group Parents at Work this is putting 'the nation's health, wealth and happiness at risk' (Evans, 1995: 1–3). There are a number of reasons for this. Mention has been made of technology changing the speed at which we work. In addition these new technologies have involved major restructuring in the workplace with many companies downsizing their workforce. This has resulted in flatter structures with fewer people undertaking more diverse roles. Handy (1994); a business writer, puts these changes into a simple equation: $1/2 \times 2 \times 3 = P$, meaning employ half as many people, work them twice as hard and they will produce three times as much. At the same time jobs have become less secure. Increasing global competition has meant that companies are having to work harder in order to survive, while individual customers have become more demanding. In today's marketplace the customer not only has product prices in mind, but also quality, flexibility and innovation of products and services.

In 1994, for the first time, an employee successfully sued his employer for a stress-related illness induced by work. This could be the first of many cases unless employers take the problem in hand. Enlightened employers are responding to these workplace changes by introducing a range of measures to combat stress. These measures include counselling, employee discussion circles, fitness centres, and a range of therapies (massage, aromatherapy, reflexology etc.) to combat stress.

Those organizations that tackle the problem of employee stress and actively seek to enhance employee health are most likely to ensure the well-being of the individual as well as the company as a whole.

Handy (1994) points to a future where fewer people will be in full-time and long-term work. He suggests people will need to develop 'portfolios' of social and work activities. Some will have several part-time jobs, while others may work part-time and be involved in a range of other social and/or educational pursuits. In a world where jobs for life are no longer guaranteed, and with companies increasingly developing part-time working or buying in specialist time for a fixed period, rehabilitation programmes face new challenges.

Psychosocial programmes play an increasingly important role through their emphasis on integrating people within the communities in which they live. These programmes recognize their clients as people first and respond by providing individual 'needs driven' rehabilitation. Psychosocial work programmes aim to enable people to identify their strengths and weaknesses. They aim to help the individual to evaluate their work performance and develop skills, and to set realistic future goals.

Some clients will achieve the level of work and communication skills needed to cope with and achieve integration into competitive employment. For others, more sheltered settings will be required which, while offering greater support, still confer worker status and provide a commercial rather than a clinical or therapeutic orientation. Psychosocial work programmes are in a strong position to provide both short and longer term types of service. At the heart of their philosophy is the principle of helping people to reach their fullest potential and that this can only be achieved by recognizing that work, social and welfare needs all have to be addressed. This holistic model is well suited to the changing nature of work and in responding to individual needs.

What is psychosocial rehabilitation?

In seeking definitions for this chapter it has become clear that the terminology is imprecise and that the terms 'psychosocial rehabilitation' and 'psychiatric rehabilitation' can apply to a wide range of services and are sometimes used interchangeably. However, the use of the word 'rehabilitation' in both terms emphasizes the development of skills and creation of supportive environments to improve the client's ability to function. 'Rehabilitation' is used instead of 'treatment' which is taken to refer to pharmaceutical or psychoanalytic interventions to reduce symptoms.

In the period since the Second World War, these terms have been applied to programmes developed as an alternative or complementary to standard hospital treatments for mental illness. In the United Kingdom, therapeutic communities were established, and independent work projects were created beyond the hospital walls. Vocational rehabilitation programmes originally set up for people with physical disabilities were extended to those with psychiatric disabilities. These all contributed towards a *psychiatric rehabilitation* approach. Bennett described this as: 'the process of helping the psychiatrically disabled person to make the best use of his or her residual abilities in order to function at an optimum level in as normal a social context as possible' (1978: 209).

In the USA the concept of *psychosocial rehabilitation* arose from the foundation of clubhouses in the post-war era. Fountain House is the most famous one. Psychosocial rehabilitation does not contradict the definition given by Bennett, but rather suggests a particular consumer-led approach to how psychiatric rehabilitation is achieved. The clubhouses were created to promote the social and vocational rehabilitation of their members who had previously spent time in psychiatric institutions. Emphasis is placed on what the member has to offer, on the necessity of each member's contribution, and on celebrating each member's presence and efforts. Social, housing and vocational needs are all addressed by this programme. Staff and members work alongside each other to keep the various parts of the clubhouse running.

Psychosocial rehabilitation recognizes the effects of social isolation, often compounded by inappropriate social behaviour, that both result from and reinforce mental health problems. Psychosocial work programmes address the social context in which the client is expected to perform as well as the skills needed to perform in that context. The goals of psychosocial rehabilitation for these clients are to participate as fully as possible in competitive employment and to achieve independence in their daily lives. Rutman sets out the following core qualities of psychosocial rehabilitation:

1 Normalizing roles and relationships.
2 Dealing with practical, realistic elements of an individual's needs.
3 Facilitating social learning and behavioural change through experiential activities.
4 Minimization of the differences in role, authority and status between the user and the professional. (1994: 4–6)

Additional features listed by Rutman are:

1 Programs are based in non-clinical locations.
2 Functional assessments of strengths and weaknesses are used and the client's existing abilities are recognized.
3 Staff come from a variety of backgrounds and have flexible roles.
4 Realistic expectations for clients are created around the goals of social competency and personal independence. (1994: 6)

Anthony lists the concept of psychosocial rehabilitation as one of the contributing factors to the model of *psychiatric rehabilitation* developed at Boston University's Center for Psychiatric Rehabilitation.

> The overall goal of psychiatric rehabilitation is to assure that the person with a psychiatric disability can perform those physical, emotional, social, and intellectual skills needed to live, learn, and work in the community, with the least amount of support necessary from agents of the helping professions. (Anthony, 1994: 18)

The following section will examine how this model has been applied to psychiatric vocational rehabilitation.

The vocational rehabilitation context

A traditional vocational rehabilitation model uses a sequential process of *evaluation, work adjustment* within a sheltered setting and *vocational counselling*, possibly followed by *job placement*, to enable clients to work towards employment. Clients are not placed into open settings until any behavioral problems or skill deficits have been addressed successfully within the workshop environment. At the evaluation stage, a range of tests may be used including psychometric tests, work samples, and simulated work environments. Assessment continues during the work adjustment phase within the workshop. During work adjustment a number of approaches may be used including: behavioural modification, counselling and skills-building techniques. In many facilities, a work acclimatization or work hardening approach is used, whereby the programme becomes increasingly demanding and more like the conditions found in open employment. As clients progress vocational counsellors and work-placement staff help them to identify their next step.

Although this approach has drawbacks, there are also benefits:

1 Staff working in a rehabilitation centre may be able to supervise more clients at any one time than can those working with individual clients in an integrated setting.
2 Clients vocational aspirations and potential can be explored in relation to a range of jobs, whereas many of those offered to clients placed in open employment settings tend to be entry-level positions in fairly basic service or manufacturing occupations.
3 A sheltered environment can allow clients to deal with disturbing symptoms at a manageable pace.

The disadvantages of this train-then-place model include the following:

1 The skills taught may not be relevant to the potential jobs available in open employment.
2 Where learning has taken place within the rehabilitation workshop, clients may experience difficulty in transferring it to other situations.
3 The closed and segregated nature of the workshop may lead to a low level of expectations by both clients and staff.
4 The segregation of people with mental health and other disabilities does nothing to dispel the prejudices and mistaken ideas held by the general public.

A particular approach to vocational rehabilitation for people with mental health problems is the Psychiatric Rehabilitation Model developed by Anthony and colleagues (1988) at Boston University. This model can be applied within work programmes ranging from the sheltered workshop to placement in a competitive employment environment. The development of the model was influenced both by the psychosocial rehabilitation movement and by models developed in the rehabilitation of people with physical disabilities. This approach is based on the premises that psychiatric diagnoses and symptoms are not predictive of vocational rehabilitation outcomes and do not correlate with the client's skills, whereas training in critical vocational skills can improve outcomes. The process consists of three phases.

1 In the *rehabilitation diagnosis* phase, the practitioner works with the client to produce a practical description of their current level of skill functioning and environmental supports in relation to the client's preferred work environment.
2 In the next phase the client and practitioner draw up a *rehabilitation plan*. This takes into account the individual's needs, skills, values and interests in order to write individual rehabilitation goals. The plan specifies how to improve the client's skills and/or the person's work environment in order to achieve the client's vocational rehabilitation goals.
3 In the *intervention phase* the vocational rehabilitation plan is carried out and the effectiveness of the interventions are monitored.
(Anthony *et al.*, 1988: 65–66)

For the client the psychiatric rehabilitation process will address the following psychosocial/psychological work performance components:

1 Identifying and developing values, interests and self-concept.
2 Identifying, maintaining, and balancing the functions that are required to perform the role of a worker.
3 Interacting by using manners, verbal and non-verbal communication, active listening, and self-expression appropriate to the social context of the work environment.
4 Managing stress by developing coping skills.
5 Maintaining a balance of work, leisure, rest and self-care by using time management skills.
6 Exercising self-control by modifying own behavior in response to the requirements of the work environment, personal aspirations, and feedback from others.
(American Occupational Therapy Association, 1994).

These components require corresponding skills from the rehabilitation practitioners in order to facilitate the progress of clients towards their vocational goals; and will be considered later in this chapter.

Employment models and psychosocial components

Over the last twenty years there has been a trend towards greater community integration and the provision of more open work settings for people with mental health problems in both Europe and the USA.

In the USA, changes have emphasized an 'individual placement' model of helping people into paid competitive employment with appropriate support. While the traditional sheltered workshop model exists, it is no longer felt to meet people's needs adequately (Anthony *et al.*, 1984; Bilby, 1991). Also, 'work evaluation' using work samples is being replaced by the assessment of clients within real work settings (Hursh *et al.*, 1988). A number of vocational rehabilitation models have developed, which are helping people with mental illness to secure and maintain employment. The most widely known are two USA models: the Supported Employment, Choose–Get–Keep model developed at Boston University and the Transitional Employment model, associated with the Clubhouse psychosocial movement.

A third emerging model is that of the *affirmative* or *entrepreneurial* business, which has developed both in the USA and in Europe. Enterprises in this category range from user-run cooperatives to more traditional business organizations. In common with the other two models, affirmative businesses offer real work in a non-institutional location, but with less potential for integration into the non-disabled workforce.

Psychiatric rehabilitation is seen as part of the recovery process focusing on individual needs and building on abilities. The vocational models described next adhere to this principle, offering a comprehensive range of services to support clients in achieving and sustaining employment.

The Supported Employment model

The Supported Employment model is characterized by its *place–train* approach, rather than the more traditional train–place model of vocational rehabilitation, where individuals are trained in a workshop setting before moving to competitive employment. The place–train model emphasizes placing the client directly into open employment and teaching the necessary skills in that setting. The training and support continue at an intensity, and for a length of time, determined by individual needs.

Supported Employment programs have the following features:

1. Participants receive wages for the work they do which should be at the going rate.
2. Integration is a key aim. The work setting should allow for contact with non-disabled workers and members of the public.
3. Support is ongoing and may take place both on and off the work site.
4. Supported programs are targeted at individuals with severe disabilities, such as long term mental illness, who have experienced difficulties in maintaining open employment.

(President's Commission on Employment for the Handicapped, 1987)

The Choose–Get–Keep model of supported employment

The Choose–Get–Keep model of supported employment (Anthony, Howell and Danley, 1984) specifically helps people with psychiatric disabilities in choosing, getting and keeping a job. It emphasizes that these three areas of competence are critical to a person's vocational success. Integral to the philosophy of the model is the emphasis on client choice and in setting clear rehabilitation goals and plans.

The pre-employment 'choosing' phase is thorough; clients are helped to identify personal and work-related values, interests and skills and ask the question 'do I really want to work?'. In the second 'getting' stage the client is asked what supports they need in getting a job; this may vary from help with a curriculum vitae to attending interviews. Clients continue to develop job-seeking skills and are provided with peer support. The 'keeping' phase centres on helping the client, once a job is found, to overcome the interpersonal and environmental problems of the workplace that often pose the greatest challenge. A job coach or employment specialist works closely with the company and the client on an 'as needed' basis providing the necessary support. Increasingly, employment specialists are making use of 'natural supports' in the workplace, developing supervisors'/employers' skills to support the client.

Observations

As described by Danley *et al.* (1987) the 'simplicity and common sense' of the Choose–Get–Keep model of supported employment has much to recommend it. This model is clear and can be easily understood by clients, their families, and practitioners alike. It focuses on individual need and choice, making it flexible in its application. If a client is unsure whether they want to work, feel they need further education or training, or if they do not feel ready to take up the challenge of competitive employment, then these needs can be met in various other ways which act as assessment guides and stepping stones to achieving the client's goals. This model, therefore, embraces other employment rehabilitation models such as Transitional Employment.

The presence of a job coach in the workplace can have the effect of singling out the client as someone who is different to the others and may lessen the potential interactions between the client and coworkers. A case has been made by Hagner *et al.* (1992) for using 'natural supports' in the workplace, i.e. line supervisors or fellow workers. They looked at promising practices in agencies that took the approach of minimizing professional interventions in supported employment. The study resulted in the identification of strategies for encouraging the natural supports within supported employment that would be used by any 'normal' worker. The client is encouraged to identify personal contacts who can provide leads in the job-seeking stage. The supported worker should participate in the working day in as similar manner as possible to coworkers, including joining in with social activities. The job coach should adopt a consultant role, providing information and support to the host firm, enabling their own supervisors to manage the client. Where possible, the job coach should allow the client to learn the job through the mentoring of a coworker or by other in-house techniques.

The supported employment model depends on skilled and experienced practitioners, on trusting and lasting relationships among staff, clients and employers, and on economic factors, such as the availability of employment. Some supported employment agencies have found that retention of job coaches is a problem and their services can be costly when supporting people with chronic and persistent problems in open employment. On a study tour of the USA, one of the authors (Hallam, 1994) found that this view was supported by several service managers and practitioners. While employers spoke positively about clients working with them and their involvement as 'natural supports', one summed up what many others articulated: that, 'we are not here to provide a social service'.

The Transitional Employment placement model

This model guarantees every client the opportunity to work in competitive employment for regular wages in non-subsidized jobs.

Transitional Employment (TE) originated from the psychosocial clubhouse movement, developed at Fountain House, New York. The clubhouse model developed to provide 'a restorative environment', where individuals who have been socially or vocationally disabled by mental illness could 'be helped to achieve or regain confidence and skills necessary to lead vocationally productive and socially satisfying lives' (Beard *et al.*, 1982: 47–53).

The Fountain House TE model incorporates a prevocational programme where clients become involved in contributing to the everyday running of the clubhouse. This involves all aspects of its work, therefore providing a good range of opportunities for skill development while building confidence. Clients can participate in educational programmes, including literacy and numeracy. Successful participation in the prevocational programme encourages individuals to look at future employment possibilities.

The TE programme is designed to help clients develop work skills and habits and develop a job record. This is achieved by securing job positions in industry. In a survey of 135 TE programmes, Malamud and McCrory (1988) found a number of common features:

1. Normally jobs are at entry level positions requiring only basic training and work skills.
2. Employers pay wages at the going rate for the job.
3. The majority of jobs are worked on a part-time basis (20 hours per week). This allows two people to use one placement, it increases the chances of success, allows time for participation in clubhouse activities and can avoid problems with social security benefits.
4. Most placements are individual rather than in a group.
5. Placements are temporary or 'transitional', providing employment from three months to a year. Clients can therefore maintain temporary entry level employment through a series of TE placements or use the placements as a step to independent employment.
6. Failure on a TE placement is seen as a legitimate part of the total learning experience in securing employment. Equally, the celebration of success in making steps forward is implicit to the clubhouse TE philosophy.
7. Job placements are only maintained if the individual meets the work requirements and there is an absolute guarantee to the employer that the job will always be filled.
8. Staff are familiar with the job positions and working environment and it is with this knowledge they are able to place and train clients successfully and maintain a mutually beneficial relationship with the employer.
9. The evaluation of vocational potential was enriched by having access to a range of normal work environments.

Observations

The TE model has much to offer clients with severe and persistent mental illness – those individuals who the clubhouse movement has sought to help. It is a holistic model; vocational success is part of a philosophy which recognizes that people's employment goals can only be achieved when they have secure housing and their social needs are met. Employers have a real incentive for participating in this model due to the guarantees that accompany it.

Hallam (1994) visited three clubhouses, including Fountain House, during a study tour of the USA. A number of issues were noted. They were:

1. Staff reported difficulty in securing TE places. Partly this was due to the economic climate but often it reflected a lack of staff expertise. Those succeeding were using people with marketing and business experience.
2. Staff mentioned the personal 'burn-out' factor due to the extensive demands of the job.
3. Clients with higher level qualifications and professional backgrounds may not have their needs met due to the entry-level nature of jobs.
4. The focus on staff maintaining TE placements appears to detract from helping clients to achieve permanent independent employment. This was acknowledged and programmes were developing to focus on these needs.

Despite these problems the visits to clubhouses were a positive experience; clients felt valued, had a sense of hope and many were clearly achieving employment goals.

The affirmative or entrepreneurial business

This more recently recognized model often incorporates elements of the models previously described. It is best described as arising from the traditional workshop approach, but with a very different focus. The choice of work activity has a very strong community focus, repetitive industrial therapy is replaced by a small business environment providing goods and services to the public. Often in these services creative activities are used with jobs that provide high levels of satisfaction in a 'real work' yet supportive setting.

The structure, development and staffing of these businesses shows great variance, but all provide work that allows individuals to develop and progress. For some people these businesses offer long-term job opportunities, while for others they are a stepping stone to open employment. Clients are usually paid the going rate for similar work in competitive settings although there can be large differences. Most clients work part-time to maximize their earnings potential without jeopardizing social security benefits. The businesses maintain close links with other rehabilitation support services and clients have access to other vocational services, such as job coaches:

These 'affirmative' and 'entrepreneurial' business often have a high level of client involvement and some (especially in Europe) are run as cooperatives.

A version of this type of affirmative business is the 'Social Firm':

> A Social Firm is an ordinary business structured to provide goods or services under normal business terms and conditions, however, it has a fundamental difference from other enterprises in that the majority of its employees will be recovering from mental illness and will therefore need a carefully planned and sympathetic working environment. (BIIT, 1993: 47–53)

Social Firms have been run successfully in the Republic of Ireland since 1989 following a European Community sponsored initiative. In an evaluation of their effectiveness for the individual, Coughlan (1993) outlined a number of benefits:

1 Individuals were empowered through the process of making their own decision to join the firm and to negotiate their role within it.
2 Staff teams were encouraged to take a positive philosophy, viewing workers in terms of their future potential rather than their current limitations.
3 A safe and positive environment was created in which the individual could make positive developments and become more productive.
4 The emphasis on becoming a profitable unit helps the individual to grow through improving their work performance. This helps them to move on from the self-perception of themselves as a patient or disabled person that could be maintained within a hospital or traditional rehabilitation setting.
5 The individual grows in confidence and security as they find that their positions are held open for them despite their health difficulties. Team members were found to spend fewer days in hospital after joining a Social Firm.
6 A real work ethos was created by on-the-job training, through contact with customers and location within commercial areas.

Observations

The affirmative and entrepreneurial business in many ways complements the Transitional and Supported Employment models. It is well designed for people who need long-term sheltered work and for others who require a transitional setting. Its success depends on a strong business orientation. Unlike the other models, it need not rely on securing places in competitive employment. It appears to be an embryonic model, but with a clear direction of making the business as client-run and professional as possible.

A report commissioned by the National Institute on Disability and Rehabilitation Research, Washington DC to survey these businesses showed that these programmes were rapidly growing and 'proving to be a viable and potentially valuable vocational rehabilitation model' (Granger and Baron, 1992: 47–53). The semi-sheltered, supportive nature of these organizations offers an advantage to people who frequently relapse yet have periods of good work functioning and ability. For the enterprise to be successful it must compete and coexist with the commercial sector, therefore offering a very real mainstream work experience. This model provides integration of mental health services into the community that can make the skills and abilities of individuals with mental health problems become visible and attractive.

The value of choice

Each of the models outlined has something to offer. Ideally clients with mental health problems should be offered a continuum of services to match their level of need. There should be movement between the different programmes as a person's circumstances change. Each model can improve the psychosocial functioning of users by:

1 Offering a more normalized environment.
2 Allowing for choice and user empowerment.
3 Enabling the self-development of clients through practical work experience.
4 Avoiding the creation of dependency through sensitive and appropriate professional staff input.

As the provision of such schemes increases there will be an increased demand for rehabilitation staff with appropriate skills.

Staffing of work programmes

Whatever the work programme model adopted by an agency, staff have a crucial part to play in ensuring the effectiveness of that programme.

In all the programmes mentioned, practitioners need to be skilled in helping clients set realistic goals that take account of their interests, values, functional abilities, and support needs. Staff will need to facilitate the process of breaking these goals down into specific objectives within achievable time-scales. They will need to develop a good rapport with clients and to be creative and inspirational in their approach to problems. Practitioners need to be able to evaluate the existing skills and limitations of clients and to help the clients assess their functional abilities within their chosen work environment.

Once the client has achieved entry into their chosen work environment they are likely to need the services of one of a number of practitioners.

Within a rehabilitation workshop or prevocational setting, a work adjustment specialist or work supervisor will be employed. This person will perform a wide range of functions including: skills teaching, job analysis, behavioural observation and management, giving feedback on performance, organizing work activities, developing group dynamics, supporting individuals, and liaising with others. Staff should be able to reduce their teaching and supportive input as the client becomes established.

Vocational counsellors and work-placement staff have to possess a thorough knowledge of the job market and an awareness of the skills needed to perform different occupations. They need to be able to help clients achieve their chosen goals and to be able to suggest alternatives where these goals are not achievable.

Staff employed in affirmative business will need all the above skills plus others linked to the commercial aspects of running a business. They must be flexible in their roles and be good at developing community relations.

Within supported and transitional employment programmes, the client is usually supported by a job coach. The fact that the job coach will be operating within a range of open employment environments means that he or she needs to be particularly adaptable. They will need many of the skills required of staff in a workshop setting in addition to being able to support the client in their relationships with coworkers and supervisors in the host firm.

Menz (1993) considers competent and trained staff to be a resource that must be developed as a matter of urgency for supported employment schemes. He outlines a 'quality nucleus' of seven attributes that should be held by staff: humaneness, competence, intelligence, leadership, diversity, flexibility and commitment.

Lessons can be learned from research into supported and transitional work programmes by those working in more sheltered settings. The psychosocial approach values the input of all members of a programme and they can be encouraged to take responsibility for passing on skills and offering support to fellow workers within the workshop or prevocational setting. The aim for all staff should be to help clients to develop their skills and natural supports to the level at which the need for professional involvement is at its minimum.

The future

The future holds real challenges for work rehabilitation programmes. There have been positive developments in recent years, with programmes increasingly responding to individuals' needs and recognizing that people with mental health problems are capable of work. But the rate of unemployment within this group remains unacceptably high: 'Much more needs to be done to improve opportunities for persons with psychiatric disabilities to establish and sustain a long-term attachment to the nation's labor market' (Baron, 1994: 1–2). Even for those fortunate to be in employment, there remains the problem that people with mental health disabilities, regardless of their skills and abilities, can often only obtain and stay in low-level and low-skilled jobs.

As noted earlier, the demands of the workplace increasingly necessitate technically and socially skilled individuals, who are adaptable and able to produce high-quality work. Psychosocial work services will need to address these difficulties and challenges. Support and active help is needed to enable people to choose, get and keep a job, whether it be in an open or sheltered employment setting.

The National Institute on Disability and Rehabilitation Research, Washington DC (1993) stresses four fundamental aspects in developing effective rehabilitation services: the practitioner, the process, the programmes, and the principles. We would like to add a further four essential factors: the people, the policies, the place and the partnerships.

In describing these aspects in more detail, it seems appropriate to begin by looking at who the service is for, and then to take the list in a logical order.

The people

Before psychosocial work programmes can develop, they need to consider: Who it is for? What are their needs? Living with a severe and enduring mental illness can be devastating. Unlike many disabilities, mental illness is often an extremely unstable condition, requiring careful management. This can be a slow and painful process, but if successful, makes an enormous difference to an individual's life. People need to develop strategies and skills to cope with the effects of their illness.

The concept of 'recovery' from mental illness has become strong in the USA. This concept does not imply that people will be cured, but as in the case of physical illness a person severely disadvantaged by a disability may still be able to recover to a point where they can assume the roles of everyday life. Anthony (1994: 567–90) describes recovery as 'a deeply personal, unique process of changing one's attitudes, values, feelings, goals, skills, and/or roles'. Recovery is all about finding a meaningful and purposeful way of life and being able to cope with the devastating effects of mental illness. It is not just recovery from the illness either, but also from all the other traumatizing effects accompanying and following on from a mental illness. This includes dealing with the stigma, the negative effects of unemployment and hospitalization. This health-conscious approach, where the individual takes 'control' of their illness, can be time consuming and difficult but clearly contributes significantly to a person's chance of successful social and economic integration.

People need to feel valued and involved in programme service development. The potential for developing consumer-run services needs greater recognition and support. User empowerment has become a familiar phrase, but needs further work to promote understanding of what it really means and how it works in practice. The mechanisms and processes need to be in place before it can be truly effective.

The policies

Without effective policies, mental health work rehabilitation programmes will continue struggling with uncertain and insecure funding and clients will continue to face barriers to social and economic independence. National and local policies have been slow to develop. Where policy does exist, it often focuses on the disabled group in general. While this can help some people, others with more severe conditions often seem to lose out. However, a number of countries over the last few years have seen new legislation develop aimed at more specific help for the individual with a disability. Much of this has come about through the lobbying efforts of disability advocacy groups. Undoubtedly this effort needs to continue.

The process

The rehabilitation process needs to be 'comprehensive, dynamic, and adaptable, not limited to standard programming'. The process must be able to cope with wide-ranging demands and needs. 'In effective agencies, vocational counselling, assessment, job development, placement, training, and follow-along services are flexible enough to respond to the characteristically varied and changing needs of the population' (National Institute on Disability and Rehabilitation Research, 1993: 1–4).

The principles

A number of important principles need to be adopted when planning or providing psychosocial rehabilitation services. First, the focus must be on the individual and their needs. Then come a number of principles which are all important to programme effectiveness. Some services will undoubtedly hold some of these principles more strongly than others but all need attention.

Programmes should have a strong and positive culture. They also need to have a strong and positive community image, be well integrated and able to provide public education and relations work. Programmes need to focus on consumer empowerment and to recognize and make use of natural supports in the client's environment. Flexible support is needed and not just for the consumer, but also for employers. Support should be given throughout the rehabilitation process and beyond.

Psychosocial rehabilitation services need to work closely with other agencies providing help and support. An approach encouraging partnerships ensures the concept of the 'seamless' service in which the clients can access help when they need it and are offered smooth transitions.

The practitioner

For psychosocial rehabilitation programmes to succeed they must have highly skilled and dedicated staff. Staff who can recognize and respond to the changing world and see potential for change in the individuals they are working with. Rehabilitation practitioners need to respond to changing employment conditions and work creatively in helping clients achieve their employment goals. This means that rehabilitation staff must continue to learn and to develop themselves. This is the challenge, but also the excitement confronting future rehabilitation practitioners.

It is suggested that practitioners can be most effective when they work from a team approach. The makeup of teams is another essential factor. Teams need to have a range of skills and specialists, both rehabilitative and business.

The programmes

Programmes need to revolve around people, not people around programmes. It is essential they should offer choices, 'geared to different interests and different levels of ability' (Shepherd, 1993: 1–19). No one programme or programme model is likely to suit all individuals. There will need to be sheltered work opportunities as well as help to return directly to competitive employment. Barker (1994: 57–65) views programme development on a continuum, to 'a multiple access network of attractive programmatic and employment directions'. Hirsch (1989: 26–31) shares this view and suggests a continuum of employment opportunities with various levels of support is more important than the type of supported employment used. In a world that is so constantly changing, programmes must continuously evaluate and review their services, 'programs that are in the business of changing people must be constantly in the business of changing themselves' (Anthony, 1993: 51–3).

The importance of staff training has been emphasized. The training and education needs for clients must also be high on the programme's agenda. Securing employment may be dependent on having basic numeracy and literacy skills and on having a specific accredited skill. Training needs to be offered in sheltered as well as open environments. There should be a focus on developing skills and abilities that are directly relevant to the jobs in the economy. Some psychosocial programmes will need to offer high levels of support, others more discreet flexible support.

The place

The environment in which the person with a disability operates plays a crucial role in their overall well-being. Community integration is an essential aspect. It is not just the person needing assessment but also the environment, both on a micro and macro level. While local issues such as labour market information, transport and support structures all need evaluation, so do national conditions such as social security systems and legislation, that may act as an opportunity or deterrent for people with mental health problems.

Pfeffer and Salancik (1978: 117) wrote that: 'Organisations are inescapably bound up with the conditions of the environment'. Psychosocial programmes need to consider their environments carefully if they are to have a positive impact on their local community. The way they interact and what they add to the community they operate from can make a critical difference. Programmes should be well integrated into the community, an essential concept that easily gets overlooked in the planning stage. Barker (1994: 57–65) identifies three particular aspects of importance:

1 Programmes should be responsive to the specific individual needs within a particular community.
2 Programmes should build on the strengths, resources, relationships, and unique aspects of a particular community.
3 Programmes should develop relationships with businesses in the particular community rather than adopting a single market approach.

The partnerships

Anthony and Farkas, (1989: 226–39) wrote that: 'Vocational rehabilitation is a lengthy process that requires a comprehensive approach and a great deal of cooperation from many systems.'

A complex world that places great demands upon the individual worker also places increased demands on psychosocial work programmes. Programmes cannot work in isolation nor rely on psychiatric professionals to do all the work. Wide-ranging relationships are essential. Dynamic networks with other psychiatric agencies, social welfare organizations, and the community as a whole, especially with employers, are crucial if programmes are to succeed. Developing these interagency links takes time and persistence.

Funding rehabilitation services and helping clients with mental health problems return to employment should also be considered in partnership. So many agencies have a stake: health, social welfare, employment and training. Unfortunately, all too often no one takes the lead or works jointly together. With no clear strategy this can result in duplication or it creates gaps in service provision and makes transitions from one service to another difficult and frustrating.

Conclusion

Psychosocial programme development is in a dynamic state. New programmes are developing all the time and increasingly users' views are being listened to and acted on. There is a growing recognition that people with mental health problems have a right to 'normal' educational, social and vocational opportunities. Programmes need to develop that respond to different needs and 'economic realities'. Successful psychosocial programmes offer comprehensive and professional services and have a strong commitment to the concept of rehabilitation and recovery. These programmes acknowledge people's failure as part of a learning process and celebrate success joyfully. Successful programmes have strong and lasting partnerships with members of the business community and play an important role in educating the public on mental health issues. Anthony (1992: 164–70) provides an excellent definition of future rehabilitation needs: 'effective integration of psychiatric rehabilitation into mental health systems depends on the skills, knowledge, and attitudes of the various personnel who interact with the client; the programs used by the personnel; and the service systems that support the people and programs.'

There is still much to learn and a continued need for research, evaluation and information sharing. It is paramount for vocational services to deliver effective future programmes and for rehabilitation staff to develop the necessary expertise. In the future an increased understanding of the jobs and work environments that best sustain and enrich the quality of life for people with a mental illness would be of great benefit.

While national policies will inevitably largely determine the success of community work schemes and mental health integration, Handy (1994: 271) reminds us of the actions we can take ourselves. 'Change comes from small initiatives which work, initiatives which imitated become the fashion. We cannot wait for great visions from great people, for they are in short supply at the end of history.'

Case history

Introduction

Psychosocial work programmes can appear very different from each other. The largest and perhaps best known is the Fountain House Clubhouse in New York City (USA). It was developed in the 1950s and pioneered the Transitional Employment Program (TEP). Many other innovative programmes and models have developed over the years often with a similar philosophy based on social and vocational factors, but running programmes that are delivered very differently. One such psychosocial work programme is Restore in Oxford, UK.

Restore (Rehabilitation Services Trust for Oxfordshire Re-Employment) Oxford, UK

Restore developed in 1976 as a new approach in helping people recover from mental illness. It developed in response to the need to find additional and alternative forms of work to hospital-based industrial therapy. The work rehabilitation model pioneered by Restore offers clients creative work opportunities within a business-like setting, producing high-quality goods, sold directly to the public. The initial aims were to restore confidence and pride, utilize skills and abilities, provide purpose and confer all the social advantages of the workplace. For some people this can offer a pathway back to competitive employment, while for others it provides appropriate longer-term support.

Restore provides places for 55 clients who attend either full or part-time. Clients become involved in one of four main work areas: woodwork, printing, horticulture and marketing and sales, including computing. All design work is carried out in-house and workers sell their work both directly to the public through a shop attached to the workshops and through a number of outlets in Oxford. The business relies on effective team work and communication. This aspect in particular emphasizes the psychosocial approach to Restore's work.

Structure, culture and approach

Restore is a charity as well as a company limited by guarantee. This organizational structure gives a clue to its status and standing within the community. As a charity, it is an independent organization, quite separate from other health and social welfare organizations. But it is also a manufacturing company. Clients referred to Restore view themselves as coming to work to assume the role of worker. 'Patient' and 'client' are alien terms and never used. Being small and quite separate from the bureaucratic constraints of large institutions has enabled Restore to evolve and develop continuously in response to people's needs. While partially relying on statutory funding, Restore has had to depend on its own efforts to raise much of its funding and particularly to fund new initiatives. Product sales have been essential as have the relationships formed with organizations and people in the community, providing funding, contributions in kind, and services free of charge. These associations have added significant and essential benefits. Restore has strong community relationships with businesses, colleges, other service providers, and with the countless individuals who purchase its products, volunteer their time, and give donations. All this adds quality to the rehabilitation provided. Workers have access to a range of educational, training, social, health, and information services, which encourage and support people in their struggle towards independence and integration within the community.

As a company, Restore designs, makes and sells an extensive range of well-made handcrafted products and homegrown produce. Restore takes a professional approach to its business. Like any company, it must be able to sell its products and compete with the open market. Restore's workers are involved in all aspects of the business. Creative people apply their skills to design work. Others use reasoning and practical skills to build new prototypes, or in product manufacture. Others work in sales and marketing, are involved in promotion, market research, wholesale and retail sales, or provide the clerical and administrative backup. Within these activities, workers develop work habits such as: regular and punctual attendance, concentration, motivation and the confidence and self-esteem needed to pursue a more independent and satisfying life.

Workers are consulted and encouraged to share ideas at all levels within the organization, both daily and, more formally, at its annual planning meeting. Workers thus experience all aspects involved in the running of a professional company and know their individual and team efforts are essential. Young (1987: 16–17), President of the College of Health, summed up these important aspects of Restore's culture and approach:

> Costs need to be kept down and standards of workmanship up if the products are to sell. The overall purpose is restorative but it can best be achieved by being highly professional about the work that is done. The emphasis is all on health and abilities rather than illness and disabilities. The clients need to have pride in their own workmanship, and most of them do. Their morale would put many ordinary companies to shame.

An attractive and enterprising business not only has a positive impact on its mental health users, the benefits for the community are great too. Restore provides a valuable community education service where the stigma of mental illness can be faced and overcome. Few places in Oxford offer such a range of environmentally friendly handcrafted products and produce. The first image Restore's customers have when they enter the Restore shop (based in a busy commercial and residential area) is often a lasting one. The products engage people: 'Bright, vivid gifts and toys line the shelves,their vibrant colours clamouring for attention' (Rees, J., 1991: 8–9). The depressing and often frightening image of mental illness is replaced by something positive and engaging.

Restore makes no secret that its workforce is made up of people with mental health problems. A local school has become regularly involved and a group of 11-year-old students work alongside Restore's workers. Without the education and support of local communities, people with mental health problems would be disenfranchised from society.

The group of workers whose members have the most severe and enduring mental health problems, of whom a number have spent most of their lives in institutions, run a horse-and-cart delivery round in their local neighborhood. They sell their chemical-free, freshly picked produce. The horse-and-cart round offers this group's members positive contact with a wide spectrum of the community. Older customers receive a service reminiscent of the days when there was a strong 'community' spirit, while parents of small children can enjoy selecting vegetables with a child engrossed in meeting the horse! It is this sort of activity in a psychosocial work programme that can really make it work. The process is two way, everyone benefits and enjoys it.

Working at Restore – referral, selection and induction

The process of joining Restore is very like that of any job. Initially a mental health worker suggests Restore to a client, or a person may self refer. Restore's referral coordinator is contacted, application forms completed and a visit to Restore is arranged. At the visit, the client sees the different work areas, has a chance to discuss the placement and choose whether to take up a place. The client's immediate aims and needs are identified along with their longer term goals. A key worker is appointed; someone outside Restore who knows the client well and who remains involved throughout that person's stay. The key worker is involved in worker reviews, can be contacted in a crisis and ensures a person's needs beyond those of work are met and coordinated. The Restore supervisor provides a comprehensive induction for new clients which serves to reconfirm the aims of the placement.

The continuing process of self-development

Restore has a strong culture and belief in the value of training and self-development. All workers meet with their supervisor regularly to monitor progress, identify difficulties and strengths and to develop and maintain an 'action plan' that responds to their individual goals. This takes time, but is essential in ensuring that aims are clear and needs are met.

Restore has two sites, each of which have different emphases. At one site, the emphasis is for workers to move on to further training or employment. No time limits are set, but worker and supervisor actively work on these goals together. As well as working in one of Restore's main work areas, workers can also access a range of training and development opportunities both within and outside the organization. Restore's training and development worker or work group supervisors will help clients make these choices. This may include developing literacy and numeracy skills, taking a recognized qualification or developing job-readiness skills through attending Restore's Employment Group. Some workers need career guidance and this is offered through other agencies. A work placement officer becomes involved when a worker feels ready to start considering work in competitive employment. For many workers, a period of work experience in an open employment setting is appropriate; others choose to take up a voluntary work opportunity or find a part-time job. The work placement officer offers support and guidance to the client and is guided by them in the extent of contact they make directly to a potential employer. It is important at this stage to explore welfare benefits to ensure the worker is sufficiently informed about them and to prevent financial problems arising through changes in employment status.

Restore's second site offers workers a longer-term work setting. There is an emphasis on personal development, increasing independence, and community integration. Even those people institutionalized for long periods can, when given the right opportunities, reach a stage where they no longer need to depend on psychiatric services

Psychosocial factors

Earlier in this chapter, the comment was made that work is a social activity. This is entirely true for Restore, where productivity and overall effectiveness is determined by good team activity, and a positive culture is so dependent on social interactions. Staff and workers can become involved in a wide range of social interactions, such as appearing in the media, speaking to groups of visitors or organizing outside events. Restore staff and workers are frequently out visiting retailers, holding sales at universities, hospitals and companies' premises. There is frequent contact with customers at the Restore shop and garden centre, where workers need to be knowledgeable about the plants and products. There is always too much to do and so, as in the clubhouse model, workers are relied upon for all aspects of the operation, bringing their skills and abilities to a wide range of needs-,both commercial and rehabilitative. Like any other good company, there are times for social events too.

Not all the workers feel comfortable with social contact and therefore the range of environments they work in at Restore are important. Some workers prefer the space that the allotment setting can offer, others prefer the shop environment but each can offer opportunities for progression. The small working groups facilitate positive social interactions. There is a dependence on inter-group working for production purposes and this means that workers meet their colleagues and learn to appreciate other's working practices. Problem solving can be approached differently in the groups, thus workers learn to appreciate different approaches and practices, acquiring for themselves new problem-solving and decision-making skills.

Questions

1 List three key features of Supported Employment.
2 How does Transitional Employment differ from Supported Employment?
3 What are the three stages of the Supported Employment Model developed by Anthony, Howell and Danley?
4 What characteristics make an enterprise an 'affirmative business'?
5 Describe two advantages of the 'place–train' approach over that of the 'train–place' model.
6 Describe three characteristics of a psychosocial approach to rehabilitation.

Answers

1 Any three of the following would count as key features of Supported Employment:
(a) The client is placed directly into open employment and taught the necessary skills in that setting.
(b) Participants receive wages for the work they do at the going rate.
(c) Integration with non-disabled workers and members of the public is a key aim.
(d) Support is ongoing and may take place both on and off the work site.
(e) The training and support continue at an intensity, and for a length of time, determined by individual needs.
(f) Supported programmes are targeted at individuals with severe disabilities.

2 (a) The majority of jobs are worked on a part-time basis.
(b) Most placements are individual rather than in a group.
(c) Placements are temporary or 'transitional', providing employment from three months to a year.
(d) Many programmes are linked to a 'clubhouse' which provides additional activities and supports.

3 (a) In the 'choosing' phase clients identify personal and work-related values, interests and skills and ask the question 'do I really want to work?'
(b) In the 'getting' stage the client is asked what supports they need in getting a job. Clients continue to develop job-seeking skills and are provided with peer support.
(c) The 'keeping' phase centres on helping the client once a job is found to overcome the interpersonal and environmental problems of the workplace. A job coach or employment specialist works closely with the company and the client on an 'as needed' basis providing the necessary support.

4 (a) The choice of work activity has a very strong community focus.
(b) It is often a small business providing goods and services to the public.
(c) The enterprise is situated in a commercial environment.
(d) Often creative activities are used to provide high levels of satisfaction in a 'real work' yet supportive setting.
(e) They provide work that allows individuals to develop and progress.
(f) Clients are usually paid the going rate for similar work in competitive settings.
(g) The business maintains close links with other rehabilitation support services.
(h) These businesses often have a high level of client involvement.

5 (a) The skills taught are relevant to the potential jobs available in open employment.
(b) Where training has taken place within the workplace, problems with the transfer of learning are avoided.
(c) A more realistic level of expectations by both clients and staff is possible than in a sheltered setting.
(d) The client is able to develop a real job record.
(e) The approach allows for much greater integration with non-disabled people.

6 (a) An emphasis on normalizing roles and relationships.
(b) Dealing with practical, realistic elements of an individual's needs based on the goals of social competency and personal independence.
(c) Facilitating social learning and behavioural change through experiential activities.
(d) Minimization of the differences in role, authority and status between the user and the professional. Staff come from a variety of backgrounds and have flexible roles.
(e) Programmes are based in non-clinical locations.
(f) Functional assessments of strengths and weaknesses are used.

References

American Occupational Therapy Association (1994). *Uniform Terminology*, 3rd edn.

Anthony, W. A. (1992). Key issues and future policy. *J. of Psychiatric Rehabilitation*, 164–170.

Anthony, W. A. (1993). Programs that work: issues of leadership. *The Journal*, 51–53.

Anthony, W. A. (1994). Recovery from mental illness. In *An Introduction to Psychiatric Rehabilitation* (L. Spaniol *et al.*, eds) pp. 560–7, Publication Committee of the IAPSRS.

Anthony, W. A., Cohen, M. R. and Danley, K. S. (1988). The psychiatric rehabilitation model as applied to vocational rehabilitation. In *Vocational Rehabilitation of Persons with Prolonged Psychiatric Disorders* (J. A. Ciardiello and M. D. Bell, eds), pp. 59–80, Johns Hopkins University Press.

Anthony, W. A. and Farkas, M. (1989). The future of psychiatric rehabilitation. In *Psychiatric Rehabilitation Programs: Putting Theory into Practice* (M. D. Farkas and W. A. Anthony, eds), pp. 226–39. Johns Hopkins University Press.

Anthony, W. A., Howell, J. and Danley, K. (1984). The vocational rehabilitation of the psychiatrically disabled. In *The Chronically Mentally Ill* (M. Mirabi, ed.), SP Medical and Scientific Books.

Anthony, W. A. and Jansen M. (1984). Predicting the vocational capacities of the chronically mentally ill. *American Psychologist*, **39**, 537–44.

Barker, L. (1994). Community-based models of employment services for people with psychiatric disabilities. *Psychosocial Rehabilitation Journal*, **17**(3), 57–65.

Baron, R. (1994). Editorial on employment issues. *Psychosocial Rehabilitation Journal*, **17** (3), 1–2.

Beard, J., Propst, R. and Malamud, T. (1982). The Fountain House model of psychiatric rehabilitation. *Psychosocial Rehabilitation Journal*, **5** (3), 47–53.

Bennett, D. H. (1978). Community psychiatry. *British Journal of Psychiatry*, **132**, 209–20.

Bennett, D. H. (1983). The historical development of rehabilitation services. In *Theory and Practice of Psychiatric Rehabilitation* (F. N. Watts and D. H. Bennett, eds), John Wiley & Sons.

Bilby, R. (1991). Transitional employment – supported employment: a response to the criticisms of transitional employment. Paper presented at the 6th International Seminar on the Clubhouse Model, South Carolina.

British Institute of Industrial Therapy (1993). *Social Firms Handbook: A Beginner's Guide*. BIIT.

Danley, K. S. (1987). Training and personnel issues for supported employment programs which serve persons who are severely mentally ill. *Psychosocial Rehabilatation Journal*, **11**(2), 87–102.

Evans, M. (1995). Long hours threaten health and family life. *Oxford Times Business Supplement*, 25 August, pp. 1–3.

Granger, B. and Baron, R. C. (1992). *A National Survey of agency-sponsored Businesses employing Individuals with Long Term Mental Illness.* Matrix Research Institute, October 1992, pp. 1–6.

Handy, C. (1994). *The Empty Raincoat*, p. 271. Hutchinson.

Hirsch, S. (1989). Meeting the vocational needs of individuals with psychiatric disabilities through supported employment. *Journal of Rehabilitation*, 26–31.

Hursh, N. C. (1988) Vocational evaluation with people who are psychiatrically disabled: results of a national survey. *Vocational Evaluation and Work Adjustment Bulletin*, Winter, **21**(4), 149–155.

Malamud, T. J. and McCrory, D. J. (1988). Transitional employment and psychosocial rehabilitation. In *Vocational Rehabilitation of Persons with Prolonged Psychiatric Disorders* (J. A. Ciardiello and M. D. Bell, eds), pp. 150–162, Johns Hopkins University Press.

Menz, F. E. (1993). *Who Should be Doing Job Coaching?* Focus.

National Institute on Disability and Rehabilitation Research (1993). Strategies to secure and maintain employment for people with long-term mental illness. *Rehab Brief,* **XV** 10, 1–4.

Pfeffer, J. and Salancik, G. (1978). Cited in *In Search of Excellence,* T. Peters and R. Waterman, Harper & Row.

President's Commission on Employment for the Handicapped (1987). Fact sheet on supported employment.

Rees, J. (1991). Out of the forest, *Limited Edition Magazine, Oxford Times,* **57**, 8–9.

Rutman, I. D. (1994). What is psychiatric rehabilitation? In *An Introduction to Psychiatric Rehabilitation* (L. Spaniol *et al.,* eds), pp. 4–8. Publication Committee of the IAPSRS.

Seyfried, E. (1992). Integration into open employment. *Rehab. Network,* **27**, Autumn 1992.

Shepherd, G. (1993). Providing work opportunities – the policy context. Paper presented at RDP Conference. Why Work? College of Ripon and York St John, 21–23 Sept. 1993, pp. 1–19.

Watts, F. N. (1983). Cited in *Theory and Practice of Psychiatric Rehabilitation* (F. N. Watts and D. H. Bennett, eds), p. 219, John Wiley & Sons.

Young, M. (1987). Restoring pride and purpose. *Self Health,* **16**, 16–17.

8

Work Programmes to Enhance Cognitive Performance Components

Gary Donaldson

Learning objectives

Upon completion of this chapter the reader will be able to:

1 Define the emerging trends and the evolving role of the vocational rehabilitation practitioner in provision of employment services.
2 Compare the influence of four value systems on patterns of beliefs, expected nature of transactions, cognition, and the perception of worthy performance within a work setting.
3 Describe the structure, function and enhancement of cognitive components in relationship to work performance.
4 Relate the use of socio-technical systems analysis and value-added services to identifying and creating employment opportunities.
5 Identify a four-phase consultation process and eight corresponding roles used by a vocational rehabilitation practitioner when working with business to create and sustain employment opportunities.

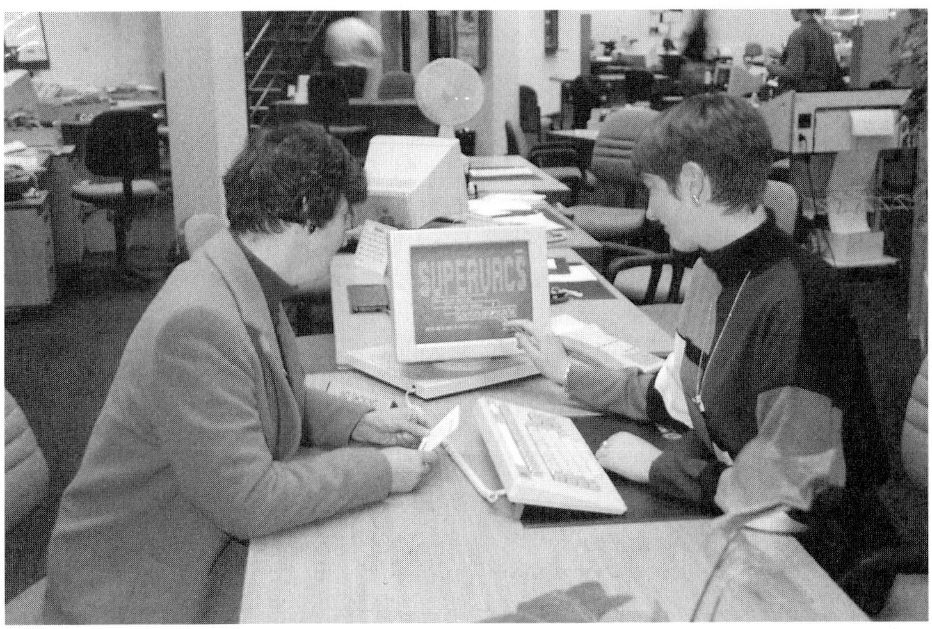

Abstract

Emerging trends reveal an evolution in the role of the practitioner. Movement is toward incorporating socio-technical system interventions with human performance technology. The enhancement of cognitive performance components will increasingly be delivered within actual work environments and will be dramatically influenced by the culture of the specific business environment. The practitioner will serve in the role of organizational and human-resource development consultant. Both the clinical support needs of the client and the financial performance needs of the employer will be the focus. Advocacy for employment opportunities will be framed in terms of value adding.

Introduction

New directions

Employment services for persons with severe disability in the United States are rapidly moving toward a new horizon that will eventually redefine, transform and realign the industry. A major portion of employment specialists will join the mainstream of organizational, business and human-resource development professionals. A new identity will emerge (see Fig. 8.1). Trends suggest that the employment specialist will increasingly focus on performance and value engineering. Consultation to business and industry will dramatically increase. New concepts will serve as a professional frame of reference such as: whole system architecture; virtual networks; self-organizing systems; socio-technical process; and smart technology. With whole system architecture, the practitioner will be required to look beyond the specific job the client holds to the broader concerns of the employer. Understanding and working with the dynamic alignment and interdependence of organizational elements such as market forces, organizational culture, structure, strategy, skills, team work, and reward systems will be of vital importance in crafting rehabilitation solutions. Virtual networks will serve as the fundamental division of labour for business. This form of structure will transcend traditional work-unit boundaries. Employees will form transitional partnerships, affiliations, and project teams in order to bring a product to market. In essence, the web of collaborations and project teams will serve as the framework for organizational structure. This will create a flexible, constantly changing configuration of resources and tasks. Organizational structure will be in constant

EMERGING TRENDS

BUSINESS ENTERPRISE & ORGANIZATIONAL SYSTEMS FOCUS

- Economic interests take priority
- Case work success measured by enhanced economic performance of a specific employer
- Increased concentration on design of socio-technical systems
- Evolving expertise in performance & value stream engineering
- Merging with organizational & human resource development professionals

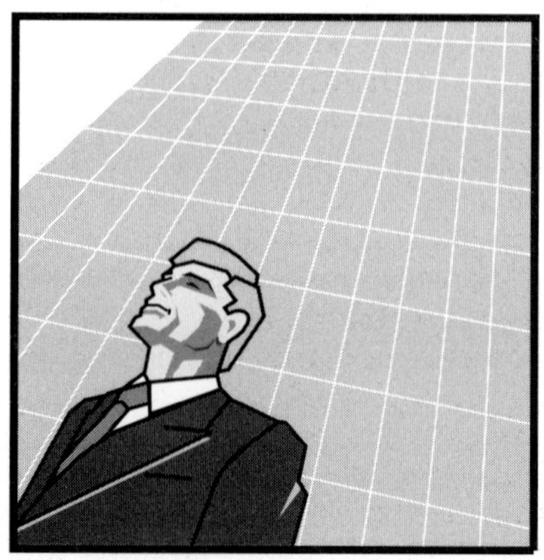

Figure 8.1 Emerging trends.

'far from equilibrium' states. Rapid and frequent changes in roles, routines, and relationships will create a tremendous challenge for practitioners. Individuals with a limited set of skills, who require stability and predictability, will need creative support systems in order to perform and survive in the competitive market. Continuous realignment of resources will reduce vertical chains of command and control. Each project team will rely upon self-governance. The teams will operate as a self-organizing system. Hierarchical control will be replaced with horizontal commitment between members as the principle for regulating resources for a common purpose. Natural supports for persons with disability will increasingly be dependent on coworker, team and interpersonal dynamics. The practitioner will be intimately involved with work process design involving the synthesis of linear and non-linear technical work procedures with social factors. This socio-technical aspect of the work environment will serve as a central focus for the practitioner. Rapid advances will take place in the use of computers, artificial intelligence software and other related smart technology. This will radically alter options available to persons with severe disability both positively and negatively. The advances in technology will simultaneously create and eliminate jobs. It will also open the door to new occupations yet to be discovered (Ashkenas *et al.*, 1995; Fabian *et al.*, 1994; Goldstein, 1994; Lewis, 1990; Miller, 1994; Morton, 1991).

Diversity and accommodation

As the United States population continues to increase in complexity business appears to be more concerned with diversity than with disability. The future workforce will offer multiple challenges from cross-cultural dynamics to a basic lack of functional skills. The notion of disability will be overshadowed. Building and harnessing the capabilities of a diverse workforce will demand the attention of most employers. Business will increasingly encounter workers with a behavioural repertoire that is in conflict with the established blueprint for success in existing work environments. Designing work environments that build on different abilities and support needs will take on increased significance. The concept of being 'disabled' will be replaced with an awareness that everyone requires a specific configuration of supports to meet the challenges of a work environment and the tasks assigned. Examples exist in everyday activities. An accountant needs to work at home two days a week in order to cover child-care obligations. An information systems administrator needs access to a technical support line 24 hours a day for a complex software product. A machine operator speaks Spanish but cannot read in Spanish or speak English. Work instructions need to be taped in Spanish and given to the employee along with a cassette player. A stockbroker needs a doorknob lowered in order to enter and leave an office with a wheelchair. A night watchman needs special binoculars that enhance light in order to patrol dark areas. A data entry clerk needs to take five minute breaks every thirty minutes in order to tolerate performance pressures and cope with severe anxiety. In these examples, each employee receives functional support in order to successfully complete work assignments and achieve performance goals. The design and management of support mechanisms will be the issue, not disability. As business faces the challenge of diversity, reasonable accommodation and individualized support will be considered a component of every employee's performance strategy.

Performance and value

Value perception

Ultimately, value is recognized in economic terms by business and industry. The source of value can be directly from the performance of an employee or more indirectly because of the presence of the employee. Revenue earned as a result of the direct output of an employee is a measure of value creation. Targeted tax credits and value-added performance engineering and consultation offer an indirect source of value.

Similarly, value can be perceived as tangible and intangible. Tangible value is 25 units of work produced per hour by an employee. Intangible value relates to issues such as morale, team spirit, cooperation, dependability, reliability and consistency. Intangible factors contribute to the achievement of effective and profitable work outcomes. They surround the production process and facilitate the probability of success. No matter how well a production process is designed and streamlined, it is the intangible aspect of production that can support or sabotage the ability to achieve desired financial goals. Intangible factors influence the perception of value. They have profound consequences for the longevity of employment and the focus of employment specialists.

Performance measurement

Performance is the perceived and measured accomplishments of the interaction between a person and an environment. It is within the person/environment relationship that the concept of performance comes to life. For business and industry, accomplishments need to create or add value for its customer base and economic value toward the company's bottom line. When the value of the accomplishment exceeds the cost to achieve the results, it is deemed commendable, worthwhile, and competent performance. Measurement of performance is typically associated with quality, quantity and cost. Each environment has specific requirements along these three dimensions that signify profitable and acceptable levels of performance. Valued performance can be defined by any single factor or by combinations of factors (Gilbert, 1978).

Quality is reflected by the accuracy of the accomplishment. It is the comparison of the actual with the ideal. Focus is on the degree of match between the measured result and the specified requirements. Errors of omission or commission indicate the degree of separation from the expected profile. Quality is concerned with the comparative superiority of the accomplishment with similar outcomes that could be considered equally acceptable and could serve as a substitute. For example, two brands of modems may both transmit and receive data at the same rate, however, one may have less difficulty negotiating the complex network of phone lines resulting in clearer transmission and reception performance. Comparative superiority can be based on objective physical measures or through more subjective terms, such as judgement, opinion or originality.

Quantity refers to the rate, timeliness and volume of performance. The focus is on number of units of production in relationship

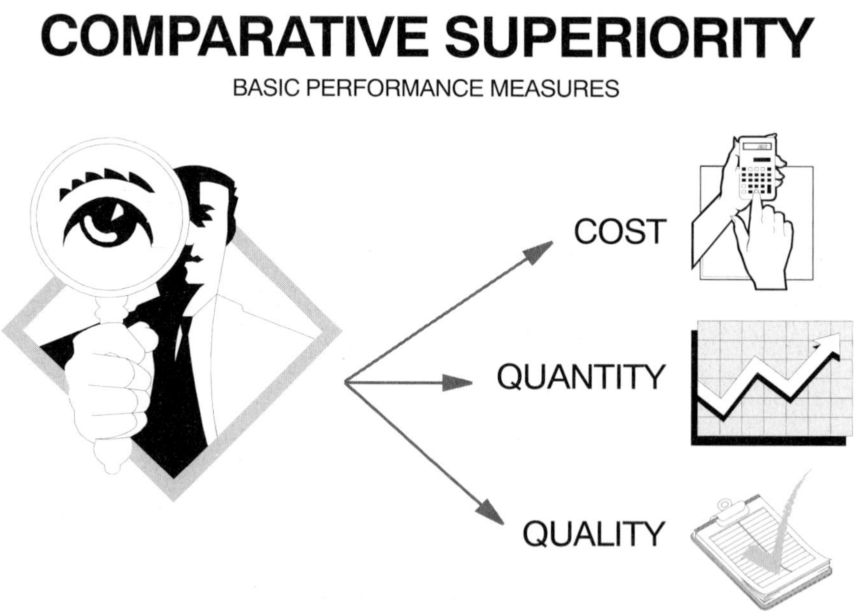

Figure 8.2 Comparative superiority.

to a time period or to the total magnitude of output. Each dimension holds value depending upon the requirements of the perceiver. As with quality, each factor may stand alone or in combination.

Value and cost

Cost to obtain and cost to use are considered critical factors in defining the value of accomplishments (DeRose, 1989; Nilson, 1992). Cost to obtain may include labour, management, supervision, overhead, benefits, insurance, handling, shipping and taxes. Cost to use reflects the maintenance expenses related to possession of the accomplishments. In most instances, performance accomplishments are valued if cost is less than the perceived worth. There are times when maintaining a loss leader (cost exceeds direct return) if the accomplishment opens opportunity to gain in other areas. It may cost more to make flowerpots than the price at which they can be sold. However, customers are likely to buy plants and fertilizer at a rate that more than compensates for the loss. Without the flowerpots, the volume of sales with the high-income producing articles would be less. The flowerpots, in essence, become value adding.

Competent performance

The perception of competent performance is in direct relationship to the context of how value is defined within a given environment. A perceiver judges and assigns worth to the impact of observed behaviours. To assign worth, the perceiver compares the impact of observed behaviours against an acceptable standard. That which is identified as worthy or desirable reflects that which is recognized, considered relevant and viewed as important (Gilbert, 1978). To be considered worthy, the impact of behaviour has to make sense to the perceiver. It must be meaningful, significant, important and held in high regard.

Value adding

Value adding is the process of providing desired accomplishments beyond that which

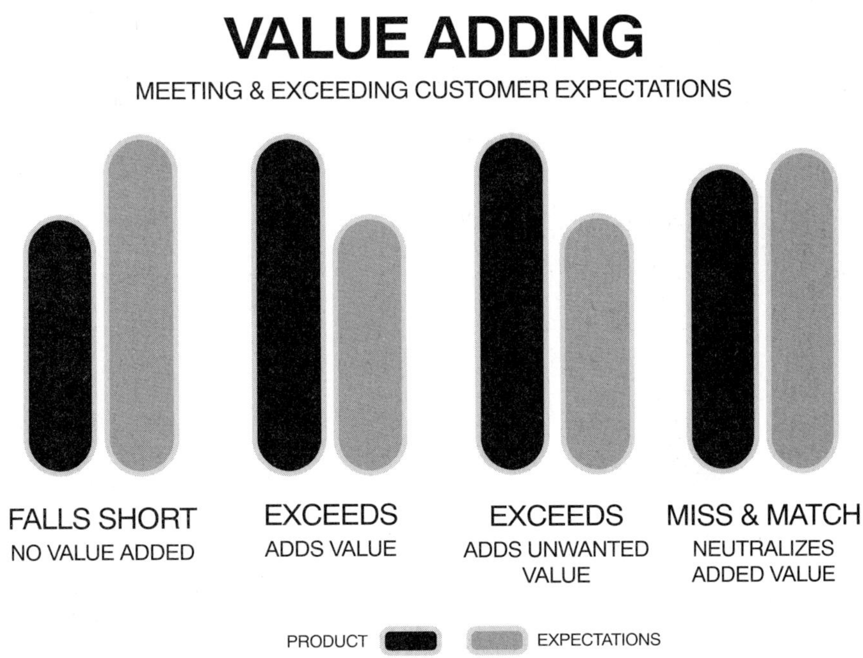

Figure 8.3 Value adding.

is expected (see Fig. 8.3). The accomplishments need to be relevant. Exceeding expectations is not worthwhile when non-relevant accomplishments are delivered. Worthwhile value-added accomplishments exist when expectations are exceeded in relationship to relevant preferences (Band, 1991; Lawton, 1993). Purchasing a computer system with pre-loaded software, at no additional charge, may make the package more attractive to the buyer. The computer system is viewed as exceeding expectations and thereby enhancing value. If the same computer system did not come with software but with passes to a local amusement park, the added value may be viewed worthless.

Contributing value

To obtain and maintain employment, a person needs to be perceived as contributing value directly, indirectly, tangibly and intangibly. Since value is in the eye of the beholder, effort spent on enhancing individual cognitive performance becomes intimately connected to addressing the social cognition of a work environment. Attempting to enhance cognitive performance without a person–environment interactional framework leads to less than acceptable results. Enhancing cognitive performance of an individual is more powerful and practical when functionally linked to the definition of worthy performance within the culture of an organization.

Organizational culture and social cognition

Cognitive consensuality and knowledge systems

Cognition can be viewed as a networked biopsychosocial structure and process that a person relies upon to perceive, interpret, problem solve and act in order to function and survive within an environment. Individual members of a work environment have their own distinct patterns and processes of cognitive performance. However, as a whole, members tend consensually to share a preferred and dominant cognitive strategy for:

1 selecting what to perceive;
2 interpreting perceived data;
3 problem solving;
4 selecting acceptable solutions;

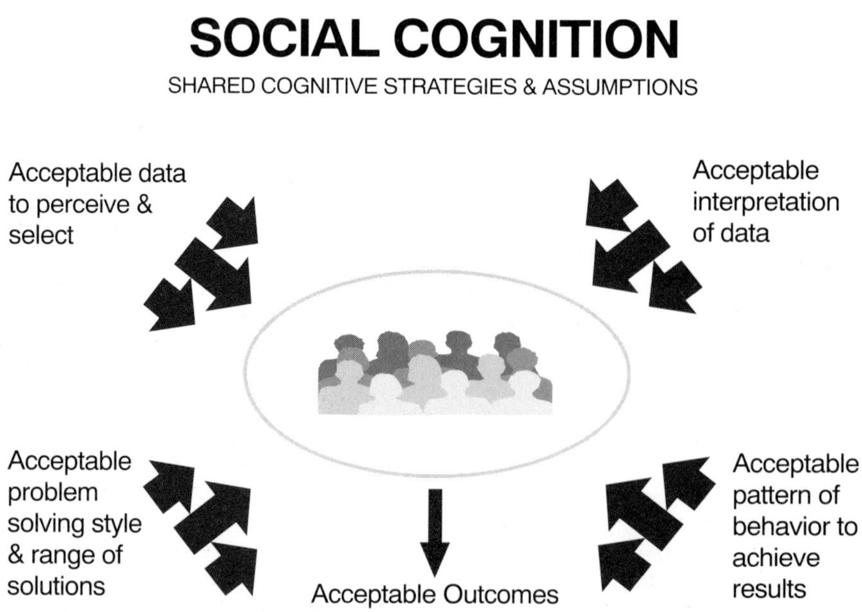

Figure 8.4 Social cognition.

5 performing an acceptable pattern of behaviour to achieve results; and
6 evaluating acceptability of outcomes (see Fig. 8.4).

Work settings are complex information environments. Members are not passive responders to the stimuli. They actively read the situation and take action based on their analysis (Sims Jr. *et al.*, 1986; Lovett, 1985).

Members use filters to sort out essential from non-essential information relevant to the specific context and task at hand. This cognitive process is frequently accomplished with little conscious awareness, attention, or significant forethought. The information processing takes two basic forms: controlled and automatic (Sims *et al.*, 1986). During controlled processing, the individual actively focuses attention on the situation and task while consciously screening out other data considered non-relevant. Reading a book on a bus is an example. Noise from passengers and the bus engine are blocked and set aside while concentrating on the process of reading comprehension. High demands are placed on the capacity of the person to pay attention and concentrate. Focus is on one activity at a time. Without controlled focus, cognitive functioning is subject to overload and derailment. The person explicitly gathers relevant information, then thinks through the assessment, planning and execution of appropriate behaviours. Controlled processing is very significant during the acquisition and application of new skills.

Automatic processing demands less attention, handles more familiar situations and can be applied to several activities at the same time. Previously learned skills and knowledge operate without the need for highly focused attention and problem solving. There is less strain on the cognitive information processing capacity of the individual. Routines are carried through without the need to be as vigilant as in controlled processing. Automatic knowledge bases are more difficult to alter or suppress. Driving a car while listening to the radio, responding to traffic signals, looking for street signs and carrying on a conversation with a passenger serve as an example of the automatic process. If an ambulance were to suddenly appear with lights flashing and the siren blaring, then there would be a shift back to controlled processing to avoid trouble or failure.

To filter, simplify and manage the overwhelming amount of available information, members rely upon pre-existing, shared knowledge and behavioural systems known as social cognition (Sims Jr *et al.*, 1986). Through a culturally accepted frame of reference, members rely upon a shared information processing strategy to reduce uncertainty and anxiety. Social cognition facilitates a personal and a group sense of control, stability and predictability. The day-to-day experience of a shared and dominant pattern of social cognition serves as an unspoken and preconscious social contract. Within this social contract, there exists an assumed formula for success the group can rely upon to achieve desired outcomes. The knowledge systems are composed of patterns of information that infer meaning and provide direction for behaviour. These patterns of information form cognitive structures identified as schemata. Schemata represent organized knowledge regarding a stimulus and the rules that direct interpretation, action and expectations.

Cognitive schemata types

There are four basic types of cognitive schemata:

1 self
2 person
3 script
4 person in situation
(Sims Jr. *et al.*, 1986).

Self schemata contain information regarding one's own personal characteristics such as personality, appearance and behavioural data. Self schemata are represented by the statement: 'I'm usually easy going and enjoy being with other people.' Person schemata focus on generalizations regarding trait and behaviours common to certain groups or types of people. Person schemata are reflected by the statement: 'Australians are a hearty and fun loving people.' Script schemata include knowledge concerning the typical unfolding and sequence of events in a given situation. The daily routine of operating a binding machine in a print shop serves as an example.

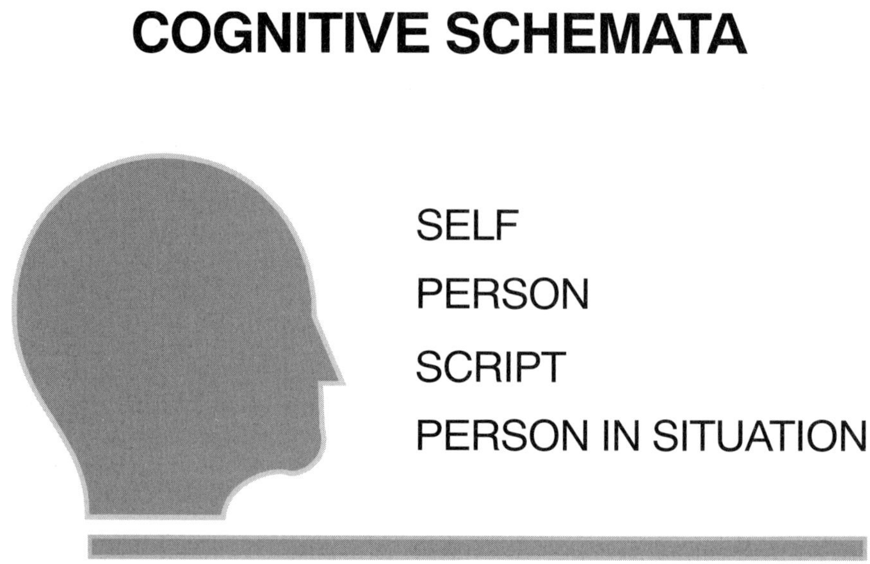

Figure 8.5 Cognitive schemata.

Person-in-situation schemata refer to knowledge related to people and behaviour typically found in a specific social situation. This type combines person and script schemata. Sitting quietly in a movie theatre during presentation of the film reflects use of this knowledge base.

Self schemata

Self schemata are derived from past experiences. For a person with severe and persistent mental illness, the schemata may reflect a self-attribute that one does not have the ability to succeed under pressure. This is used to search, filter and judge incoming information in relationship to the attribute, and to note and process information regarding the same attribute in others and various situations. If coping with pressure is a significant self-attribute, then the person will search for information regarding pressure across many circumstances and in most people. Practitioners work with persons with severe disability to reframe and alter self schemata into positive images related to worthiness, success and achievement. They also work with coworkers to facilitate an awareness of common ground with persons with severe disability.

Self-relevant information is highly affect-laden and resists change. A person can partially transcend the egocentric point of view of seeing the outside world primarily through one's own attributes. This usually occurs as one becomes closer and more familiar with a situation or other person. The egocentric point of reference remains firmly intact for those unwilling or unable to reach out and connect.

Person schemata

Person schemata are part of the categorization process. Individuals sort other persons into clustered groups or types based on essential features and similar characteristics. Person schemata are not closed sets. Boundaries remain 'fuzzy' permitting overlapping of features in common with members of another related category. For example, Italian and Spanish cultures share a common characteristic of being expressive when discussing feelings. Yet, both cultures simultaneously have separate identities and characteristics. Abstract features of each category are formed resulting in a cognitive prototype. The prototype serves as a model by which other people are compared and assessed for similarities and differences. The prototype becomes a benchmark standard and resides in long-term memory. Features of an individual are compared to the idealized features of the prototype. Similarity of features between a person with disability and the prototype of a targeted work environment increase the probability of acceptance, natural supports, and success. This underscores the importance of the person–environment match in job development and placement.

The 'point-of-view effect' is characteristic of person schemata labelling and memory. A person may be observed as generally friendly to coworkers. When the observer looks back to previous interpersonal contact, information will be retrieved to reinforce this notion. Although contradictory information may exist, the memory of the observer will tend not to find examples to counter the proposed notion. However, if the observer looks at the person from another point of view, such as aloofness, examples will be retrieved from memory that demonstrate that trait.

Basically, people see what they want to see and believe what they want to believe, regardless of the empirical reality. These perceptions and beliefs are base inferences and judgements that are set in motion by person schemata. Person schemata are based on information that is easily observed and easily retrieved from memory. Public and easily observable behaviours are given significant causal importance. They become the basis for judgement. The deeper, inner world of an individual typically is not referenced for construction of the person schemata. As the time between observing performance and frequency of judgements widens, reliance on the person schemata also increases. People are seen less as individuals and more as stereotypes. Person schemata are used by observers to manage complex social information prudently and efficiently but not necessarily accurately. Shaping and facilitating images of the person with disability within a work environment is a fundamental task for the practitioner. Positive images are created by demonstrating behaviour that is consistent with the environment's definition valued performance.

Script schemata

A script schemata is a cognitive structure that describes the appropriate sequence of events for a given situation. Script schemata facilitate the implementation of task and role performance by mapping step-by-step linear and nonlinear activities. Script schemata are directly related to functional requirements a person faces in every-day situations. There are both weak and strong scripts. Weak scripts give guidance to general behavioural requirements for situations. However, they do not provide guidance for the exact sequence of these behaviours. For example, a weak script schemata may provide global information related to safety routines and protocols when it comes to crossing streets. A strong script schemata provides the specific steps that need to take place at a specific intersection. Practitioners focus on developing script schemata with coworkers in order to ensure long-term, successful natural support mechanisms.

Person-in-situation schemata

These schemata combine the characteristics of the person and event schemata. Generalizations about categories of people involved in scripts provide a rich source of information. For example, when discussing how to help persons with mental retardation learn to wash dishes in a restaurant, images come forth regarding the challenges that will be faced and the best strategies for success. Quick inferences can be made regarding the type of task, environmental demands, and the instructional style that will be most effective in expediting learning. More vivid, concrete data is available due to the increased number of characteristics that combine synergistically. Person-in-situation schemata are more widely used than either person or script.

Person perception distortion

A variety of perceptual distortions can exist in cognitive schemata. The most frequently observed are:

1 'halo-effect'
2 stereotyping
3 selective perception
4 projection
5 expectancy.

A *'halo-effect'* takes place when an attribute is generalized to classify and describe a person.

An individual may place back tools in the original storage rack before leaving from work each day. The person is perceived as orderly. This perception is then attributed to how the person probably manages her personal finances outside of work. The observer has no first-hand knowledge that this may or may not be true. However, the person develops a reputation as orderly in all aspects of daily living. This is a false generalization.

Stereotyping obscures individual differences. The observer may not have the capacity, motivation or ability to sort through the wealth of information available regarding a single person or situation. If not understood and handled carefully, stereotyping can cause errors in selecting and retrieving information. This could result in less than successful consequences. Although a person may be viewed as carrying characteristics of the stereotype, lack of attention to detail regarding the observed individual can be detrimental.

Selective perception is the process of paying attention to only those aspects of data that reinforce a preconceived notion, need or belief. A person with a strong background in mental health may selectively look at everything through the lenses of pathology. A counsellor may label a person's behaviour as resistance, when, in fact, the client is trying to give feedback to the professional that the direction of therapy is off course.

Projection is the assignment of one's own attributes to another individual. Projection is typically associated with an unconscious splitting-off of unwanted characteristics or feeling states. An individual may see another person as constantly angry and critically judging. Upon closer examination, it may actually be the perceiver that has these feelings but is unable to face them directly. It can also cover more benign attributes. An individual may assume another person has the same training needs as oneself when in fact it is not true. At times, the person who is the object of the projection may own the attribute and act it out without knowing, therefore reinforcing the premise of the projection.

Expectancy is the foundation principle for the self-fulfilling prophecy. An individual may have such a strong desire or need that through unconscious behavioural activities, the person may actually cause a situation to occur. For example, an individual may anticipate and predict that a job interview is going to turn into a disaster. Through subtle and unconscious behaviours, the person actually creates the very situation that was feared. On the positive side, the person may envision being offered the job. Through positive imaging, the event unfolds as wished and the person is hired.

Attribution theory

Closely related to the notion of cognitive schemata is the concept of attribution theory. It is concerned with how people attempt to understand the cause of an event, assess responsibility for the outcomes of the event, and assess the personal qualities of the people involved. Behaviour is analysed to determine if the outcome of the event is internally generated or externally caused. If locus of control is internal, then a person is considered personally responsible and is held accountable for the impact. If not, then it is assumed circumstances that surround the individual are the cause. Understanding this dynamic aides the practitioner in diagnosing and correcting underlying assumptions that either the client or others may hold.

Perception of the locus of control is influenced by the factors of distinctiveness, consistency and consensus. Distinctiveness and consistency refer to the usual and customary performance of the individual across a variety of circumstances and situations. If a person typically performs well or poorly with most tasks then the locus of control is viewed as internal to the individual. If performance on a specific assignment varies from the individual's usual and customary results, then an external locus of control is considered the source of the outcome. Consensus factors compare how a typical person facing a similar situation is likely to perform. If most people tend to do well or poorly with a task, then it is assumed the locus of control is external when the person achieves the same range of outcomes. When results differ from the norm, the locus of control is assumed to reside within the individual.

Two basic errors are associated with the process of attribution. They are fundamental attribution error and self-serving bias. Fundamental attribution error exists when there is a tendency to underestimate the influence of situational factors or overestimate the influence of personal factors. Self-serving bias is the tendency of an individual or group to deny personal responsibility for failure, but claim personal responsibility for performance success.

Collaboration and performance requirements

Designing and implementing employment services that enhance cognitive performance requires a clear understanding of how valued performance is defined within the target environment. Valued performance is reflected through the corporate culture. Corporate culture forms the drawing board upon which a series of spoken and unspoken collaborative operating agreements are established between coworkers. The operating agreements specify tangible and intangible outcomes expected between members, including styles of behaving and thinking. This knowledge becomes a rich source of information for the practitioner to successfully create a plan of action to develop and enhance adaptive cognitive functioning.

Value orientation and influence on cognition

Value systems

The culture of a work environment shapes social cognition. Culture is a system of assumptions, beliefs, values and norms that bind and influence the behaviour of individuals and the members of the work environment as a whole (Kilmann, 1989). Culture can be viewed as the 'personality' of an organization, with characteristic styles and patterns. It plays an integral role for the practitioner in person–environment matching and facilitating inclusion.

Organizational culture is typically composed of four dominant value systems:

1 A support orientation, with the dominant focus on interpersonal commitment, human relations, staff cohesion and morale.
2 A role orientation, with the dominant focus on stability, control, consolidation and continuity of existing operations.
3 An achievement orientation, with the dominant focus on productivity, efficiency and maximization of output.

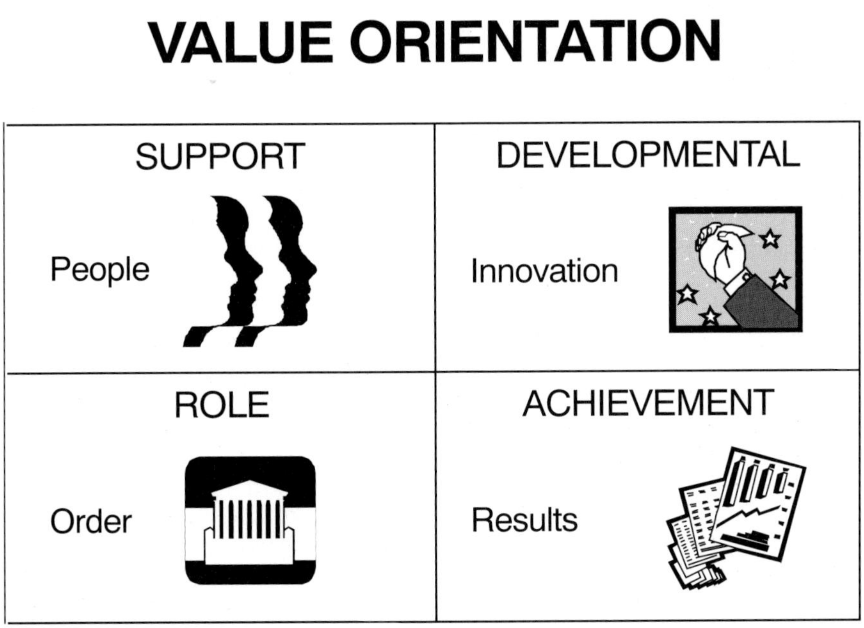

Figure 8.6 Value orientation.

4 A developmental orientation, with the dominant focus on innovation, growth, resource acquisition, external support, expansion, and adaptation.
(Frost, *et al.*, 1985) (see Fig. 8.6).

Each of the value systems operates simultaneously. Although the value systems coexist within the same organization, one value system tends to be favoured over another. For example, an organization may have a rank ordering that suggests the dominant value system is a role orientation followed by a support orientation, achievement orientation and finally a developmental orientation. Within this configuration, order, stability and staff morale take precedence. The centre of attention is the internal environment of the firm. The demands of the outside world are buffered. Maintaining a high level of comfort is valued over productivity and innovation.

Value configurations

Whatever the configuration of value orientations, there is a resulting cultural style that dynamically influences behaviour and social cognition. Within the same organization, departments, divisions, work teams or strategic business units may have a different rank ordering of value systems. Yet, all parts of the company share a common link to a central corporate culture that sets the tone for the organization. When a strategic business unit, division, department or team does not form a common link, there is usually a restriction of allocated resources, a gradual isolation of the unit, a spin off or discontinuation of the aberrant operation. The same can be said for individual members.

The configuration of the value systems can change at various times in the life cycle of the company. During the first stages of entry into the market, a business may be positioned in the developmental orientation, where flexibility and creativity are required to introduce a product line. Once the business is established and growing, it may shift to an achievement orientation in order to maximize output efficiently and effectively. During the mature phases of a product line, a role orientation may emerge to standardize and routinize operations.

Regardless of the stage of a product line, over time, a company establishes a core

PATTERNS OF BELIEF

APPROPRIATE NATURE OF TRANSACTIONS

- Direction of cognitive mapping
- Flexibility & control
- Appropriate motivations
- Information processing style
- Time frame for action
- Decision making process
- Power & influence
- Evaluation of members
- Compliance

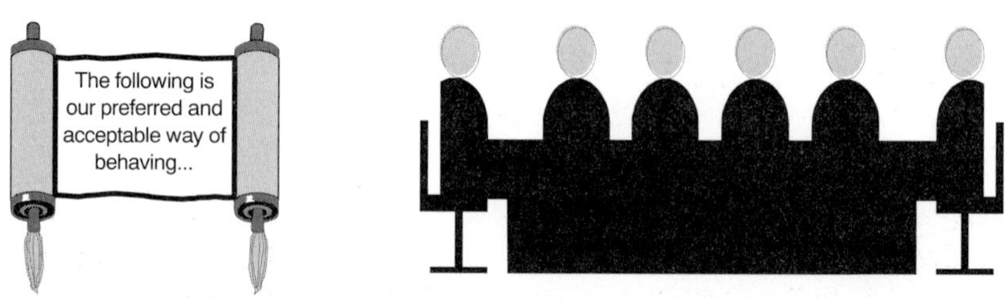
The following is our preferred and acceptable way of behaving...

Figure 8.7 Patterns of belief.

configuration of values that represent the unique cultural identity and orientation of the firm. Successful organizations develop a strategic ordering and balance between the competing value systems that both facilitate adaptation and ensure continuity.

Patterns of belief

Within each value orientation are embedded beliefs and assumptions regarding the appropriate nature of transactions and the acceptable style of cognitive performance. These govern such issues as:

1 direction of cognitive mapping
2 flexibility and control
3 appropriate motivations
4 information processing
5 time frames for action
6 decision making
7 power and influence
8 evaluation of members
9 compliance.
(Frost *et al.*, 1985; and Quinn, 1990).

Cognitive mapping

Cognitive mapping is the process by which an individual takes in representations of the environment for use in thought, reasoning, judgement and problem solving. The achievement and developmental orientations prefer cognitive mapping that is directed toward the external world of the organization. Members are valued for constantly scanning the environment outside of their work unit, division or company. From this scanning, members adjust their behavioural repertoire to be consistent with critical success factors in the environment. Data from the external focus is used to guide thought and performance within the organization.

The developmental orientation encourages members to look to the future for information, direction and growth. This value system uses creation of vivid images, language and metaphors to understand and communicate. A shared vision is nurtured. Cohesion is around ideas and what they reflect. Shared vision is used to pull the present thinking and performance toward a new idealized future. Members are focused and driven by 'the big picture'. Focusing on detailed bits of data is not valued as a method for constructing meaning and understanding. Grasping and sensing the whole is considered more utilitarian. Notions, intuition and hunches have equal weight with logical reasoning.

Thinking, communicating and behaving coalesce around a vision of what is possible. Vertical, creative and non-linear thinking are valued as tools to use with cognitive mapping. An assumption exists that there is no absolute reality. Reality is defined from the perspective of inquiry and the interconnection of elements within the inquiry.

The achievement orientation system encourages members to look to the present and immediate future. It stresses a focus on current competitive market forces, competitive positioning and the immediate impact on production. Logical connection of facts are used to cognitively map meaning, direction, strategy, goals and timetables. Hard data is used to represent the outside world. From the hard facts, logical conclusions and plans of action emerge. Cognitive mapping is centered around information and facts that are related to current realities, history and trends.

In contrast, role and support orientations promote cognitive mapping that focuses internally within the firm. Data and behavioural repertories relevant to maintaining harmony, order and stability between coworkers, management and the company are valued and reinforced. Members are valued for cognitive styles and functions that promote a sense of serenity and peacefulness.

Within the role orientation system, members are reinforced and valued for gathering and managing information that contributes to a steady state of operations. Cognitive mapping scans for standard operating procedures and information that contributes to meeting deadlines and completion of assignments. Mapping is directed toward factors that strengthen or threaten well-defined structures, systems, stability, control and continuity. Maintaining an orderly environment is paramount. Rule consciousness is valued. Variability from established operating procedures is not valued.

Members tend to compartmentalize information and problem solving. This results in suboptimized solutions at the expense of the whole. A clear understanding of boundaries, chain of command and authority are expected to be part of the mapping process. The need for reducing confusion and conflict focuses the information gathering process toward identifying data that will promote clarity and harmony. New and different ideas or concepts are generally not welcomed unless they can fine tune the present order.

The support orientation stresses a cognitive mapping process that focuses on concern and consideration of individual member's subjective feeling states. Maintenance of the social climate is foremost. Scanning the internal environment for data related to non-verbal feeling states is expected. This system encourages members to search for the personal meaning of events and issues. Although interpersonal cohesion is highly valued, there is an emphasis on the individual. Each person is viewed as having a valid point of view that is relative to one's subjectively experienced situation. Subjective experience is honoured as truth. Whereas the role orientation system stresses that there is one absolute point of view, the support orientation value system is more flexible regarding how meaning is defined.

Seeking information and displaying a behavioural repertoire that facilitates individually tailored caring, support, and inclusion in the larger group are considered the underpinning of the support orientation. Taking time for the individual outweighs a focus on productivity and the world external to the firm, unless there is a perceived injustice that interferes with the individual. Focusing on data related to justice for the individual is a worthy cognitive process. The external world is expected to accommodate to the individual. Interpersonal relationships and bonds are given the first priority.

Flexibility and control

Both the developmental and support orientation systems value decentralized operational structures that provide for flexibility and freedom of thinking and performing. In contrast, achievement and role orientation systems prefer work environments that are controlled, centralized, integrated and uniform.

In support orientation environments, mutuality and equality of coworkers is considered more important than concern for the chain of command and control. Direct control of others is avoided. There is more reliance on collaboration. Members are expected to read between the lines when scanning for interpersonal information and meaning. Non-verbal cue reading is valued. It is perceived as caring and supportive. Indirect communication styles are frequently used. Direct communication does occur. Yet there is a conscious attempt not to use it as a way to control others. Through indirect communication, members replace direct controlling with the more subtle mechanism of alert watchfulness. Indirect communication styles require an acute awareness of individual members and the surrounding events. Meaning is derived from deciphering subjective feeling states. With this information, support is provided that validates the experience of the individual. Communicating empathy is expected and nurtured. Control is through informal channels. Although there is a conscious attempt to be viewed as non-controlling, communication styles within a support orientation can be as demanding and potentially more powerful than the formal control structure in the role orientation system.

Freedom from control is a cornerstone within the developmental orientation. Maximum flexibility is valued in order to rearrange the status quo, discover new ideas, invent new structures and create new futures, all at the speed of real time. Control is typically imposed externally. It is viewed as a respite for the fatigued, frightened or numbed individuals outside of this value orientation. To members within the framework, everything is considered temporary, unfinished and behind schedule as everyone journeys to an unknown destination. Continuous evolution and improvement drives the system.

Role orientation environments value centralized control, high degrees of structure and minimal variation. Clear standard operating policies and procedures attempt to dictate and confine the range of thinking and behaviour. Innovative or 'outside the box' thinking is not valued. Role expectations and official problem solving procedures serve to provide stability, order and continuity. Consolidation, coordination and management of information serve vital functions in maintaining the internal environment. There is an assumption that human behaviour can be channelled as if it were part of a smooth running machine.

Achievement orientation value systems also support centralized command and control in order to minimize error rates and achieve maximum efficiency. Flexible, non-linear approaches are not valued. They are viewed as a threat resulting in wasted motion, lowered yields, increased costs and missed target dates. Through centralized control, there is an assumption that predictability of outcomes is assured.

Appropriate motivation

Growth, adaptiveness, risk taking and idealism are deemed appropriate motivations within a developmental orientation. Members value constant stimulation in a never-ending quest for transformation and evolution. Letting go of the status quo is more than acceptable. It is expected and reinforced. Inventing creative solutions is viewed as an important process. Performance directed toward resource acquisition is valued and supported.

In contrast, security, stability and predictability are considered suitable motives within role orientation environments. Perpetuating the status quo is valued and supported. Cautious, conservative and skceptical perspectives dominate. There is an initial distrust of anything new or different. Holding on and maintaining that which currently exists is preferred. Standardization and routinization of activities are honoured and revered.

Similarly, the achievement orientation values the ability to use familiar and historical solutions to contemporary challenges. Results speak louder than words. Practical and functional approaches that can deliver 'here and now' results are favoured. Striving for a solution that does not result in an immediate remedy is considered unacceptable. This, in turn, restricts the focus of cognitive functioning to obvious cause-and-effect relationships. This may be done without considering root cause or long-term implication information. Individual initiative that is clear, focused and rational is viewed as the proper motivation toward work. Closure is expected in the problem solving process. Members are encouraged to think in terms of a 'beginning, middle and end' in relationship to tasks. Open-ended assignments are not valued. If they do exist, they are divided into component parts and solved as if they were a series of separate projects with deliverables and end dates. Quick, decisive performance is expected. Members motivated by 'doing more with less' are held in high regard. Efficiency is viewed as essential.

The support orientation values motivations that focus on increasing connections between internal members and not on efficiency. Creating an environment that facilitates affiliation, interpersonal cohesion and positive morale are viewed as essential. Within an achievement or developmental orientation the rallying theme is 'customer first'. Within the support orientation it is 'staff first'. It is assumed that comforting staff is required to create the proper conditions for high productivity or customer satisfaction. Tactfulness and diplomacy are the preferred mechanisms for dealing with conflict-laden situations. Compromising a person's self-respect or self-esteem is not acceptable. Diverse opinions are welcomed. Time is taken to process and integrate divergent positions into a unified whole. 'Win-win' solutions are encouraged. Consideration of the individual is viewed as a noble motivation and obligation.

Information Processing Strategies

Achievement orientation systems value rational information processing. Logic and factual analysis are preferred over internal feelings and emotions. Members are expected to be precise and stay focused on the issue under review. The process is built on sound, detailed numbers, statistics and perceived facts. Strong recognizable cues are sought that can lead to conquering problems through old and familiar means. New or novel means of information processing are not preferred. Members look for patterns and select an appropriate past strategy to solve problems. Situations involving an unexpected turn of events are confronted head-on in an attempt to re-establish order. Continuity is valued.

The reduction of uncertainty begins with goal clarification. A clear sense of direction, purpose and desired results are established upfront. Members search for evidence before engaging in analysis. Practical solutions are sought. Rewards and payoffs are identified before analysis is initiated. A systematic, structured and methodical approach is taken toward gathering, processing and acting on findings. Logical consistency is paramount. Members tend to build an airtight case for positions taken. They are quick to justify findings and solutions. Recognizing patterns and choosing a solution that has worked in the past under similar circumstances is the preferred method for problem resolution. Command and mastery over details is valued.

Role orientation environments also share a preference for building solutions with old and familiar tools. Continuity of the present order is a major objective. When faced with uncertainty, members prefer to isolate, compartmentalize and separate the source of tension from the environment. Observable and measurable facts are used to construct solutions. A methodical parts-to-whole approach to problem solving is followed. Documentation and computation are methods relied upon for correct processing of information. There is a tendency to classify data in black-and-white terms with little tolerance for in-between positions. Control of outcomes is important. Data is drawn from the way things are now, not in terms of what they could become. The boundaries for problem solving are drawn around a single issue frequently without linking it to other interdependent relationships. As a result, solutions tend to be suboptimized and centered on fine tuning the present order. When processing information, there is a search for the one best-fit solution. The assumption is that there is only one right way and it needs to be discovered. Solutions that provide for a secure, orderly and routinized environment are valued. Criteria for successful information processing include preserving the status quo and protecting the work unit or company from the stressors of the outside world.

Developmental orientation systems are in a constant state of changing the rules. Curiosity and creative juxtapositions of information serve to facilitate innovative solutions. There is a focus on multiple issues and interrelationships simultaneously. Reliance is on intuition and insight rather than pure logic. Quick, global analysis is the first step in solving problems or facing challenges. An attempt is made to grasp the whole first and then move toward the parts. Information is rapidly gathered in an action research method. Scenario building is used to tie information together in a macro perspective. Transformational solutions frequently emerge. When this is not possible, the issue is reframed and tackled from another point of view and possibly with a different targeted outcome. There is a preoccupation with the future and all the possibilities that can exist. Members within a developmental orientation are constantly searching for ways to discover and release untapped potential.

Support orientation environments look for opportunities to reinforce affiliations, interpersonal connections and mutual interdependence between members. Meaning and understanding are unlocked through the process of human interaction. Overly practical solutions are not valued. As with the developmental orientation, there is a focus on multiple issues and perspectives at once. Support orientation systems often have elaborate goals as opposed to the single focus of the role and achievement orientations. There is more of a reliance on subjective feeling states instead of fact-based logic. Solutions are based on soliciting and integrating multiple perspectives. Each discrete perspective maintains its integrity while merging ideas and positions into an acceptable whole. Every situation is defined as unique and not subject to predetermined or previously used solutions. Custom tailored, flexible information processing that is conducted toward others with respect, dignity and consistency is considered worthwhile. Information processing without the support of colleagues is avoided.

Time frame for action

Developmental orientation environments prefer immediate action, even at the risk of chaos. Experimentation and rapid responsiveness facilitate an open-ended, discover and adapt-as-you-go style. Personal initiative is valued and encouraged. New and innovative strategies are encouraged without a need for immediate results.

Achievement orientation systems also prefer personal initiative and immediate action. The major difference is that behaviour is directed toward clear, reachable goals. Practical outcomes are sought that can be immediately felt. There is an exhaustive, unrelenting dynamic competitive style to reach desired outcomes that relies on application of previous learning and past strategies.

Support and role orientations do not encourage immediate action. With the support orientation, cooperation is valued over immediate results. Time is given to establish and nurture relationships, build trust and eventually extract performance demands. Long time horizons are accepted in order to allow concern, support and consideration of others to take the lead in directing behaviour. Within a role orientation environment, no action is taken until the facts are gathered and the best solution found. Systematic, cautious, conservative action is expected.

Decision making

Developmental orientation systems focus more on strategic visioning and planning than on tactical problem solving. Decisions are based on a reasoning process that begins with a general notion or premise. From the premise, specific conclusions are drawn and translated into actions to be taken. The detailing of actions may be delegated to others more comfortable in that realm. The flow of decision making is from the 'whole to the part'. Decision making is based more on leaps of insight than on hard data. A grasp of the whole picture is preferred to immediate details. Decisions are arrived at after an open exchange of ideas. This leads to dreams of what is possible. 'What if' questioning is used to draw out ideas and develop future scenarios.

Achievement orientation environments approach decision making as a series of undisputable pronouncements on a course of action to be taken immediately. Individual decision making is favoured over group process. Use of logic, orderly analysis, evidence and hard data are stressed. There is a constant focus on the end objective to be obtained. Decisions are expected to have a linear connection between the objective and the course of action. The most direct, 'no frills' route to a solution with the least amount of effort is valued. Individuals are expected to convey decisions clearly, firmly and concisely. Once a decision is made, it is considered the final word. Steadfast adherence is expected. Lack of confidence or doubt is held in contempt.

Support orientation environments approach decision making as an interactive, face-to-face process between members. It is built on empathy, emotional support, self-disclosure of feeling states and impressions, sharing of vulnerabilities, personal anecdotes and respect for multiple points of view. The decision making process is dependent on close collaboration. There is a dislike for decisions requiring pure factual analysis, lack of emotions and quick solutions. Inclusion and synthesis of multiple points of view are valued and honoured. Members feel most at ease when focusing on the well-being of each other and long-term interpersonal commitments. Decisions related to building and liberating the talents of each person serve as a major source of strength. Members seek freedom and flexibility to find their own means to succeed in decision making and problem solving. There is a lack of harsh pronouncements. Listening, gaining rapport and joining members in a common cause are tools used to facilitate decision making and arrive at consensus.

Role orientation systems approach decision making as a methodical, objective process based on rigid, unyielding tradition, procedures and factual analysis. Decision making is viewed as a technical process that utilizes measurement, documentation and detailed information. Ongoing collection of data plays an important role. The flow of the decision making process is from the 'part to the whole'. Short, direct and factual discussions are preferred during deliberation. Flaws, contradictions and inconsistencies in thinking are quickly grasped. There is little tolerance for impractical or fuzzy ideas. There is a tendency to hold firm to a position and take minimal risk. Little concern is directed toward spending time nurturing support and commitment to decisions. It is assumed the rules, procedures or traditions supersede the need to focus on personal issues. Everyone is expected to comply regardless of feelings.

Power and influence

Within support and developmental orientations, power and influence are obtained by fostering feelings of trust and faith. Performance that increases healthy interdependence and mutuality gains influence within the support orientation environment. Power exists through relationships. Members that demonstrate empathy, caring and maintenance of the group gain influence. Those who facilitate and develop internal relationships are viewed as powerful. The wider and more intimate the network of friendships, the stronger the influence.

For the developmental orientation, feelings that convey a sense of hope and an anticipation of a better future gain power and influence. The developmental orientation uses connection power. Members that gain and maintain favourable access to resources outside of the work unit, division or company are considered influential and valuable. Openness and flexibility combined with passionate values, a strategic vision and the ability to facilitate growth and improvement are performance traits that enhance power and influence for members.

Performance that establishes structure and exercises authority over others is perceived with reverence within role and achievement orientations. Access to and control of information have power within the role orientation environment. Delivery of tangible, bottom-line results and use of rational persuasion gain influence within the achievement orientation.

Legitimate power holds the most influence with achievement orientation environments. The relative formal position of the member determines the degree of power. The higher the member is in the chain of command, the stronger the influence. However, individuals hold significant informal power when they:

1 take initiative
2 perform with a clear sense of direction
3 set obtainable yet challenging objectives
4 proceed in a structured, orderly fashion with deliberate speed
5 achieve bottom line results.

Members in positions of legitimate power are strongly influenced by successful front-line achievers.

Role orientation environments support expert and information power. The more skill, knowledge, information and expertise in the field, the more respect is bestowed upon the member. Skill, information and knowledge refer not only to a trade or work process but also to social cognitive abilities within the environment.

Evaluation of members

Members within an achievement orientation are formally evaluated in terms of tangible output. Measurement is quantitative and typically covers volume, quality, speed and cost. Efficiency and effectiveness are central to analysis. Informally, members are critiqued on individual initiative, task focus, loyalty to the boss and dedication to the mission of the firm. Predictability and dependability are closely monitored. Fundamentally, members are measured in terms of their accomplishments.

Support orientation environments focus on qualitative dimensions. The informal connection between people within the environment takes on more significance than the formal tasks. The depth and breadth of interpersonal relationships measures the degree of member effectiveness. Performance that facilitates or inhibits human development, support, social inclusion, mutual interdependence, interpersonal cohesion and morale are monitored and judged.

Role orientation environments measure members' performance through formal criteria. Rating scales and other similar instruments are used to control for standardization of measures. Formal procedures are followed to ensure objective and even-handed treatment of members. Members are evaluated in terms of their ability to contribute to the stability and control of the environment.

Members within a developmental orientation are evaluated by the degree of innovation, growth, expansion and resource acquisition brought to the environment. The ability to envision a better future, open opportunities for advancement and obtain the necessary support to achieve goals is rated favourably.

Compliance

Role orientation environments rely upon surveillance and centralized control to keep members within the bounds of acceptable performance. Gathering and managing information are strategies used to maintain order. A chain of command and span of control are the channels through which information and directives flow in order to maintain stability, control, and status quo. Top-down directives authorize and direct behaviour. There is an underlying lack of trust or faith that members have the internal ability conscientiously to self-regulate. Members are given information on a need-to-know basis. Understanding of the total system is held only by those in the senior level of the chain of command. Members have a compartmentalized view of the environment. They are encouraged to specialize in a particular aspect of the total operation and leave the synthesis of the component activities to authorities further up the chain of command. Members, in part, are controlled by the degree of access to information and authority over others. Flow of information is unbalanced. Higher authorities demand and expect the information to flow upward. Only select information flows downward accompanied by a directive or command. Reasoning and higher order problem solving are done for the member further down the chain of command. Members violating the range of acceptable behaviour tend to be singled out and psychologically isolated from others to prevent 'contamination' of the general membership. Various levels of fear are used as tool of control.

Achievement orientation environments rely upon contractual agreements. Each party commits to deliverable outcomes. A clear understanding of goals, objectives and results is established. The understanding is mutually binding. Control is achieved through a mutual pledge and individual accountability. Personal responsibility and self-initiative are standards by which members approach obligations. Self-regulation is valued. Failure to meet obligations is subject to confrontation and acts of domination by the aggrieved party.

Developmental orientation environments build on shared values to which members commit to uphold. Values are used to guide behaviour more than to control actions. Ethics, ideals and principles are the basis of binding members toward a common mission or purpose. Trust of members' intentions and follow through with commitments are assumed. There is an honour system. Commitment to the shared values is viewed more on the level of a sacred covenant. A member's conscience serves as a personal regulator of performance. Members are gently reminded of their shared values when performance drifts from desired outcomes. Serious violations of the covenant result in social isolation and rejection.

Support orientation environments achieve compliance and control through mutual commitment to a process that safeguards the self-esteem and self-confidence of its members. Reaching consensus through discussion is the preferred method for resolving conflict. Parties strive to develop 'win-win' solutions. Members are given the opportunity to synthesize divergent positions into an acceptable course of action that addresses each person's individual needs.

Inclusion and natural supports

Facilitating membership within the social fabric of a work environment and utilizing natural supports requires building on the existing organizational culture. Any thoughts of modifying the basic orientation of an organizational culture or changing the basic nature of a client to fit into a work environment will end in frustration. The most fundamental strategy of the practitioner is to begin with the maxim: 'Birds of a feather flock together'. Person–environment congruency is central to effective social inclusion. Effective practitioners build on the basic vocational and lifestyle preferences of the client. This includes preferred activities, world views and behavioural patterns. The information is compared to the value system of a company to search for a natural match. For example, individuals that are blunt, practical and task oriented would have a tendency to feel alienated in a support orientation environment. Yet, the same person would feel at home in an achievement oriented culture. Once a match is made, the practitioner frames each intervention in terms that respect and reflect the culture of the work environment. For example, requesting that a group of coworkers meet daily to process their feelings and experiences with the client would be perceived as congruent with the way people interact in a support orientation. Trying the same approach in an achievement oriented environment would be viewed as 'out of touch' and a waste of valuable time. Within a developmental orientation environment, experimenting with creative work flow designs would be greeted with open arms. The same process would never be launched within a role oriented culture. Members would perceive the intervention as a threat to the stability and predictability of the work setting.

Cognitive functioning

Cognitive framework

Cognitive activities can be framed according to:

1 Content
2 modality
3 phases
4 operations
5 level of complexity
6 level of abstraction
7 level of efficiency.
(Feuerstein, 1979).

This serves as a platform for assessment and planning of enhancement strategies. Understanding the means by which the client processes and acts on information assists in determining the nature, configuration and extent of support required. Determining when and where cognitive processes succeed or perform ineffectively provides valuable insight into the medium, strategy and tactics that will facilitate remediation, training and reasonable accommodation. Assessment is performed through a series of personal, interactive contacts with the client, in a variety of natural community environments. Direct observation, interviews with significant others, file reviews, and related assessments, can assist in an understanding of the client's cognitive skills and process in applied settings. Using the cognitive framework provides a systematic and disciplined manner in which to collect and organize the data generated.

Content

Analysis and planning begin with understanding the subject matter that is the object of the cognitive process. Within a work environment, the client is addressing issues such as task skills, routines, corporate culture compatibility, social skills, and the physical environment. Task skills relate to primary and secondary job duties. Job routines are concerned

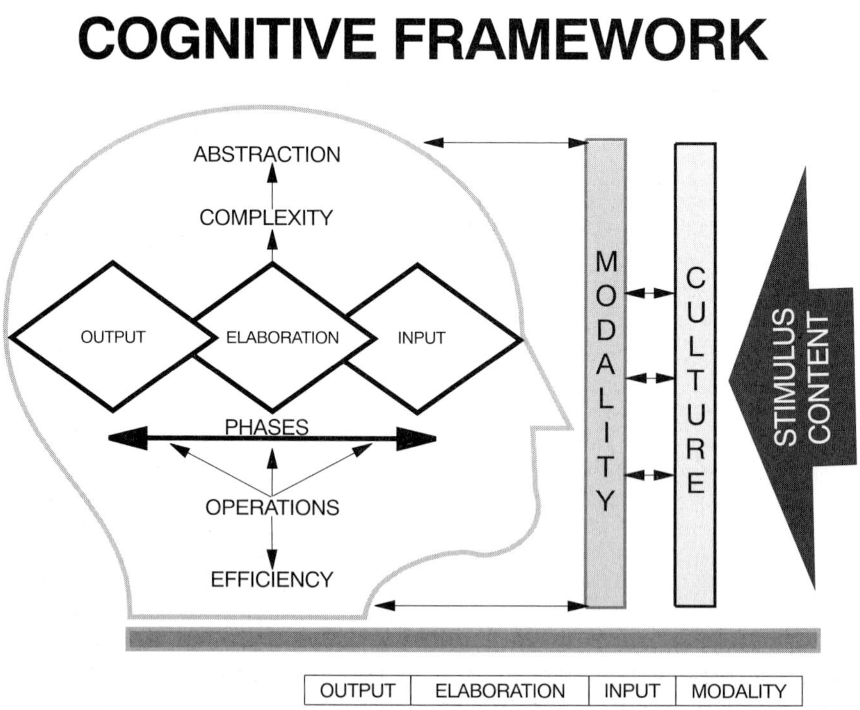

Figure 8.8 Cognitive framework.

with the various steps involved in carrying out job-related responsibilities. Routines include both linear and non-linear activities. Cultural compatibility addresses the natural social-psychological match between the individual and coworkers. Compatibility is based on the degree of harmony and congruence that exists around basic values, preferences and world views. Social skills focus on the ability to connect and participate with coworkers in a manner that is normative and productive for the target setting. Social cognition skills are an important component of this factor. The physical environment dimension is concerned with location (indoors or outdoors), temperature, light, vibration, noise, physical capacity requirements, and other related factors.

The degree of familiarity with the content areas is important. Content provides an understanding of what a person needs to know in order to be successful. First-time exposure may not give a true reading of inherent ability, compatibility and skills. It does suggest how the person deals with incorporating unfamiliar information and experience. When the degree of familiarity is high, then important information is obtained on how the person applies previous knowledge, skills and experience. The degree of familiarity with the content and context influences what is observed. The individual's existing strategy and process for managing new learning integrates both task and social issues. A person may be at ease around strangers yet challenged to incorporate new task routines.

Social cognition content plays a critical role in job matching and on-the-job training. Learning the social and cognitive tasks of the job setting flow more easily when there is a natural compatibility. The focus of remediation or training is to strengthen and develop the cognitive skills and style of the client that are inherently congruent with the performance requirements of the setting.

Modality

Modality addresses the means by which a person takes in information through the senses. Understanding the preferred modality of the client provides an important source of information for structuring the learning process, designing reasonable accommodations, and establishing ongoing supports. Information and instruction can be presented through a variety of means that include but are not limited to verbal, non-verbal gestures, pictorial, numerical, figural, smell, touch, sound or a combination of these and other sensory means. For example, a 27-year-old male with moderate mental retardation combined with a severe behavioural disorder was referred by a case manager for mental health services to an agency specializing in dual diagnosis (Mental Retardation/Mental illness). The client had a history of destroying property, physically threatening harm to others, and impulsive self-destructive behaviour. His special education experience had been chaotic and unsuccessful. He had never been able to secure and maintain employment. He had been discharged from two sheltered workshops and one day activity centre since he left school at the age of 22. The clinical treatment in the new agency included individual psychotherapy and medication. After an initial period of psychotherapeutic treatment, the clinician referred the client to a vocational rehabilitation practitioner. The therapy and medication stabilized the client somewhat but did not eliminate his impulsive and explosive behaviours. The clinician felt participation in a structured vocational experience would accelerate treatment gains.

During the vocational assessment phase, the practitioner identified the client's preferred sensory modality. Talking about career preferences with the client did not work. He had to see a job first hand in order to determine his likes and dislikes. When the client and practitioner went into the community to visit various types of employment to identify vocational preferences, the client exhibited behavioural episodes immediately following the excursions. It was discovered that each time the client saw a job he automatically assumed the job was his. He could not differentiate between viewing a job and being hired. He did not respond well to verbal dialogue when it came to understanding and learning. The client preferred and relied upon visual information to the exclusion of most other modalities. Further investigation revealed that this was true for other parts of his life as well.

The job seeking process was modified to incorporate the preferred use of the visual modality. The practitioner prescreened potential employers, instead of taking the client. The prescreening was based on known preferences and needs learned through interviews with significant others, record reviews and direct observations. It was learned the client wanted work in a restaurant where employees wore a uniform with a shirt, tie and slacks. The client wanted to dress for work like his older brother. In terms of a job position, he specifically wanted to be a dining-room attendant, removing dishes and cleaning tables. When a site visit was necessary to determine a job match, it was done not as a job interview but as a field trip to eat lunch. The client did not enter the site with the intention of choosing or interviewing for a job. The experience was reframed to a neutral task to avoid any potential disappointment resulting in dysfunctional behavioural episodes. The practitioner made prior arrangements with the manager of a restaurant to pass by the table and ask if they were pleased with their food and engage in light conversation. This allowed the manager to ask questions causally and observe the client to determine hiring potential. It also gave the practitioner an opportunity to observe the interaction to determine if there was potential for a natural working relationship. The employer agreed to a reasonable accommodation in his hiring process by using a 'stealth' (invisible) interviewing approach.

The practitioner made a prearranged agreement to have the manager ask the client if he would like to work at the restaurant if there appeared to be a good match. The manager and practitioner prearranged a mutual signal if both thought a job should be offered. This gave both parties an opportunity to gracefully decline further involvement, if warranted. If both parties were in agreement to proceed, then the manager would ask the client if he would like to 'see' a room-attendant job and work at the restaurant. The client then had the opportunity to accept or decline. The process worked around the preferred visual modality in order to prevent misunderstandings during the job interview by appearing invisible to the client. However, when the time came for client choice and control in job selection, the visual modality was engaged by the employer through having the client see the job and determine if he would like to work at the restaurant.

Once the client chose to work at the restaurant, the clinician, vocational rehabilitation practitioner and employer designed a ten-point behavioural self-management plan. The purpose of the plan was to prevent, reduce or eliminate behavioural problems that would result in job loss. The behavioural plan included a series of photographs of the client successfully controlling his behaviour step by step. The first step began with a photograph of the client recognizing that he was frustrated. It showed the client with an angry facial gesture and body posture. The very process of eliciting a demonstration of the behaviour typically used by the client induced paradoxical effects. It gave the client an opportunity to take control over a behavioural expression he frequently experienced as beyond his control. It also taught him to recognize his own early warning signs when a situation was heading for trouble. The second step showed a picture of the client going to a table in a quiet place to get away from the immediate situation. This gave a concrete action the client could prescribe to himself to head off a problem situation and use to control his own behaviour. The third step showed a picture of the client sitting down at the table. The fourth step showed a picture of the client setting an ordinary cooking timer for ten minutes as indicated by a red line drawn by the practitioner. The fifth step showed a picture of the client placing his head on his folded arms on the table. The sixth step showed a picture of the client resting with his eyes closed. Clouds were drawn coming from his head as if he was dreaming peacefully in his sleep. The client was taught to self sooth using a basic biofeedback technique. During the time he had his head was on his arms the client was instructed to begin breathing slower and slower like he did when he was falling asleep at night. This relaxed the client. The seventh step showed a picture of the client sitting upright with a smile when the timer was at zero and a ringing sound was heard. This was noted by wavy lines coming from the timer. If he did not feel calm and rested at the end of the ten minutes, he was instructed to set the timer for ten more minutes. He was told to keep repeating the sequence until he felt calm. The eighth step showed a picture of the client smiling while going back to his job station. The ninth step showed a picture of him successfully doing a job task with a smile. The tenth step showed a picture of the client successfully completing his task with a smile and a 'thumbs up' gesture.

The pictures were placed in the proper order in a photo album and given to the client to use while at work to teach and remind him what to do when upset. Next, a video tape was shot that followed the sequence of the photos. The client acted his own role. The tape was then viewed with the client and related to the photos. The client kept the video to watch at home whenever he wanted to see how he could be successful at managing his behaviours at work. In addition, the employer and practitioner designed a process to resolve conflicts and underlying causes of frustrations experienced by the client. This gave a message to the client that the cause of his disappointments did not always reside with him.

Phases

Although cognitive functions may be divided into phases and associated functions, all are highly integrated and interdependent. This makes phase distinctions somewhat arbitrary. With this in mind, cognitive activity can be divided into three basic phases:

1 Input, receptive functions involving areas such as sensory stimulation, awareness, recognition, discrimination, selective perception, patterning, data gathering and initial encoding.
2 Elaboration, concerned with activities such as reasoning, memory, recall, ordering, comparing, computing, abstracting, generalizing, concept formation, judgement and planning.
3 Output, activities related to expressive activities such as speaking, writing, interpersonal behavioural patterns, physical gestures, gross and fine motor activities, facial expressions and bodily movements.
(Feuerstein, 1979; Heinseen and Glass, 1990).

The benefit of isolating cognitive activity within phases is that it assists the practitioner in identifying points of entry for enhancing and supporting cognitive functioning.

Input phase

The input phase is concerned with how the client gathers and takes in data at both the controlled and automatic information processing levels. Exploring, selecting and initially registering incoming data from the surrounding environment are primary activities. This is accomplished through a preferred sensory modality or combination of modalities such as sight, hearing or touch. Understanding how many sources of data and instructional steps can be handled at one time is useful information for constructing an enhancement strategy. The practitioner is particularly interested in identifying the conditions under which data gathering and initial registration are most effective and least effective. Exploratory behaviour ranges from planned and systematic to impulsive and scattered (Feuerstein, 1979).

The type of data the person tends selectively to perceive and map provides valuable insight into how the person constructs personal meaning. A practitioner looks for patterns across a variety of activities that include:

1 learning
2 performing new and routine tasks
3 problem solving
4 conflict resolution
5 individual and group interpersonal relationships.

Effective cognitive performance builds on accuracy and precision of data gathering. Motivation, training, self-discipline and capability influence the process. Once data has been collected by a person, then it is organized into initial meaningful information. The practitioner evaluates the ability of the person to recognize initial and basic patterns in the gathered data. It is useful for the practitioner to identify the type of data the person can immediately understand and not understand in order to design the support strategy.

Critical to data gathering is the ability to know essential from non-essential information in relationship to the task at hand. The practitioner evaluates the person's ability to go after the right data. Reasons and motivations are identified that influence the choice of selectively perceived data. The practitioner pinpoints the conditions that facilitate the person's ability to gather data and initially register the data into meaningful information. From this understanding, the practitioner determines if compensatory mechanisms or reasonable accommodations are required and the form they may take.

Elaboration phase

The elaboration phase is composed of a complex network of discrete activities that are highly interdependent. These activities work through a set of cognitive operations that operate individually and in concert with each other. The classification of operations varies with the perspective and techniques of various professional disciplines. For the purposes of this discussion, the following constructs are identified as cognitive operations:

1 Reality testing, the process of verifying the accuracy of perceptions.
2 Judgement, the process of anticipating consequences and choosing the proper course of action.
3 Sense of self, other and situation, the process of social cognition.
4 Regulation and control of drives, affects and impulses, the process for adaptively modulating feelings, thoughts and behaviours.
5 Thought processes, the activities associated with reasoning, level of abstraction and concept formation.
6 Adaptive regression, the process of controlled partial and temporary lowering of cognitive functions.
7 Defensive functioning, the process of using cognitive skills and mechanism to buffer against threatening, painful or overwhelming emotional information.
8 Stimulus barrier control the processes related to filtering sensory data to adaptive levels.
9 Autonomous functioning, activities associated with sensory perception and performance, attention, tracking, concentration, orientation and intention.
10 Mastery and competence, the process of skill performance in relationship to capacity, competency and effectiveness.
11 Synthetic–integrative functioning, the process of binding together the multiple cognitive activities and functions into a coherent and effective whole.

(Bellak and Small, 1978; Feuerstein, 1979; Heinssen and Glass, 1990; Lekak, 1976; Lovett, 1985; Mirsky, 1987; Wolf, 1988)

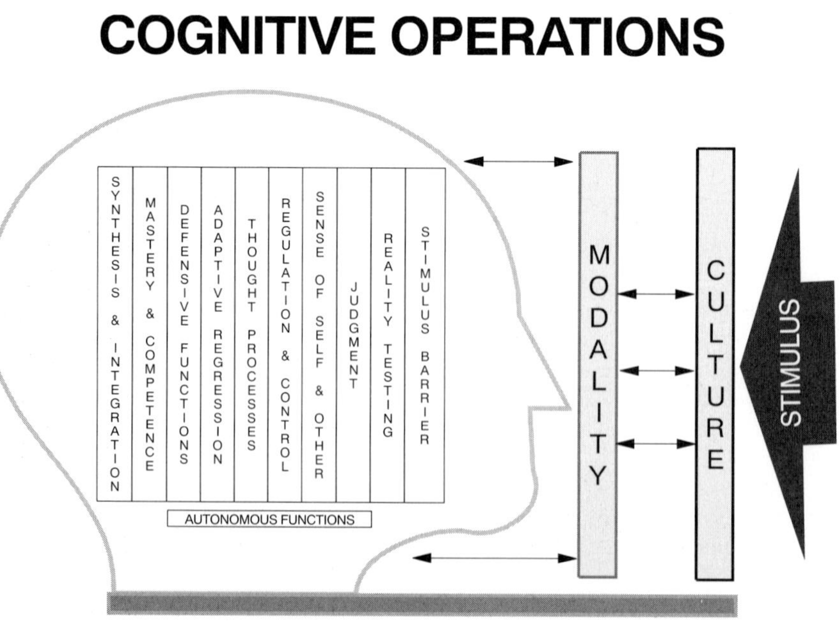

Figure 8.9 Cognitive operations.

Reality testing

Reality testing involves three key processes that operate automatically and seamlessly in normal circumstances. The first process is the continuous selective scanning process to locate the source of cognitive stimuli. Its purpose is to determine if the stimulus is external or internal to the person (Bellak and Small, 1978). External stimuli are located in the physical and social environment. Internal stimuli are located within the affective, cognitive and physiological states of the person.

The second and third processes determine the perceptual accuracy of the external and internal events respectively (Bellak and Small, 1978). The process involves double checking the data across a variety of the senses and prior knowledge to compare findings and look for patterns, consistencies and meaning. The purpose is to determine if the perceptions reflect a true reading of the information generated by the stimuli. The external frame of reference includes orientation to time, place and situation while the internal frame of reference is concerned with the degree of accurate self-awareness. Culture, norms and values influence what is considered relevant to scan in the external social environment. Having the ability to observe one's self in a situation while simultaneously attending to events in the situation is important for internal scanning.

Cognitive impairment, psychological dysfunction, emotional disturbance, behavioural disorders or physical states influence the ease, deliberativeness and accuracy of the three processes. Reality testing is a useful concept when facilitating a person's ability to cope and adapt to the social-psychological aspects of a work environment. For example, an employer observed one of her employees acting increasingly frightened and withdrawn. Absenteeism had been on the rise. There was a general sense that the person was avoiding job tasks and routines. Performance was unacceptable. A practitioner was summoned to rectify the situation. The employer valued the employee and wanted to help. A practitioner was contacted after the employee burned her hand while using a press machine that makes rubber soles for boots. The practitioner learned that until the previous month the employee was doing fine. Performance had been so good that she had been promoted from a custodian to the machine operator position. Since the promotion, everything seemed to have taken a downward spin.

Upon completing a discussion with the employee, the practitioner learned the employee never finished high school and

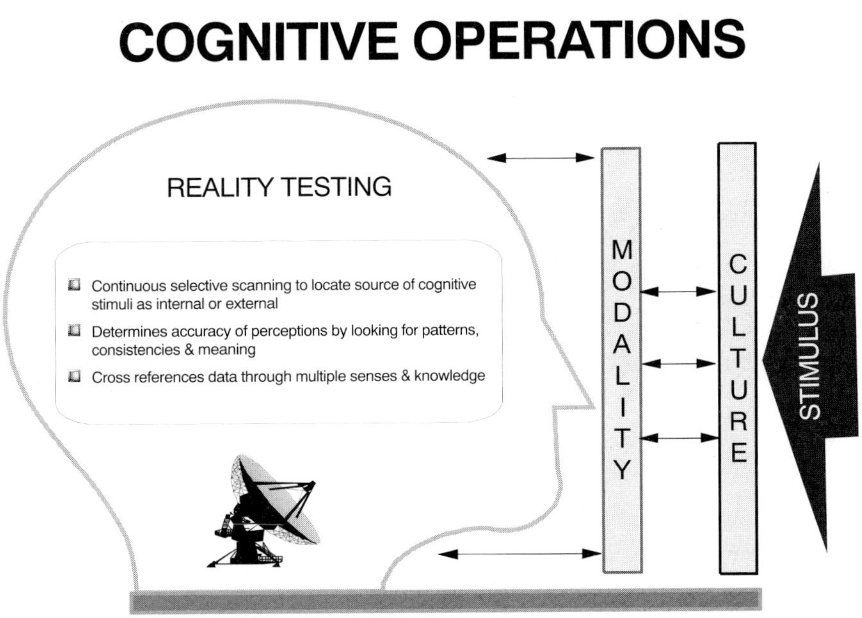

Figure 8.10 Reality testing.

generally did not do well academically or socially. She had been working as an entry level, unskilled worker since she dropped out of school three years ago. She had been with the current employer for six months. She had obtained the job through a friend of the family. The employee really wanted to please her boss. The boss had been very good to her, more so than anyone else. When exploring the difficulties at work, the employee was not aware of what was causing her problems. She had a great deal of difficulty understanding or articulating why she had been doing poorly. It became evident during the discussion that the employee was a very concrete thinker and not introspective. It was hard for her to see the connection between inner feelings and outward performance. Essentially, the employee did not want to let her boss down. She was afraid to fail. She was afraid to disappoint someone who had become important to her and had faith in her.

The employee reported she had been avoiding work because she thought the boss was angry at her for not learning the job faster. Every time the boss had come around to check on the work, the employee thought the boss was angry. When the practitioner asked her how she knew the boss was angry, she was not able to identify any concrete evidence. She stated she just knew. She had been making mistakes as she learned how to operate a fairly complex machine. The production line was shut down four times because of errors made by her. She had never been reprimanded but she just knew the boss didn't like her as much now that she had seen her for what she was ... a major disappointment. The mistakes were evidence, once again, that she could not learn well and that she did not deserve to be promoted. As the practitioner provided counselling and emotional support, a link between the burned hand and the employee's self hate was revealed. The burned hand had been an unconscious, self-inflicted punishment for not doing as well as she would like for her boss and coworkers. Each time the production line was shut down, it reminded her of all her previous failures in school. It provided evidence, once again, that she simply couldn't make it. Hurting herself was an unconscious way to resolve the conflict. The employee never checked her assumptions. She didn't ask the boss if everything was OK when she made mistakes. She didn't check to see if her coworkers were disappointed and angry at her. These were accepted as fact. Because of a lack of self-awareness, the employee did not have the tools to deal directly with her problem. She did not have an accurate perception of her internal and her external world. Nor did she take time to check the facts.

The practitioner worked with both the employee and employer to establish a feedback system between each other. The employee was taught to check out her thoughts with her boss whenever she was feeling uneasy. She was taught to ask for feedback. In turn, the employer was coached proactively to schedule intermittent feedback encounters so the employee did not have to second guess how she was doing. The employer was also encouraged to facilitate connections between the employee and other coworkers to prevent the sense of isolation the client was experiencing. Coworkers were asked to let the client know she was valued. They were asked to give feedback both when performance went well and when it needed to be corrected. In other words, they needed to be real with their coworker. This way, the client did not have to second guess her status with her peers nor feel she was being handled as if she were fragile and incompetent. The workers were also encouraged to normalize the client's feelings and role model problem solving and coping strategies. They were taught to engage in verbal self-disclosure regarding their performance struggles, as they were happening. The coworkers were asked to share their internal dialogue when they were dealing with their own frustrations and disappointments.

A coworker was identified to serve as a performance mediator (Feuerstein, 1979). The performance mediator was taught how to work with the employee to teach and provide guidance on how to:

1 Monitor and recognize internal thoughts and feelings.
2 Link the internal thoughts and feelings to the source of conflict.
3 Problem solve while keeping self respect.

By strengthening the cognitive function of reality testing while arranging external supports with her boss and coworkers, the employee was able to return to work and become a productive worker.

Judgement

Judgement is primarily concerned with the ability to:

1 Anticipate the consequences of intended behaviour.
2 Choose a course of action that is appropriate to the situation.
3 Learn from one's actions in order to improve judgement skills.
(Bellak and Small, 1978; Heinssen and Glass, 1990; Lovett, 1985).

Anticipating the consequences of intended behaviour is the key distinguishing feature of judgement. It provides a future vision that simulates a range of options available for action. Central to scenario building is the capacity to identify and understand critical success factors, their inherent properties and how they dynamically influence events accurately. The more accurate the anticipation matches the actual consequences the more effective and efficient judgement is. The ability to learn from experience influences the efficiency and effectiveness of judgement. The process of 'expect–check–correct' supports the continuous improvement and accuracy of this cognitive function.

Motivation overshadows whatever judgement skills may exist. For example, a person may have an overwhelming desire to wear a uniform. This could potentially weaken judgement regarding the right company with which to become employed. Factors related to company culture and work practices may be ignored, only coming back to haunt the person once the glory of the uniform wears away and is replaced with the somber reality of the situation. Judgement can also vary according to topic area. A person may have superior judgement regarding the stock market, but may be disastrous when applied to interpersonal relationships.

Appropriateness of judgement is closely related to the cognitive consensuality of the environment. What may be appropriate in one circumstance may backfire in another. For example, a clinical social worker left a private practice to work in a for-profit health-care company. Within private practice, broad goals for treatment had been established with patients. The focus had been primarily on a long treatment process that explored multiple aspects of a person's life. The depth and

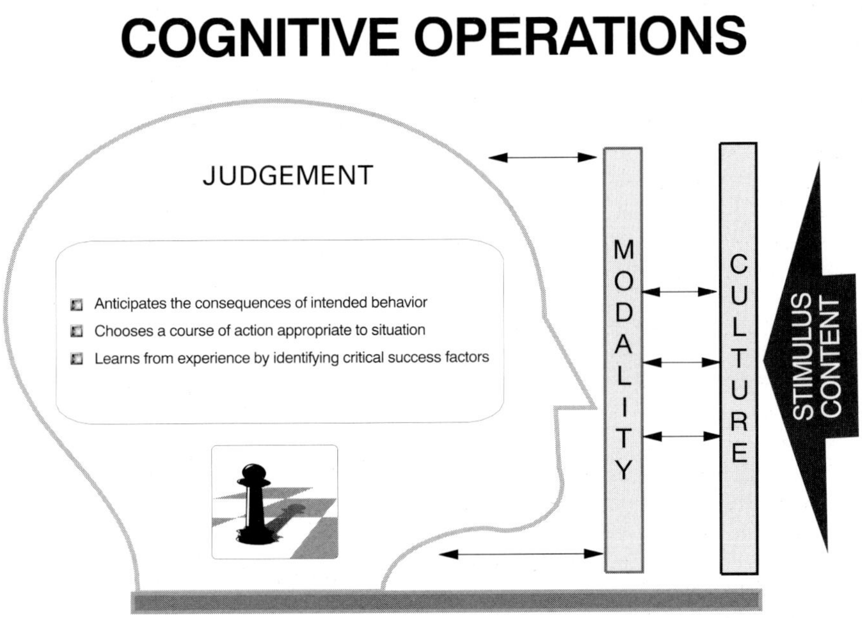

Figure 8.11 Judgement.

quality of the relationship between the social worker and the patient had been viewed as the centre piece for the treatment process to be effective. Within the for-profit, high-volume environment of the health-care provider, appropriate treatment was considered very time limited at 10–12 sessions, with very specific behavioural objectives. If the social worker continued to focus on long-term treatment approaches, it would be considered inappropriate and more than likely, employment would be short lived.

Enhancement of judgement tends to focus on the underlying issues affecting the cognitive function. Lack of knowledge, skill and experience, congruency with the surrounding culture, feeling states, time constraints, unclear expectations, external pressures, double binds, intellectual and cognitive impairments, self-concept, fatigue, impulse control, personal motivations and needs, physical well-being, socialization and other related factors all contribute to enhancing or interfering with performance. If judgement is impaired to the degree the person is not able to develop the skill, then compensatory arrangements are made. Another person may be paired with the individual to serve as an alter ego and make judgements on behalf of the person. Smart technology may be designed using artificial intelligence (AI) programming. The person is taught to press buttons in a certain sequence. The buttons to be pushed automatically light up in the proper sequence. By pressing the button, a series of activities are set in motion to complete a work task or portion of a task. Although the person cannot anticipate the more complex implications of activities, the AI technology is able to compensate.

In terms of social judgement, modelling, feedback, guidance and performance mediation serve as ways to learn appropriate cues and behaviours. The natural influence of corporate culture cannot be over stated. Through systematic exposure and support, many persons learn naturally how to behave in ways acceptable to the environment. The closer the match between the natural personality, style and values of the person with that of the environment, the higher degree of success is likely. Judgement is dependent on the data gathering activities of the input phase.

Sense of self, other and situation

Sense of self, other and situation is a cognitive operation that links self-awareness with awareness of the surrounding physical and social environment. This juxtaposition provides the platform for defining socially relevant meaning and appropriate performance requirements (Bellak and Small, 1978; Heinssen and Glass, 1990; Kegan, 1982; Lovett, 1985). Self-awareness and self-perception provide valuable information on how one's behaviour is experienced, interpreted and judged by other persons within current surroundings. Observations focus on people interacting with each other and tasks being performed. By observing and noting the pattern of behaviours and the functional results they create, a person is better able to learn the language and meaning of performance within a specific context.

Information is collected that gives the person a sense of self (self schemata), other (person schemata) and situation (script schemata and person-in-situation schemata).

Having a sense of self is understanding what is 'me', 'you' (not me) and 'us' (shared me). The self-definition guides behaviour. For example, if a person has a self-identity as one who cannot tolerate sustained performance, then the person will more than likely tend to behave accordingly. Self-concept directs a person's behaviour toward a self-fulfilling prophesy. This includes idealization of a preferred self. The content and stability of the self-concept is important to nurture in order to achieve high performance, both with the job duties and as a respected and valued social being within the company.

Sense of self and situation is also concerned with the extent to which the external events in the environment are experienced as real and embedded within a familiar context. Having a stable environment is important. If the routines, rules and relationships are constantly changing, it makes successful performance more difficult to achieve.

Performance mediation is an effective strategy for enhancing sense of self and situation, as well as other cognitive operations. A performance mediator frames, selects, focuses and feeds back environmental experiences in a planned and systematic way (Feuerstein, 1979; Shea, 1994). The performance mediation builds on the uniqueness of the individual. Person-

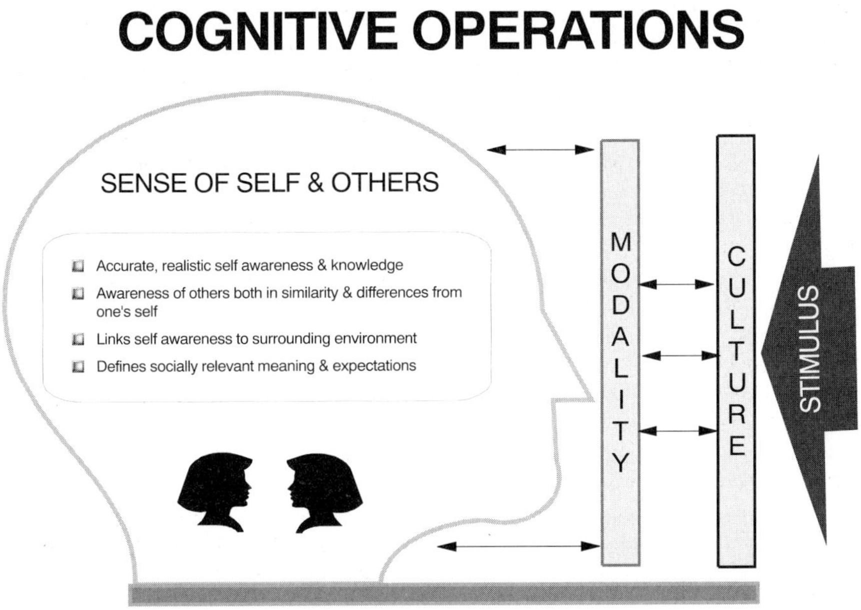

Figure 8.12 Sense of self and other.

ality style, degree of maturity, cognitive functioning, and level of cognitive complexity are all considerations in the design of the mediated learning process. Successful mediated learning experiences serve as a transitional process of learning through direct and immediate exposure to environmental stimulation.

Performance mediation begins with establishing a working relationship with the client that is built on mutual trust. To enhance the development of a healthy self-concept, the client needs to have exposure and experience with real-life situations both on and off the job. This process is facilitated by creating an interpersonal relationship between the performance mediator and client. The performance mediator is taught to:

1 Use mirroring and empathic attunement.
2 Build on the naturally occurring processes of idealization and merger.
3 Serve as an alter ego.
4 Promote personal efficacy by facilitating the client's ability to have a positive impact on others.
5 Gently use adversity to reinforce autonomy and understand how to deal with differences.
6 Create a framework for learning.
(Wolf, 1988)

Mirroring and empathic attunement Mirroring involves giving undivided attention to the person while using empathic attunement. The purpose is to provide an interpersonal experience that is stable and able to fulfill the client's needs to feel affirmed, confirmed, recognized, accepted and appreciated (Wolf, 1988). Mirroring is the process of reflectively communicating to the person through various forms of non-verbal gestures, facial expressions, bodily movements and speech. The communication conveys a non-judgemental understanding and appreciation for the client's subjective experience. Empathic attunement is the ability of the performance mediator to recognize and understand the client's subjective feeling and thinking states and verbally communicate the understanding to the client. Empathic communication exists at multiple levels. At a minimum, empathic responses convey an understanding that is equal to the level of self-expression by the other person. Content is not as important as an accurate reflection of a feeling state. A phrase such as: 'You're feeling unsure of yourself right now' is an example. Empathic communication can also be at an additive level. Additive responses convey to the person that she or he is being understood beyond their immediate level of awareness. Content is added to the expressed affective state that gives deeper meaning. For example, a phrase such as: 'You're feeling unsure of yourself right now. It feels just like it did when you were in high school and weren't able to keep up with the other students.' Empathic responses need to be genuine, warm, respectful, concrete and specific. When empathic attunement is experienced, the client will be more open to receiving help. Without client permission to help, performance mediation will not succeed.

The objective of mirroring and empathic attunement is to help the client subjectively feel confirmed, accepted and valued. The client develops a sense of security and a sense that it is safe to be ambitious. With the support and prompting from the performance mediator, the client begins to develop a personal inventory of experiences that can be used to define the 'me' in self understanding. Client storytelling develops reflective awareness. Over time, the person is able to remember: how situations were handled; what problem solving strategies were helpful; what one is good at doing; what one is not good at doing; personal likes and dislikes; and social norms that are expected within the work environment. All of these experiences begin to help the client sort out their identity and develop a stable and healthy self-image.

Idealization Over time, the client begins to feel admiration, respect and attachment toward the performance mediator. The performance mediator is seen as a reliable and trustworthy person. The client feels safe, contained and soothed. This soothing exists both in the presence and away from the performance mediator. The images and attributes of the performance mediator are idealized. The performance mediator is seen as wise, non-toxic, powerful and protective. Many of the idealized attributes of the performance mediator become incorporated into the self-image of the client. Through the idealization process, the client begins to develop a personal sense of values, a vision for the future and ideals to fulfill in action and deed (Wolf, 1988). A sense of self-identity begins to develop based on identification with the performance mediator.

The performance mediator allows the idealization to take place and remain active. During a later stage in the relationship, a natural process of separation will occur and idealization will move toward realism. It is seductive to be put on a pedestal and admired. This is a time when the performance mediator may not want to let go of being seen as a heroine or hero. As time goes on, the client will begin to see the performance mediator more realistically. The performance mediator lets the realistic reassessment take place, without taking it personally. If the performance mediator is not properly prepared, there may be an unconscious attempt to block the de-idealization. This would interrupt the separation-individuation process for the client. As the separation begins to take place later in the relationship, the performance mediator needs to accept the dethroning gracefully without projecting anger and resentment directly or indirectly. The performance mediator provides support and facilitates the client's ability to begin taking adversarial views. Reinforcement and encouragement for separate points of view is nurtured, gently. The performance mediator crafts a strategy that sends a message to the client that having a different point of view will not hurt or destroy the performance mediator or the relationship. The performance mediator needs to be acutely aware of subtle changes in the evolutionary stages of self-concept development, relationship shifts and required changes in support strategies. Progress does not necessarily follow a straight and narrow path.

Merger Idealization leads the client to begin to develop a preconscious and primitive sense of oneness with the performance mediator. The client assumes both parties are very much alike, see things the same way and have similar skills. The performance mediator does not attack this belief. Instead, the performance mediator lets the client ride on her coattails. A new sense of strength is established within the client. The client feels that together, they can handle the challenges ahead. Through the merger stage, the client gains self-confidence to explore the world and to develop mastery over the environment (Wolf, 1988).

Although the client is feeling ready to take on new experiences and exercise command over the world, the practitioner advises the performance mediator to be available to provide guidance and direction. The client still needs to work jointly with the performance mediator to deal with the reality of the situations that are encountered. Feelings of bravery may exist on the part of the client, yet the performance mediator has to be careful not to let go too quickly.

Alter ego Serving as an alter ego, the performance mediator works with the client to make joint decisions and tackle challenges together as a team. A sense of partnership is fostered. Within the safety of the relationship, the client borrows the strength of the performance mediator. This is a preconscious process. The client may not be aware that facing the challenges alone may be a risky proposition. When success is achieved with a task, the client takes most of the credit even though the performance mediator may have played a major role. The performance mediator does not dispel the myth unless it is obvious that it needs to be addressed. The best developmental learning takes place when the client approaches the performance mediator and gives credit.

The performance mediator systematically assesses, supports, trains and challenges the client. In the role of alter ego, the performance mediator begins by using a hierarchy of prompts to determine the client's ability for self-directed work. The range of prompts includes:

- no help
- non-specific verbal instruction
- specific verbal instruction
- gesture and verbal instruction
- demonstration and verbal instruction
- shadowing and verbal instruction
- partial guidance and verbal instruction
- full guidance and verbal instruction.

To determine the level of prompting required, the performance mediator typically begins with demonstration and verbal instruction such as: 'Here is the computer board, computer chips and the soldering iron. Solder the chips on to the board. Here is how I want it done.' If modelling the tasks works then the fading process begins. If the person is fearful or unable to perform either the job tasks or non-job tasks, then the performance mediator is advised to be directive, using either partial guidance or full guidance along with verbal instruction. Full guidance involves physically directing the client's motions to complete the task step. Partial guidance is a slow fading of the hands-on guidance, yet remains very directive. This is a highly structured support arrangement. The performance mediator tells the client what to do without much explanation as to why. If the person is able to master this level of support, the performance mediator then begins to challenge the client to perform more independently. The prompt level moves to shadowing and verbal redirection. Shadowing is essentially looking over the shoulder of the client to watch detail by detail how the task is being completed. When the client is off course, the performance mediator first verbally redirects using non-specific verbal prompting such as: 'Are you completing the step properly?' If that does not work, the performance mediator gives specific verbal instruction such as: 'Pick up the green chip and solder it to the board.' If the performance remains off course, then the mediator moves on to gesture and verbal instruction: 'Look at the box with green chips' (pointing to the box), 'Pick up the green resistor and solder it to the board' (pointing). If the client is able to perform well with the above prompts, then the performance mediator moves to the next level. The client may be asked: 'What needs to be done next? Let's figure out together how you will get the job done and what it will look like when it's done.'

During the last phase of performance mediation as an alter ego, the performance mediator reviews the success to date, confirms the self-confidence of the client and assesses the mastery of the job task. Together, the performance mediator and client agree that the level of support provided will be on an as needed basis. It is agreed upon that whenever possible, the request for assistance will be generated by the client instead of the performance mediator shadowing every move. Performance objectives are set and agreed upon. The client then begins self-management with the usual and customary level of supervision received by coworkers.

Over the course of serving as a performance mediator, there will be times when apparent setbacks will occur. The set backs may be a:

1 Reflection of learning struggles as the client masters new skills.

2 Communication that task or skill levels are beyond reach.
3 Developmental transitions as skills, awareness and life circumstances evolve or change.
4 Conscious or unconscious attempts by the client to signal to the performance mediator that something is wrong in the relationship and/or type of help given.
5 Conscious or unconscious pressure from the family system or significant others not to change but to continue as a symptom bearer.
6 A combination of these factors.

Performance mediators need support in understanding that setbacks are a natural part of the change process and not a reflection of failure by the performance mediator or client. If the performance mediation is administered properly, then the client will move on despite the occasional parade of symptoms. Although the focus is on job tasks, a similar methodology is taught for incorporating social skills, cultural expectations and ancillary job routines.

Efficacy During the course of support, a time emerges when the client experiences the ability to have a positive impact on others. For example, the client may buy lunch for the performance mediator. This gift-giving process is important to support and accept gracefully. It usually signals the person is no longer feeling one-down. The generosity, expressed through gift giving, is a reflection that the client is feeling 'wealthy' with positive self-images and identity. Now preoccupation with nurturing oneself can move toward nurturing and caring for others. The ability to evoke positive outcomes for others is a milestone in developing a sense of self as worthwhile (Wolf, 1988).

Adversity The relationship between the performance mediator and the client reaches a milestone when both parties begin to deal openly with conflict and differences. As the client's sense of self crystallizes and takes shape, the performance mediator begins to provide tender opposition. By taking a different point of view on issues, the performance mediator is giving messages to the client on several levels. One message is that there are different points of view and not everyone is like the client. It causes the person to begin thinking beyond their egocentric understanding of the world and others. It requires the client to stop, look and listen to others in order to develop a clearer sense of the situation. The adversarial process further clarifies the sense of self by highlighting 'me, not me' awareness. It further promotes compare-and-contrast thinking and how to synthesize contrasting positions into a workable whole.

Perhaps the strongest message that is communicated is the belief in the abilities of the client (Wolf, 1988). At some level, the client experiences the shift in the relationship as a rite of passage. In a way, it is experienced as a social diploma from the performance mediator that certifies the client is a capable person and can begin standing on her or his own. It facilitates the process of separation–individuation.

Framework for learning The framework for learning represents the basic structure, ground rules and agreements between the performance mediator and client. Areas covered within the agreement may include but are not limited to:

1 Time and location of performance mediation learning and related counsel.
2 Content areas targeted for learning.
3 Type and level of work expected of client, including contingencies if performance standards are not achieved.
4 Reciprocal responsibilities each party is expected to fulfill to make the process work.
5 Issues considered relevant and non-relevant for the performance mediation relationship and process.
6 Style of performance mediation including how truth and candor will be expressed by both parties.
7 Confidentiality issues.
8 How to handle conflict and disagreements.
9 Nature of relationship following the completion of the performance mediation.
(Langs, 1982)

This framework provides a container and holding environment to nurture the growth of the client while serving as a charter for the expected work products of the process. When the performance mediation process drifts off course, the agreement serves as a tool to realign the efforts of both parties. Symptoms of trouble in the performance mediation process usually reflect a violation of the agreement by one or both parties (Langs, 1982). Some agreements are formal, with written documents, reporting schedules, and related formal control systems. Many performance mediation relationships are informal. They are based on a personal commitment.

Regulation and control of drives, affects and impulses

The regulation and control cognitive operations are concerned with the adaptive management and channelling of physiological drives, emotional and affective states, impulses and frustration tolerance (Bellak and Small, 1978). Regulation and control is not only concerned with holding back impulses and behaviours but also with over control and inhibition. This cognitive function has a highly interdependent relationship with other functions and phases of cognition.

Lack of proper modulation may interfere with the gathering of information during the input phase. If the person is impulse ridden, it can be expected the person is not involved in systematic exploratory scanning. Information is episodic and fragmented. Over control may result in insufficient data collection. Both states could interfere with learning, memory, rational thought and difficulty in the realm of social cognition. Errors in judgment are likely to emerge resulting in development of a series of failure experiences in major learning, working and social domains (Lovett, 1985). This, in turn, results in a poorly formed self-concept leading to a self-fulfilling prophecy destined to repeated failure. Physical well-being and safety are potentially put at serious risk. The ability to form attachments to other people and situations may result in faulty interdependence and lack of collaboration with others. This leads to a life of social isolation and the emergence of egocentric communication modalities further separating the individual from the ability to function in socially valued roles. The person may be in a constant state of instability rigidity. Either position harms learning, skill development and the ability to achieve valued performance.

Enhancing this cognitive component is achieved through multiple means. If the root cause is physiological, then a variety of medications may serve to inhibit, stabilize or open channels adaptively. It may be that the cognitive function that regulates stimulus-barrier control may need concurrent strength-

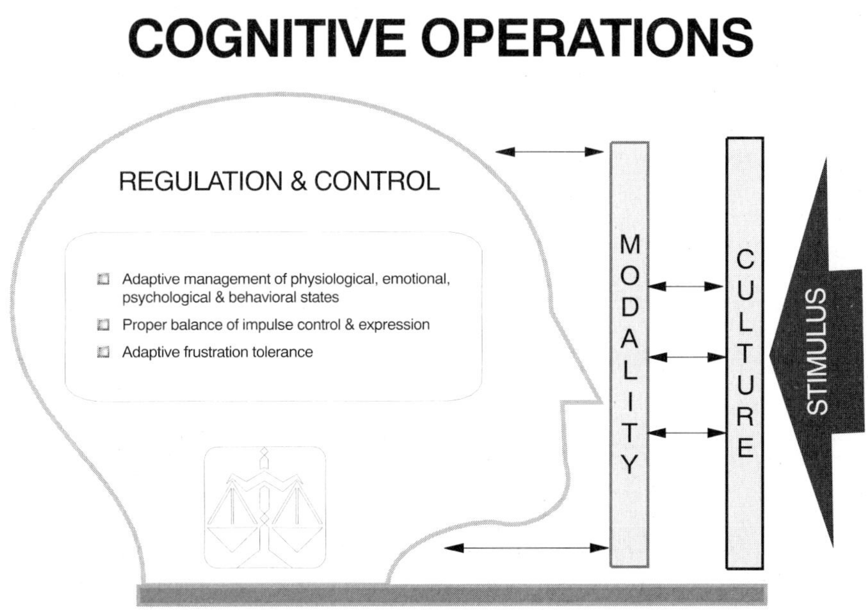

Figure 8.13 Regulation and control.

ening. From a behavioural standpoint, providing consistent structure, boundaries, and performance support mediates learning and development of this and other cognitive functions to adaptive levels. Choosing the type of environment conducive to learning may play a critical role. If the person is prone to over stimulation, more quiet, less busy information environments may be needed. This function can be enhanced by working with the person proactively to identify early warning signs that impulses are beginning to accelerate or become inhibited to levels that result in malfunctioning. Compensatory mechanisms can then be taught that aid the person to develop self-management skills. Anything from removing oneself from the situation, taking a walk, counting to ten, talking to a designated person, and biofeedback devices – and these are but a few examples. These procedures are surface-management techniques that interrupt the cycle. They need to be normative to the situation. Using a biofeedback device in the middle of a social situation may be awkward and stigmatizing. Arranging to take a brief break and use a private area may be more suitable. After the interrupt mechanism is taught, the person learns adaptive problem solving procedures.

Thought processes

Thought process operations are concerned with relating and manipulating two or more units of information through a variety of activities such as: comparing, computing, compounding, ordering, organizing, abstracting, generalizing, concept forming, analysing, reasoning, synthesizing, judging and planning. Thought is generally referred to as:

- concrete or abstract
- primary process or secondary process
- rigid or flexible
- dualistic, multiplistic or relativistic

(Bellak and Small, 1978; Knefelkamp *et al.*, 1978).

The level of abstraction is defined by the distance between the cognitive process and the object or event being acted upon. For example, sorting clothes in a thrift shop is more concrete than speculating and imaging the various categories of clothing that may be useful to sell in six months. Abstract thinking involves representing and manipulating information in more general, conceptual and representational terms. For example, at an abstract level, clothes may be viewed a representing units revenue. At a concrete level, clothes may be understood as a blouse or pair of trousers.

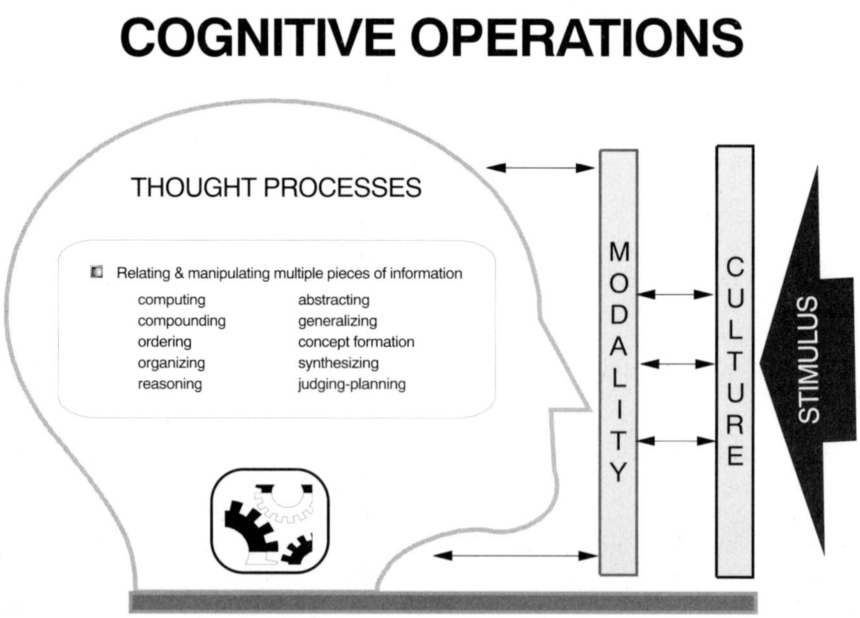

Figure 8.14 Thought processes.

Abstract thinking involves hypothetical reasoning that entertains what is possible rather than staying with the obvious 'as is' way of understanding. Managed health care can be viewed as a concrete cost containment tool. At an abstract level, it may represent a larger trend of replacing democracy with capitalism as a form of governance.

At the concrete level, individuals tend to not infer or generalize beyond the specific circumstance, to broader categories. For example, teaching conflict resolution skills to a concrete thinker would involve instructions such as: 'When he yells at you, tell him to stop it. Tell him you won't talk to him until he can stop yelling and be nice to you. Wait until he feels better before you talk. Don't talk to him when he is still angry and upset.'

With an abstract thinker, broader understanding is used. For example, in teaching concepts such as conflict resolution, instructions might be:

> The object of conflict resolution is not to win over another person. It is to form a collaborate bond to seek win-win solutions. So, when he yells at you, let him know you want to respond but not while he is in an agitated state. Once he settles down, set up a time to get together to discuss his concerns. When you do get together, let him know his needs are important to you. When you begin your discussion, ask him what's really going on? Ask where his disappointment or anxiety is coming from. Ask how you can best help him with his concerns. Don't shame him. Decide how the both of you can communicate in constructive, mutually supporting ways when under stress. Make it clear, verbally attacking you is not acceptable.

To enhance cognitive performance requires understanding the degree of abstract thinking the person is capable of managing combined with the preference of the person for abstract or concrete thinking. Intellectually, a person may be very astute and bright, yet may prefer to remain at the surface level with most issues. Generally, the more concrete the thinking, the more restricted are the sources for solutions and the more bound the person is to the present time frame. Concrete thinking leads to very practical solutions that fit the immediate circumstance. Abstract thinking, on the other hand, is less bound to the present. It may lead to root-cause problem solving that results in potentially more sweeping solutions. Or, it may lead to impractical solutions for the moment.

Primary-process thinking typically refers to loose, fragmented associations and connections between information that is more dreamlike in nature and does not appear to follow a linear, rational logic with the current reality of the external situation. Generally, it operates at a more free-floating, unconscious level. Secondary thinking is more associated with conscious, controlled, linear, rational and logical extrapolation (e.g. 'If this, then that. . .'). It builds on a consensual mutuality with other people and surrounding events.

Rigidity and flexibility of thought refer to the ability to be open to alternative perspectives. The more rigid the thinking-process style, the less open the person is to changes in the environment. Adjustments and adaptations are blocked. Interpretations of information are forced into categories and relationships that may not fit the uniqueness of the situation. Flexibility is related to entertaining and exploring new relationships of information, possibly resulting in new patterns of thinking. Flexibility opens the door to evolutionary thinking, whereas, rigidity in thinking maintains the status quo.

Memory, learning and recall After the registration activities of the input phase, information moves into immediate short-term memory called primary memory. Primary memory is the 'working memory' (Lekak, 1976). It enables a person to respond to immediate events. Primary memory is a conscious process. The person is actively aware of the content and its application. It lasts from 30 seconds to several minutes. Primary memory can be sustained for hours through continuous rehearsal, prompting and application. The information contained in the primary memory may be converted to long-term memory or it may disintegrate. This is, in part, dependent on the ability of the person's electrophysiological system to convert it into a more stable biochemical imprint. The primary memory relies upon reverberating neural circuits. An extended short-term memory exists that can maintain the memory trace for a few hours or up to several days (Lekak, 1976). Training plays a role in facilitating this effect.

The information contained in this type of memory is unstable and vulnerable to interference from competing factors.

Both forms of immediate short-term memory are of interest to the practitioner. By designing and implementing appropriate cues, supports, training and accommodations, individuals can successfully function with basic work tasks that may have previously considered off limits. This is true even if the person does not understand how all the bits of information form a more abstract process or whole.

For example, a person may have a severe intellectual impairment and still be able to perform a five-step process to wash dishes in a restaurant. This may be accomplished through the use of visual prompts. The sequence of steps necessary to complete the task are drawn or photographed one at a time. The visual prompt shows the client successfully executing each step. The pictures are placed in a clear vinyl envelope. Each picture is then put on a ring binder that allows the pictures to be continuously turned revealing the next picture in the sequence. The individual turns to each picture and copies the activity. When the sequence is completed, the person starts all over again.

The work environment may need to be adapted to avoid distractions that may disrupt immediate and extended short-term memory. For example, a client with intellectual impairment worked in a hotel restaurant washing dishes. During periods of high volume, tray after tray accumulated in the dishwashing area. The employer and practitioner designed a reasonable accommodation to buffer the load on the client. First, a rubber screen with flaps was placed in the area where the trays of dishes arrive. The screen blocked the sight of the dishes piling up. The flaps on the screen allowed the dishwasher to reach through and take one tray at a time. The client was protected from being over stimulated by the sight of the mounting pile of dishes. Secondly, the client was given a tape of soothing music that had a calming, upbeat mood. A waterproof cassette player with earphones was also provided. The client was taught to listen to the tape while washing the dishes during the busy peak periods. The screen and taped music served as stimulus barrier controls. They protected and soothed the person during stress situations that customarily would have overwhelmed the cognitive performance of the individual. The third part of the design involved arranging temporary assignment of other kitchen staff. They sorted and arranged the incoming dishes into trays. Then they lined up the trays for the client to pull through the screen. Help was also provided with putting away clean dishes during this brief period. This allowed the client to stay successfully focused on one major task. These minor accommodations resulted in a long-term, loyal employee. The intervention saved the company $4500 a year by reducing the need constantly to rehire or pay overtime for absent workers. They also received a valued service from the client.

Primary memory is followed by long-term or secondary memory (Lekak, 1976). If the individual is capable, information that has been gathered is consolidated into a pattern that is stored. Secondary memory is stored and organized by the personal meaning the information has to the individual. This may include information such as the steps necessary to cook a favourite meal, appropriate behaviours on the bus to one's work or how to read another person's intentions to see if they want to be friends. This is much different from the way information is organized and held in primary memory. Primary memory relies upon a storage system that clusters information together by sensory properties such as similar sounds, shapes or colors (Lekak, 1976). Short-term memory serves as a storage bin for immediate information and use.

Long-term memory, on the contrary, takes information and retains it for later recall and application in the same or similar situations. It expands the power of the initial information by creating a web of associations and linkages. For persons with cognitive impairments, generalization may prove to be too difficult. When this is the case, compensatory mechanisms, prompts, and related supports are designed into the job.

Adaptive regression

Adaptive regression is a cognitive operation that deals with the process of controlled, partial lowering of cognitive functions for the purpose of creativity, imagination, enjoyment and relaxation. It is the ability to:

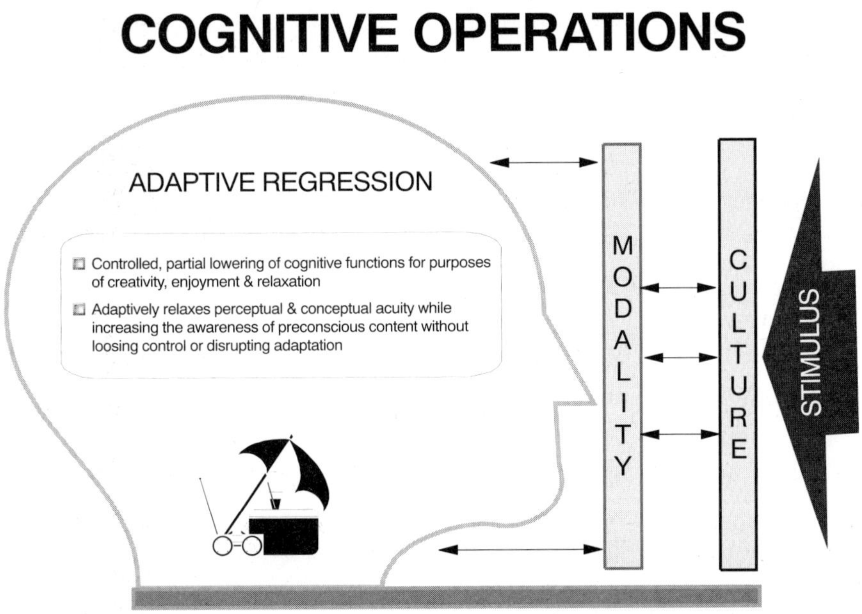

Figure 8.15 Adaptive regression

1 Adaptively relax perceptual and conceptual acuity while increasing the awareness of previously preconscious and unconscious contents without loosing control or disrupting adaptation.
2 Use primary-process thinking in a controlled manner to induce new configurations.
3 Increase adaptive potential as a result of creative integrations of primary process with secondary process thinking.
(Bellak and Small, 1978)

At the level of dysfunction, individuals may regress too frequently and to a degree that disrupts adaptive performance. A client may be so carried away with their own fantasies that there is a disruption in occupational performance. A person may also be unable to loosen and lower cognitive functioning. This might result in performing in a humourless, unimaginative, obsessional manner. Enjoyment is perceived as a threat. Spontaneous performance is defended against.

During the phase of relaxing control of cognitive functions, there may be an increased awareness of previously inaccessible feelings or thoughts that may overwhelm or frighten a client. For persons struggling to maintain secondary-process thinking, strengthening the ability to move away from regression is encouraged. Structured, obsessive concrete tasks that require an external focus and concentration are developed. This might include routinized activities such as stamp collecting, basic mathematical computations, sorting and classifying items, calligraphy, sign or letter painting, clock repair, cataloguing, data entry, library work and other related activities. A calm and stable environment may be required to avoid over stimulation.

To loosen and relax perceptual acuity, activities associated with art, biofeedback relaxation, guided imagery, artistic expression or similar activities, including an increase in leisure and recreation endeavours may facilitate performance. Participating on creative projects with other fun-loving, creative people may help the person relax, experience joy and feel support while learning through role models.

Various cognitive techniques can facilitate adaptive regression and creative thinking. A representative, yet not all inclusive list includes:

- successive abstraction
- reframing
- analogy and metaphor
- wishful thinking

- non-logical stimuli
- reversals
- brainstorming
- trigger sessions
- round robin
- wildest idea
  (Rickhards, 1974)

Successive abstraction involves varying the level of abstraction to give a different slant on the same subject. For example, a firm involved with lawn care may want to develop a new mowing machine. 'Developing a new lawnmower' is the point of departure. The next level of abstraction might be, 'Developing a grass-cutting machine', followed by, 'Developing a grass-shaping device', eventually leading the 'Methods of restricting the growth of grass'. This last abstraction may turn the solution away from development of a machine to inventing a hybrid grass that only grows to a certain height, thereby doing away for the need of a machine and seeking a biological solution instead.

Reframing changes the perspective of how to define the issue. The classic reframe involves looking at a setback as really an opportunity. Analogy and metaphor redefine the issue in less linear terms, thus promoting flexibility. The statement, 'Getting our service system ready for the twenty-first century is like preparing for life on a space station,' is an example of an analogy. It stresses the similarity of events from which new insights may emerge. 'This person is in a sea of opportunity' is a metaphor. It uses a phrase or word typically associated with something else to describe the current issue. The association is implicit and opens doors to see the situation from a different light. Wishful thinking uses fantasy to open the door to creativity. 'Building an artificial cow' may give insight on how to develop alternative forms of protein. Non-logical stimuli take a random stimulus and challenge the thinker to find a solution using knowledge of the stimulus. For example, a practitioner may instruct a client as follows: 'Tell me how the Venetian blinds on the window can help us figure out what to do next.' Reversals turn a situation or issue upside down and then looks for alternative ways to frame the challenge and search for solutions. For example, a loss may be seen instead as a new beginning. A verbal fight with a coworker may not indicate distance between each other. It may indicate each person is much closer than expected. Brainstorming and round robin seek to build on ideas generated by others. New connections and points of view emerge that a single person may never have entertained alone. Wildest idea takes issues and ideas to an extreme position to open insight: 'Libraries ought to serve as multi-purpose information centres and not just for books.' For example: 'What if the libraries had interactive video terminals that allowed access to a command-and-control centre. At the centre were customer service representatives that could dialogue with the person to obtain various forms of information regarding the services, resources and activities available throughout the metropolitan area. The customer service representatives would include persons that spoke a variety of languages, such as Spanish. All the person had to do was push a button for language preference and a representative would come online and provide help or answer questions.' This wild idea may open thinking to how a local government and business, schools and other participants could combine and consolidate resources to develop a more user-friendly, efficient and effective information support system for its local citizens.

In addition to the cognitive enhancement techniques, medication may be an option to alleviate under or over control for persons with severe challenges in this area. At milder levels, psychotherapy, counselling, and performance mediation may serve as a source of support to resolve underlying issues interfering with adaptive functioning.

During the phase of reintegration of the newly discovered material, the use of analogies, brainstorming and assignments with a partner or performance mediator may help to draw creative linkages between information. Using techniques that rely upon creative problem solving techniques, facilitate linking novel ideas with reasoning. It may be helpful for the person to connect with someone that can draw out the creative ideas and then connect with another person that is more practical and logical in nature.

Defensive functioning

Defensive operations involve the utilization of a variety of cognitive mechanisms to cope with

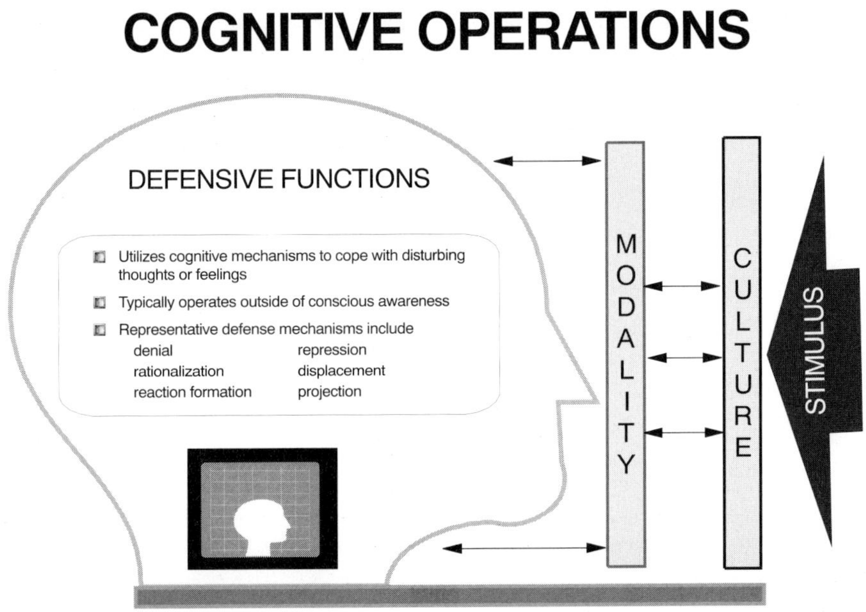

Figure 8.16 Defensive functions.

disturbing thoughts or feelings. Defences range from denial, rationalization, reaction formation, repression, displacement, undoing, projection, and a whole host of other related psychological processes. Defences typically operate outside and beyond conscious awareness. They are automatically employed to gain resolution of emotional conflict, relief from emotional tension and to prevent or mediate anxiety (Bellak and Small, 1978; Langs, 1982).

An individual in a strong co-dependent relationship may harbour deep anger and resentment toward another. The thought of displaying anger directly is unacceptable. There is an underlying fear of reprisal and loss of the relationship. At an unconscious level, the person engages in a defensive posture to block the expression of the true thoughts and feelings. Instead, the other person is idealized and praised. The distortion may be temporarily adaptive. Yet, if the conflict is serious, the blockage will eventually erupt through any variety of symptoms, including physical, emotional, psychological, and behavioural disorders.

Strategies for enhancing adaptive defensive functioning focus on:

1 Broadening the range of defences available for use.
2 Modifying existing defences.
3 Resolving the underlying conflicts so that needs can be met in a healthier way.

Defensive mechanisms *per se*, are not dysfunctional. It is when they are over-, under- or misapplied to the detriment of the individual that performance remediation may be required. Providing a stable and secure interpersonal holding environment opens the door to feeling safe, developing self-awareness, identifying defensive patterns and exploring alternatives.

The concept of embeddedness assists in understanding the process for modifying defences (Kegan, 1982). A person is typically caught up in day-to-day coping. While in the middle of manoeuvring through activities of daily living, it becomes easy to loose perspective on 'how' one actually is going about the business of living in the moment. Getting distance from the moment through reflection develops self-awareness regarding patterns of behaviour. When one's behavioural pattern is recognized and defined, it becomes the object of self-attention. Once it is an objective of attention, a person is in a position to use the information to emerge from the current state of embeddedness and begin to choose alternative coping mechanisms.

Generally, clients move between four basic states that influence the degree of receptivity to modification of defences. They are:

1 complacence
2 overconfidence
3 trouble
4 growth.

Complacence is a state in which a person feels satisfied with the results achieved through the current pattern of coping. Although defence mechanisms may not be fully adaptive to the reality of the situation, the outcomes achieved by their use are good enough for the moment. The motivation to change is low in this state.

The state of overconfidence signals that the person feels more than satisfied with results achieved by the current configuration of defences and sees no reason or need to change. This may reflect the reality of the situation or it may be a false reading. The person may be:

1 not thinking ahead
2 in high level of denial
3 setting their sights too low.

Trouble is a state in which thoughts and feelings are sufficiently uncomfortable and unsetting that there is a motivation to move away from the pain and move toward a more comfortable circumstance. Modifying defensive mechanisms is perceived as a way to remove the cause of trouble. Motivation is higher in this state. The perceived degree of urgency drives the strength of the motivation. A state of trouble takes precedence over a state of growth.

Growth is the state in which current results do not match desired outcomes. Modification of defence mechanisms is seen as a way to close the gap. The person is not avoiding pain but approaching a state of being 'better or best'. Motivation is very high.

To modify the state of overconfidence, the intervention ranges from subtle and indirect to a frontal confrontation of the position. A massive dose of reality can open the person to consider alternative forms of coping, such as witnessed in a family intervention with a member involved in alcohol dependency. Persons in this mode do not welcome information that may indicate they have been reading the situation incorrectly.

Overwhelming the person is not the usual and customary approach used by a practitioner. More frequently, a gradual process takes place in which a trusting relationship is developed that clearly communicates a respect for the person's sense of pride and autonomy. Non-patronizing mirroring and confirmation of the worth are administered. Carefully, there is probing of the facade. After time has been spent in repeated non-threatening exchanges and relationship building, questions are asked that centre around any conflicting observations and evidence regarding self-disclosed perceptions. For example, a practitioner might say: 'Bill, how comfortable are you with your supervisor and coworkers? You feel everything is fine. Both you and your work are well received. It's good to hear everything is going well for you. I am curious about a couple of issues. Do I have your permission to ask a few questions? I noticed your supervisor shook his head and looked away when you handed over your work for the day? What do you think he meant by that? Why do you think all your coworkers eat at a different table and don't invite you to join them? Are you open to exploring what might be going on?' It is essential the person feels accepted and supported, because confronting overconfidence may require dealing with the person's hidden sense of shame and doubt.

Gradually, the person begins to see contradictions. As the evidence begins to mount, the person is asked to account for the differences. This gentle and yet firm reality testing begins to move the person away from overconfidence and toward trouble or growth states. As painful as it might be, a client usually appreciates having a trusted person gently hold their feet to the fire of reality within the context of a non-judgemental relationship. The client feels comfort in the notion that difficult issues can be discussed openly without fear. This is all dependent on the level of denial the person is experiencing. High levels of denial require a process by which the practitioner:

1 Waits for a major failure or pattern of accelerating failures.
2 Chooses a strategy to work around or compensate for the rigidity of the defence.
3 Establishes environmental conditions that reduce the need to use the dysfunctional defence.

4 Makes arrangements for the person to receive intensive clinical support to work through deep-seated conflicts.

Complacency is managed in a similar fashion, yet the degree of opposition to change is less deeply rooted in shame and doubt. It is more focused on uncertainty regarding potential loss of that which is familiar, tried and true. Modifying defences may be perceived as a threat, yet this can be overcome by:

1 Assisting the person to see growth opportunities or pending trouble.
2 Pressure from a respected peer.
3 Revealing and demonstrating discrepancies that are not already perceived.

Stimulus barrier control

Stimulus barrier control operations involve:

1 Registration of external and internal stimuli impinging upon sensory modalities.
2 Sensitivity to the stimuli.
3 Threshold for the stimuli.
4 The degree of adaptation, organization and integration of responses to the sensory stimulation.
(Bellak and Small, 1978; Lekak, 1976; Mirsky, 1987).

Stimulus barrier control additionally reflects the resiliency of a person to readaptation after stress and impingements are no longer present. Flexible, automatic fluctuations in thresholds to stimulus facilitate optimal operation across a variety of situations. Stimulus barrier control serves as the precursor to defence mechanisms and serves as the primary inborn defence.

Stimulus barrier control can over-restrict the flow of sensory information or not filter it well enough, as with persons with autism. Individuals can also be under stimulated. Living an isolated disability lifestyle, where most of a person's time is spent with other people with disability and paid care givers, within a sheltered and segregated environment, offers little real stimulation related to the world of the local community. This cut-off reinforces the unproductive and maladaptive aspects of a disability. Stimulus barrier control may be inherently intact, but sheltered by external forces, thereby artificially restricting the type of stimulation required for appropriate cognitive mapping.

Environmental arrangements can enhance or interfere with functioning. Settings that are bombarded with sound, activity, or people may cause disruption in cognitive functioning.

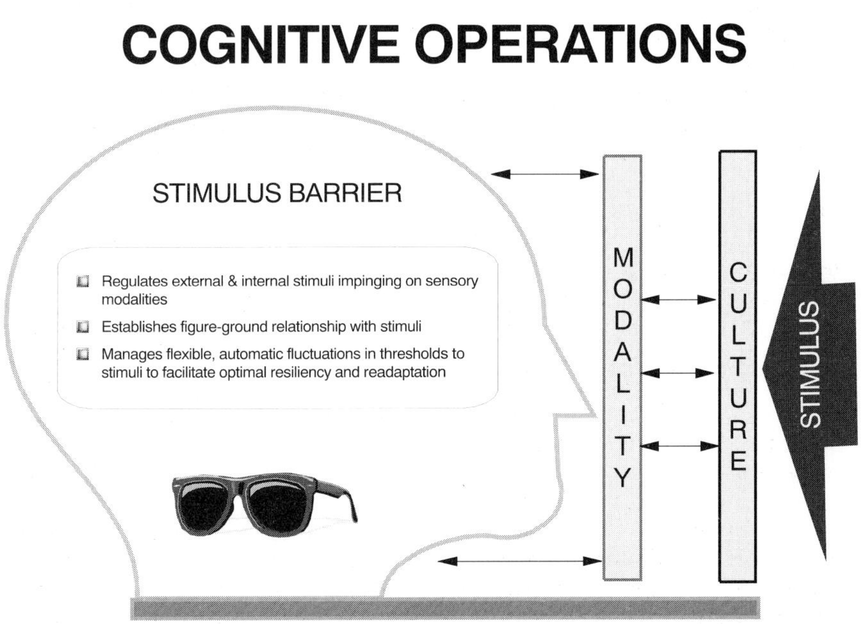

Figure 8.17 Stimulus barrier.

For example, a client with autism obtained a job as a clerical assistant in an insurance company. She worked in the claims department. The operations were laid out in a very open arrangement with all desks in one large room. The client was very sensitive to sound, light and the activity of others. Arrangements were made for her to work in an enclosed office just off the main floor. The office had been used as the mail and photocopy room. The mail and photocopy operations were moved to an area in the main room, against a wall and surrounded by dividers. To prevent social isolation, a quiet office mate was selected by the client and work supervisor. Lighting was changed from overhead fixtures to desk lamps. These minor adjustments decreased sensory stressors that would normally have interfered with successful performance.

Another client worked in a sports arena as a custodian. He had worked for the sports complex for five years as a custodial engineer prior to a work-related accident. A tool box fell on his head from the edge of a stair in a stairwell. He had left his tools on a flight of stairs just above his work area. The box was inadvertently knocked off the stair as two other workers were moving a long set of seats up to the next level. It fell down to the next flight, striking the client. It resulted in a traumatic brain injury. He was out of work for nine months before returning. He loved his job. His relationship with his employer and supervisor were excellent. The company was committed to help him return to work with modified duties. Previously, he worked very independently. Now, he needed more structure and narrower responsibilities. His duties focused on cleaning and maintaining a section of the arena before, during and after the events. His work hours were mainly during the sports and entertainment events by his request. He loved being with the fans and surrounded by the excitement of the event. This had been a dream job for him. After his first month back on the job, he told his supervisor that there were 'too many personalities' in the crowd when he worked the events. He was in sensory overload with the high volume of customer contact, the loud noise and all the activity surrounding him. As a result of his injury, his stimulus barrier control concerning threshold levels and his ability to organize and integrate stimuli had been significantly lowered. After careful consideration, arrangements were made for him to work before and after events to reduce the stimulus overload. Because of his love of the home teams and the pleasure he experienced by being around the entertainment attractions, he had his hours structured to work during home-team practice time and when the entertainment attraction were rehearsing.

A proper job match is critical. Jobs do not operate in a vacuum. Careful consideration of the influence of environmental factors on cognitive functioning is important and imperative. Everything including invisible stimuli such as sound, colour, odour, humidity, vibration and temperature need to be considered when designing an intervention to enhance cognitive functioning.

Autonomous functioning

Autonomous functioning is activities that support the input, elaboration and expressive phases of cognition. They are concerned with the degree of freedom from impairment of processes at primary and secondary levels of cognition. Primary process activities include:

- attention
- concentration
- tracking
- memory
- learning
- perception
- hearing, vision, speech, motor expression and related sensory functions.

Secondary process activities include:

- habit patterns
- learned complex skills
- work and activities of daily living routines
- other higher order cognitive functions.
  (Bellak and Small, 1978; Lekak, 1976; Mirsky, 1987)

Attention is the process of focusing on a part of the environment, as well as internal states. It involves alertness, selectivity and limited processing. Alertness is the process of proactive and reactive readiness to encounter stimuli and respond accordingly. Selectivity involves focusing on stimuli that are considered relevant and essential. Limited processing is concerned with the initial registration of stimuli that is passed on for more

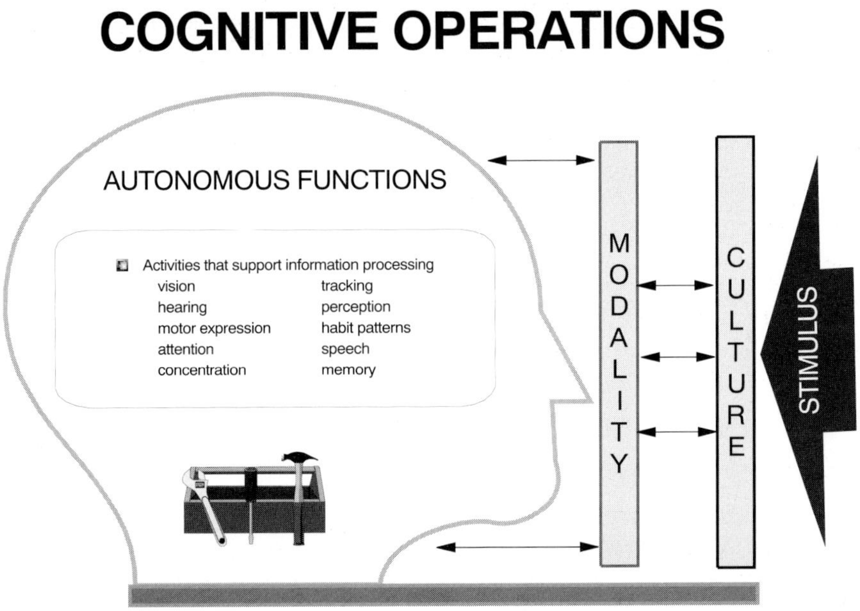

Figure 8.18 Autonomous functions.

thorough cognitive manipulation. Subfunctions include sustaining the focus for an appreciable period of time and adaptively shifting from one aspect of the environment to another. Concentration is a deliberate and heighten state of attention in which non-relevant stimuli are selectively excluded from conscious awareness. Tracking involves the process of attentively following a stimulus over a period of time, such as visual tracking or concentration on a directed train of thought. Complex tracking involves maintaining two or more ideas or stimulus patterns simultaneously and sequentially without confusing or losing the information. Enhancing this cognitive component is accomplished through a full range of interventions, from medication for attention deficit and psychiatric disorders, to prosthetic devices, behavioural training, and environmental accommodations.

Mastery and competence

Mastery and competence operations are concerned with the acquisition and application of skills across a variety of age-appropriate life tasks, including employment. The function is concerned with the degree of active striving and expertise in dealing with environmental challenges and situations, overcoming obstacles and actualizing potential (Bellak and Small, 1978; Kegan, 1982). Motivation to exert effort is influenced by personal expectations for success and certainty in one's ability. A person may have a realistic, exaggerated or undervalued sense of competency.

Realistic self-assessment indicates good judgement, intact reality testing and a healthy self-concept. Enhancing cognitive performance is focused on:

1 Identifying preferences and skill development needs.
2 Skill acquisition training.
3 Support to ensure successful implementation and maintenance of gains.

When the subjective feeling states are overinflated or undervalued, then self-assessments are unrealistic. An unrealistic self-assessment is not automatically dysfunctional. An inflated sense of competency may serve as a self-soothing defence mechanism that actually helps a person face difficult situations. When an undervalued sense of competency exists, a person may learn to take a cautionary, conservative approach to situations. Neither of these unrealistic self-assessments warrant professional attention. If an inflated sense of competency puts the individual at risk, then

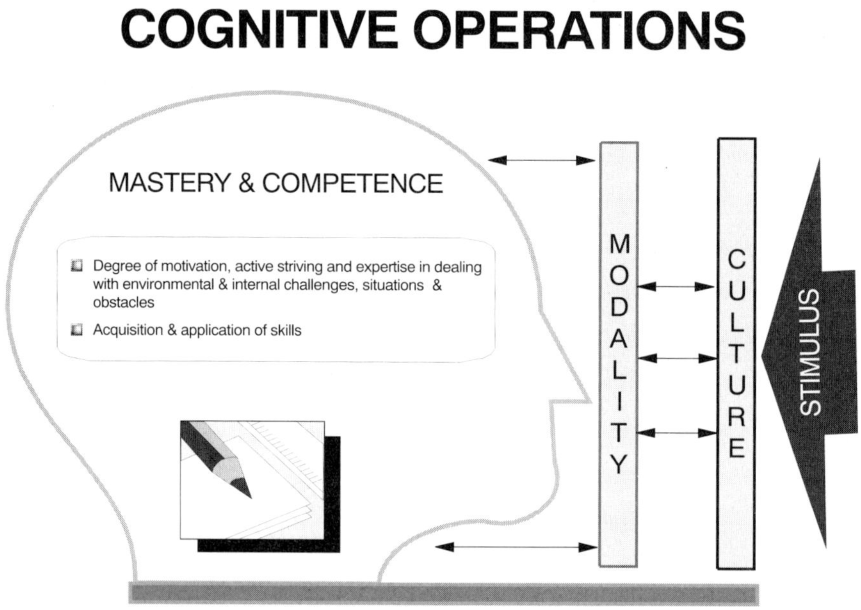

Figure 8.19 Mastery and competence.

an intervention is required. Guiding the person toward a more realistic self-assessment will not be taken kindly. The individual may need to learn through experience. After several difficult or failed situations, the person may be more open to requesting help. If the person is at severe risk, then a confrontational style may be appropriate.

More typically, a practitioner will encounter unrealistic career ambitions. For example, a worker with an industrial injury may see an advertisement on television for computer technician training. Although there may be no indication of aptitude or tolerance for disciplined training, the person may insist on pursuing the career track. Facilitating the exploration of client-driven aspirations, without being critical or harsh, promotes more realistic career objectives. It reduces the power struggle between the practitioner and client. Giving control to the client frequently results in more mature career choices. However, if judgement is severely impaired, then a more directive, reality testing process may be required. Using behaviour modification strategies that target reinforcing more appropriate choices can further facilitate the process by shaping client responses that move toward realistic self-assessment.

Clients that have an undervalued sense of competency may not be confident or may be using the one-down position for secondary gain. This may include:

- avoiding responsibility
- fulfilling a need to be comforted and affirmed
- punishing oneself
- fear of separation, loss, independence or success.

The undervalued sense of competency may also stem from a lack of exposure to successful and unsuccessful experiences. Guided exposure and experience supplemented with mirroring and other forms of affirmation can build confidence and enhance performance. When self-deprecation is at pathological levels, referral for treatment is indicated to supplement performance support at a work site.

Receiving social support from a significant person or group enhances mastery and competence when there is:

- a high degree of cohesiveness in the relationship
- anticipation of social, emotional and utilitarian gain

- norm-setting communication from the significant other.
(Janis, 1982)

A relationship has to be motivating in order to influence performance. Motivational influence is acquired by eliminating or reducing client fears of being exploited, dominated, ridiculed or rejected while building the perception of the significant other(s) as a dependable and competent source of self-esteem enhancement. The power of influence is increased when any shortcomings of the client are framed as a result of situational factors instead of inherent, irreversible traits. Influence is further enhanced by:

- Making directive statements that endorse specific actions.
- Eliciting commitment to a recommended course.
- Providing selective positive feedback on performance that moves toward achievement of targeted goals.
- Insisting the client take personal responsibility.
- Giving reassurances that both support and resources will remain available.
(Janis, 1982)

Synthetic–integrative functioning
Synthetic–integrative operations serve as a superordinate cognitive operation that brings together the discrete cognitive components into a cohesive, harmonious and flexible whole system (Bellak and Small, 1978). There is adaptive reconciliation of contradictions and inconsistencies between feelings, thoughts and behaviours. Cognitive components untie under a common purpose to achieve objectives successfully within the context of person–environment dynamics. Dynamic disequilibrium is harnessed and leveraged, not eliminated.

When synthetic–integrative functioning is not successful, there is fragmentation of cognitive operations that result in activities such as:

- disorganized behaviour
- absence of consistent goal-focused planning
- piecemeal and inconsistent performance outcomes
- fluctuations in emotional states without self-awareness
- immobilization
- discrepant self-representations
- conflict-ridden experiences

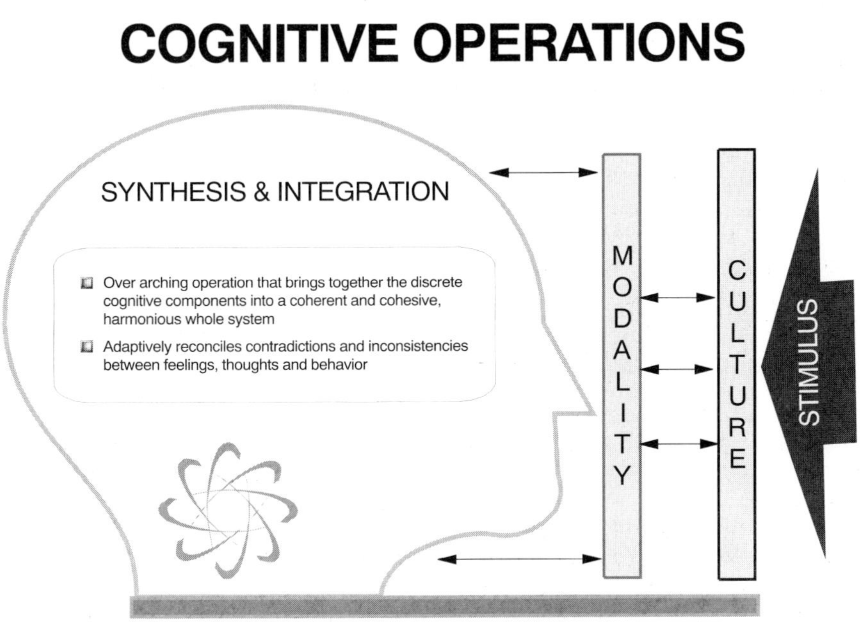

Figure 8.20 Synthesis and integration.

- high degrees of ambivalence
- inability to tolerate ambiguous situations
- gravitation to extremist positions, beliefs and groups.

Enhancing this cognitive function begins with strengthening the other operations, combined with establishment of a constant and consistent relationship with a significant other, such as a supervisor, coworker, performance mediator, counsellor, therapist or practitioner. Through the consistent relationship, a holding environment can be established between the helper and helpee. Within this framework, the helper facilitates the person's ability to target priorities, focus on strengthening and developing other cognitive functions, planning, problem solving, self-learning and emotional support.

Suggestions may also be made to decrease or restructure exposure to stressors or burdens. For example, an individual may move from a 40-hour work week, Monday through Friday, to a 25-hour-a-week schedule, Monday, Tuesday, Thursday and Friday. By taking a day off during the middle of the week, a brief break in the pressure is created. Reducing the hours from eight to five per day restructures the duration of job performance to manageable levels. The person discontinues the work day while still feeling successful and without feeling totally depleted.

Another option may be to build more breaks into the day while maintaining the weekly schedule. To reduce the financial concerns of the employer, the client would clock-out for break times that exceeded the norm for the company. Thereby, the client maintains a consistent and normative work schedule, Monday through Friday, yet has each day structured to reduce the number of hours of continuous work and stress.

Partializing the problems and tasks to be accomplished is another support strategy to alleviate a burden. Instead of focusing on the total of what has to be accomplished, the burden is broken down into smaller assignments. For example, instead of the client worrying about what has to be produced for the day, the focus may shift to half-hour increments. This way, the burden is not perceived as overwhelming. The person becomes less fragmented with a narrower performance focus. In more extreme cases, medication may be required to reduce anxiety, depression, attention deficit or other conditions.

Output phase

The output phase represents the range of cognitive operations that result in observable behavioural patterns from communication involving gesturing, speaking, writing, through physical movements and motor coordination, to interpersonal connections and relationships. Even though data may have been adequately gathered in the input phase and appropriately processed in the elaboration phase, difficulty may exist in the expressive output phase (Feuerstein, 1979). A person may be perfectly able to read and understand the content of material but may have great difficulty in expressing these ideas through writing or speaking, as may be witnessed in persons with severe cerebral palsy.

Within the domain of interpersonal relationships, expressive operations include the ability to initiate, maintain and end conversations. Conversational operations include paralinguistic activities such as voice tone, volume, pitch and pace, as well as non-verbal behaviours such as facial expressions, body movements, interpersonal distance and interactive balance.

Although maladaptive functioning may be observed in behavioural expression, the difficulty may be rooted with the prior two phases. All three phases are intimately connected and influence performance. The key is to identify the locus of difficulty. Enhancing cognitive performance within the output phase begins with defining the skill deficit, determining the location or root cause of the deficit and identifying the circumstances under which the deficit is manifested. A deficit is defined not only by physical or cognitive functioning but also by the requirements of the environment. Interventions range from compensatory mechanisms, such as communication boards and environmental manipulations such as reasonable accommodation, to behavioural prompts, modelling, micro-skill instruction, rehearsal and experiential learning.

Level of complexity and efficiency

Level of complexity is partially defined by the quantity and quality of the information contained within a cognitive operation (Feuerstein, 1979). Quantity refers to the number of items being processed. Quality is a function of the degree of novelty of the information. The more familiar the units of information the less complex the cognitive activity. The less familiar the material being processed, the more complex the task becomes. A key to enhancing performance is understanding that individuals of different personality styles, maturity and cognitive complexity experience the same environment differently. Interventions require a delicate balance of challenge and support that builds on the unique needs and world view of the individual. During the process of learning and constructing meaning, individuals tend to move through a series of sequential thinking frameworks that reflect a hierarchical increase in cognitive complexity. These developmental frameworks are:

1 dualism
2 early multiplicity
3 late multiplicity
4 contextual relativism.

Individuals may remain embedded within a developmental framework due to a variety of reasons including inherent capabilities, emotional maturity and quality of mediated learning experiences (Knefelkamp and Cornfeld, 1978).

Dualism

Within the dualistic framework, it is assumed with certainty that 'all' knowledge is known. There are right and wrong answers. The world is seen through a 'black-and-white' filter. Knowledge is viewed as a collection of information. There is only one right answer to any question and only one right way to perform. Information that flows from an authority figure is viewed as fact not conjecture or opinion.

The authority figure, whether a practitioner, work supervisor, instructor, parent or performance mediator is viewed as the source of knowledge. The expected role of the authority figure is to give knowledge to the individual as if handing over the blueprint of absolute and final truth. A good authority figure is equated with complete, accurate knowledge. The authority figure is viewed as the 'knower' of the real truth. The role of the person being helped is to imprint the information provided and demonstrate that the right answers have been learned.

Peers are not valued as a legitimate source of knowledge and learning. Evaluation of learning and performance is directly linked to sense of self. If one has the right answer, then the person is good. If one has the wrong answer, then the person is bad. Evaluation is a clear-cut process of comparing knowledge, skills or performance outcomes to the one absolute and correct standard passed on by the authority figure. There is no tolerance for grey area performance or information. It is viewed as invalid. Anxiety and anger emerge if there is any sense the authority figure is unsure, unclear and not absolutely certain regarding the final truth of the knowledge being taught. The primary intellectual task of the client is basic rote learning of facts and concepts. The dualistic thinker awaits knowledge to be poured into their mind as an unquestioning receptor. The focus is on learning parts of the whole through comparing and contrasting activities. There is only a basic effort at understanding the 'why' of the knowledge.

Dualistic thinkers are quick to reject information that may be contradictory to their belief system. Anything that may make their understanding of the world more complex and uncertain is avoided. Ambiguity, diffuseness or multiple perspectives are a major source of challenge. Conflicting information from two or more respected authorities is disorienting and perceived as a threat. Dualistic thinkers are uncomfortable when asked to make an interpretation of information through independent thinking.

Dualistic thinkers perform more effectively when provided with a high degree of structure. Performance is enhanced through the use of concrete examples of how a task is to be completed combined with experiential learning methods. Careful sequencing and timing of events that introduce more complexity are required to develop thinking beyond the dualistic framework. For example, a performance mediator may role model gathering information on different views of the same knowledge. With trust in the performance mediator as a valued authority figure, the dualistic thinker may venture forward to follow suite. Gathering information on other points of view, without being forced to accept differences creates a safe learning experience. This begins to broaden perspectives toward the more complex thinking patterns associated with the early multiplistic framework.

Early multiplicity

Persons operating at the early multiplistic level feel 'most' knowledge is known. The first view of learning as an 'ongoing process' begins to emerge. An awareness exists that there are many ways to answer questions, solve problems or view the world. The individual continues to believe, however, there is one right way. There is a realization that some knowledge domains are more fuzzy than crystal clear.

Authority figures remain the source of information for the one true answer and the 'right way' to obtain the truth. The role for the authority figure evolves to include modelling the 'way to learn' the one real truth. Early multiplistic thinkers feel their role is to move beyond the passive recipient of truth into a 'seeker and finder' of the one right way. Their role is to learn how to learn. Peers are viewed as a legitimate resource in the learning process. An interest in other points of view of peers is acceptable. There is an exchange of ideas with peers. However, the authority figure has the final say in all matters.

Early multiplistic thinkers evaluate learning and performance by their level of effort and fairness of the judging authority. Hard work, amount of time put into an effort and following the proper style of learning or performing are criteria upon which the evaluation is based. Fairness in judging, amount of work assigned and rewards are viewed as critically important.

The primary intellectual task is to compare, contrast and define multiple perspectives using basic analytical procedures and supporting evidence. An appreciation for the process of learning and performing begins to override a pure focus on content. Early multiplistic thinkers are challenged by coming to terms with the awareness that 'uncertainty' is a natural part of life and not a temporary state of affairs. They are confronted with the notion that complexity is not quantity, but is quality. There is a struggle with reconciling the multiple points of view with previously held assumptions regarding the 'one absolute truth'.

Early multiplistic thinkers perform more effectively when provided with a moderately high level of structure combined with encouragement to seek more diversity in world views and feeling more comfortable with the increasing sense of uncertainty. Clear expectations regarding evaluation procedures and criteria along with precise instructions regarding learning or work assignments provide a safe framework for performance. Individuals at this level of cognitive complexity feel comforted with the assumption that someday they will learn and know the 'one right way' through continued hard work and following orders.

Late multiplicity

Late multiplistic thinkers own the notion that the world is complex and that certainty only exists in specialized areas. All opinions are viewed as equally valid or invalid. The authority figure is experienced more as a facilitator than a dispenser of truth. Authority figures may be completely discounted. The role of the person is to begin thinking for oneself with the use of supporting evidence. Independence of thought is valued as are peers. Although peers' opinions hold questionable weight because everyone's opinion is as good or bad as that of the next person. Personal reliance increases.

Evaluation of learning and performance is based more on qualitative criteria. There is more weight given to the courage of independent thought. Game playing may emerge. The multiplistic thinker may parrot back ideas expressed by the authority figure as a form of manipulation. The primary intellectual task is to develop analytical skills and the ability to perform basic synthesis of concepts. Knowledge can be generalized to other aspects of life beyond the immediate circumstance. Abstract thinking takes form.

The late multiplistic thinker is challenged by the demand of authority to produce supporting evidence. During this stage, the thinker is learning to sort excellent resources from less reliable ones. There is a qualitative shift in accepting personal responsibility for learning and managing affairs. For some, the challenge is to build on what the authority figure has to offer instead of rejecting or devaluing. Support is most effective in enhancing performance when less structure is provided combined with more latitude to seek and create. There is great joy in experiencing diversity of opinion, thought and style.

Contextual relativism
Contextual relativistic thinkers assume all knowledge is dependent upon which point of view is taken in which specific situation. Knowledge is disconnected from any concept of absolute truth. The truth is viewed as subjective and conditional. 'The only absolute is that there is no absolute'; or 'Where you sit is where you stand' serve as axiomatic statements. Relativistic thinkers consider currently held beliefs and assumptions as a temporary truce in understanding, subject to amendment as new information is developed.

Authority figures are viewed as experts who may serve as facilitators or guides. The role of the relativistic thinker is to exercise the use of intellect by continually challenging assumptions across a variety of contexts, searching for universal principles. Peers are considered a legitimate source of learning provided concepts, perspectives and judgements are framed in terms of a context. Evaluation of work or performance is separated from evaluation of oneself. It is valued as a legitimate process and part of learning. Critique is viewed as an opportunity for feedback, improvement and new understanding. The primary intellectual task is to relate learning from one context to another while identifying both the complexity and simplicity of the situation. Abstract thought and synthesis of information are valued and sought.

Level of efficiency
Level of efficiency relates to the speed and effectiveness of the cognitive components in processing information, learning and adaptive application (Feuerstein, 1979). It is important not to confuse a person's cognitive capacity with efficiency. Improper assessment of this issue can lead to choosing the wrong intervention to enhance performance. Interference with efficient performance may stem from task-intrinsic and task-extrinsic factors. Task-intrinsic factors are related to the complexity of the task itself. Task-extrinsic factors are related to issues such as motivation, learning curve, physical well-being, energy level, metabolism, fatigue and physical environment (i.e. hot, humid, cold, wet, windy). Strategies to enhance cognitive efficiency need to be aware of the broader environmental context and the resulting influence on performance.

Interrelationship of operations and phases

All of the cognitive operations and phases are interrelated and interdependent. Cognitive operations focus on simultaneous resolution of information processing activities, problem solving and adaptation. Interdependence, cooperation and potential interference occur when the resolution of one operation impacts upon another. For example, attention affects perception, denial influences reality testing, secondary thinking conditions speech and synthetic–integrative functioning, repression obstructs memory, delay of impulses impacts judgement and autonomous functioning affects all. The environmental context establishes requirements for valued performance. Each cognitive operation needs to be indexed in terms of performance and degree of adaptiveness for a targeted environment. This requires sorting out discrete operations; understanding the effect on other components; and relating the discrete cognitive operation to global functioning.

Performance consulting

Interconnectivity and interdependence

Performance consulting is a hybrid problem solving process that combines the technologies and perspectives of human resource development, organizational development, value engineering, vocational rehabilitation, occupational therapy, ergonomics, and a host of related disciplines. Its foundation is ecological systems thinking, which emphasizes the mutual effect between an organization and its environment (Goldstein, 1994). Historically, the focus of the employment specialist has centred around the educational and clinical aspects of supporting persons with severe disability. To be successful in the next century, practitioners will need to broaden their understanding and capacity to work with a wide array of organizational systems variables. Within the context of enhancing performance, no component of cognitive functioning can be isolated from the interconnectivity and interdependence that exists on multiple levels within and outside of the immediate work environment. The process of searching for isolated, cause-and-effect relationships is being replaced with a focus on how the broader system comes together, as a whole, to influence performance. Immediate challenges and pressures experienced by a worker are linked to the challenges, pressures and dynamics experienced in the economic, social, technological and political environments of the organization. The rehabilitation profession is not immune to this shift in perspective. As business is radically changing competitive strategies and practices, so too is vocational rehabilitation. This is resulting in mutually interdependent effects that are redefining human resource development, management and work process engineering (Lynch and Werner, 1994; Risher and Fay, 1995; Robinson and Robinson, 1995; Rummler and Brache, 1995; Smith and Kearny, 1994; Swanson, 1994).

The health-care system in the United States is a prime example. A major reconfiguration of the health-care delivery system is underway as the society aligns with the productivity dictum of 'doing more with less'. Private practices are becoming linked in order to form networks. The networks are forming vertically and horizontally connected service systems that act 'as if' they are one coherent company. Membership within a network is allowing access to referrals for service, but at a discounted rate of payment. To maintain financial viability, practitioners and health-care providers are providing services to a larger volume of patients per day to earn the same money. To see more patients is requiring more focused, production-oriented, time-limited treatment regimes. This is requiring an adjustment in the type of interventions to those that generate the highest rate of return for the effort. The scope of problem solving and the strategies used to achieve outcomes are being modified. Because of time and cost restrictions, alternative forms of treatment are increasing. For example, some health maintenance organizations assume that it is less expensive and just as effective to restrict psychotherapy to 6 to 12 sessions with a behavioural focus than to use traditional longer-term, relationship-focused treatment. If longer-term treatment is indicated, then referral to a psychiatrist for medication management is encouraged. This generates accelerated research into the cognitive–behavioural, biochemical and neurological aspects of human performance.

Human performance technology

Human performance technology is an approach that adopts a systems view of how valued accomplishments are achieved. It utilizes techniques and insights from multiple disciplines to look at the dynamics that affect the individual. Human performance technology addresses the influence of three basic levels:

1 the organization as a whole
2 the work processes
3 the job/worker.
(Albin, 1992; Hupp, Polak and Westgaard, 1995; Risher, 1995; Robinson and Robinson, 1995; Rummler and Brache, 1995; Smith and Kearny, 1994; Swanson, 1994)

A practitioner defines the mission, purpose, goals, objectives and target work products of the firm. The relationship of the firm with its environment is explored to identify trends, critical success factors, and resulting performance expectations. Organizational strategy is reviewed to describe how the business, marketing and management strategies position the firm for success. Organizational structure is studied to define the link between strategy and the cross-functional division of labour. Core work process and interdependent relationships are mapped to develop a sense of work flow. Management and worker skills are inventoried to establish the match between the work demands and the expertise required to meet objectives. Reward systems are studied to characterize the congruency between

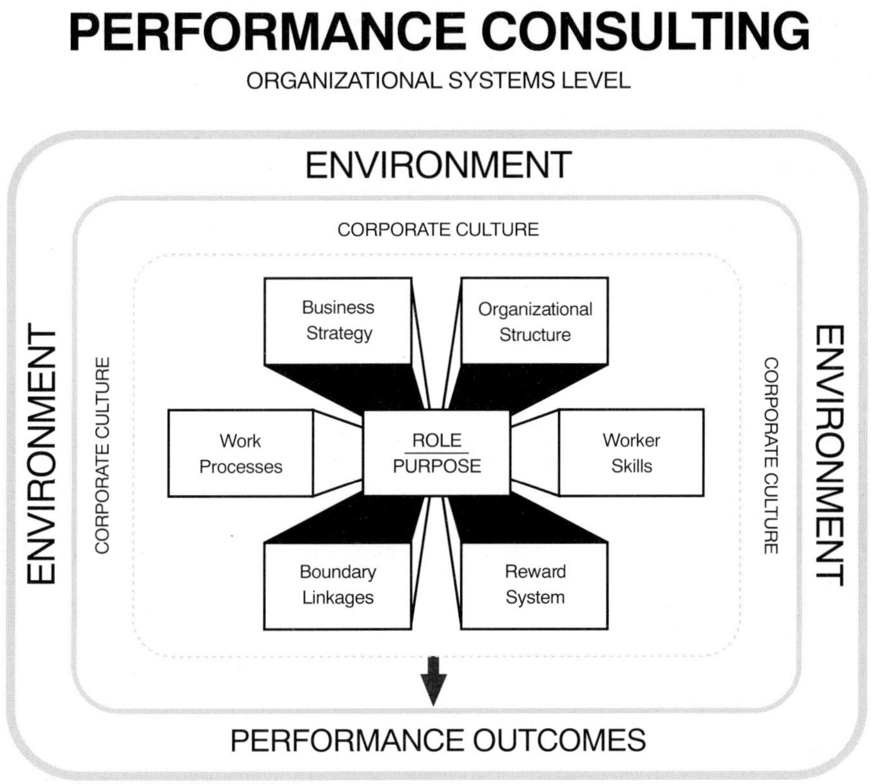

Figure 8.21 Performance consulting, organization systems level.

explicit performance goals and what is really encouraged. Corporate culture forces are distinguished to determine the influence on facilitating healthy performance (Kilmann, 1989; Quinn, 1990). At the individual performer level, knowledge, ergonomics, abilities, information, work flow, tools, resources and specifications link the macro with the micro performance factors.

Evolving relationship with business

Vocational rehabilitation service providers and local businesses have had a long-standing tradition of working together. The relationship with business has been primarily as a supplier of trained and competent personnel. The historical emphasis of vocational programming has been on pre-service training in a variety of skilled and semi-skilled areas from trade and technical jobs to office and professional occupations. Clients were sent to school, graduated, entered work and their case closed. Over the last twenty years there has been a major shift in emphasis and type of person served in rehabilitation programmes. Federal legislation passed in the United States during the early 1970s mandated vocational rehabilitation agencies to serve persons with more severe and pervasive disabling conditions. Throughout the tenure of vocational rehabilitation programming, services have been provided to persons with significant disability. Yet the majority of case loads have been filled, until recently, with clients that were able to manage formal classroom training and competitive employment while continuing on with their life without intensive ongoing support.

The last decade has witnessed a major evolution in services for persons previously considered too disabled to enter and maintain employment in real job settings. Up to the mid 1980s, services for this population had been primarily focused on prevocational issues. Programme content was concerned with life skills, personal hygiene, toileting, eye–hand

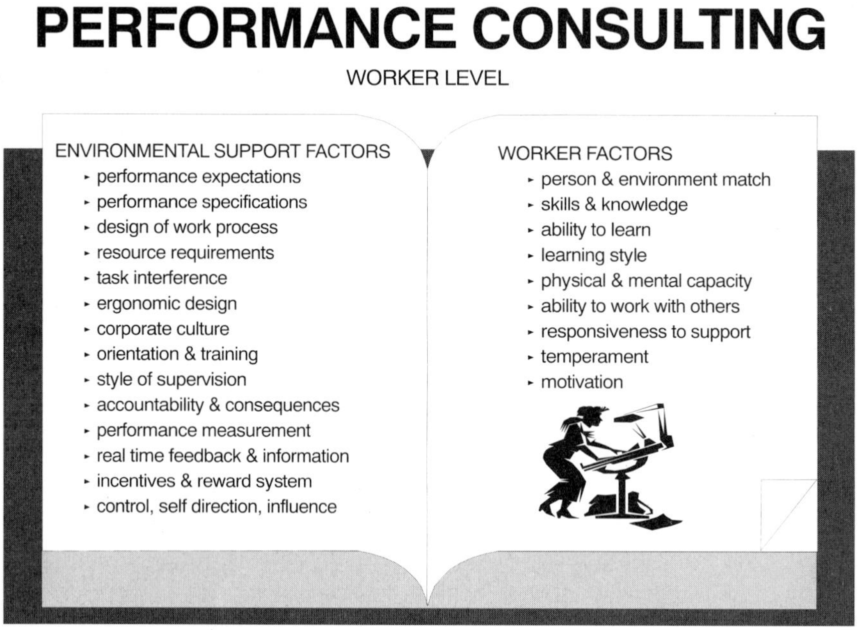

Figure 8.22 Performance consulting, worker level.

coordination, coping with the pressure of sustained performance, and other forms of readiness training. Vehicles such as day activity, work activity and sheltered workshop day programmes served as the primary method for positioning clients for employment. A very negligible percentage of persons with severe disability ever graduated to a real job. The word 'readiness' became synonymous with the word 'never'. The phrase 'day activity' turned into 'day captivity'. With low expectations and artificial environments came austere outcomes. There were exceptions. Fountain House, a psychiatric rehabilitation programme in New York, began to offer employment readiness training by using prearranged job stations in real job settings with real employers. This became known as transitional employment. Projects with industry built on a similar theme. Situational assessment emerged as a tool to pinpoint functional abilities and needs by using real situations in the community to observe performance. Real business settings were used to assess, prepare and train clients. Standardized testing took on less significance and became less relevant for the targeted population. Contextual training in real work environments began to supersede simulated training in sheltered, non-competitive employment environments (Albin, 1992).

Toward the end of the 1980s, supported employment emerged to replace the sheltered and segregated programme models. The concept of employer-based contextual training took on more significance. Supported employment moved the process a step further. Employment sites were used not only for assessment and training. They were turned into real job placements from the beginning of the rehabilitation process instead of at the end. The positions were viewed as the client's job instead of a training and assessment station connected to the service provider. As a result, the relationship between the vocational rehabilitation service provider and business changed. Up to this point, the primary relationship had been between the provider and employer. With supported employment, the primary relationship transferred to one between the employer and the employee (client). The role of the rehabilitation provider was transformed to that of a consultant to this relationship (Fabian *et al.*, 1994). Rehabilitation programmes transferred know-how and resources to employers so that the connection between client and employer could thrive and last.

The programme emphasis of the rehabilitation provider has shifted to matching persons to compatible work environments within real job settings, facilitating the design of reasonable accommodations, establishing on-the-job training, ensuring continuous onsite support, and providing ongoing follow along. The previous service paradigm of 'train, place and pray' has become 'place, train and support'.

Movement from facility-based services to employer-based settings has qualitatively redefined the connection between vocational rehabilitation service providers and business. The emerging relationship is becoming redefined as a strategic alliance and business partnership based on the principle of value-adding.

Economic value

Competition for existing jobs is increasing. It is becoming progressively more difficult for unskilled, semi-skilled or single-skilled persons to obtain and maintain employment. Many corporations are learning how to do more with less. Technology is displacing the worker who does basic, repetitive and narrowly defined tasks. Employees are expected to handle multiple and sometimes divergent responsibilities. The trend is expected to continue well into the twenty-first century. Persons with severe and pervasive disabilities are facing a hard-edged economic reality. They are competing with the general population and with individuals from other specialized work programmes. Economically disadvantaged, minority groups, welfare recipients, youth at risk, elderly, transitioning students, displaced workers, and women are receiving targeted employment services in the same market. Employers are reluctant to hire an applicant unless there is a clear, measurable, and quantifiable advantage for the firm. Potential employees are screened according to whether they are perceived as adding value to the company or as a cost that diminishes the bottom line (Fabian *et al.*, 1994).

To remain viable, vocational rehabilitation providers are beginning to reposition the discussion of value and cost. Traditional marketing of rehabilitation has primarily focused on the societal return on investment for providing services. Ratios such as '10 to 1' have been used to demonstrate that for every dollar spent on providing a service, ten dollars of value were returned to the general public in forms of reduced subsidies, taxes and earning power. This has been an important advocacy point and provides a good general guideline when discussing worth. Yet, with the focus shifting to the partnership between business and rehabilitation, a more personal statement is required with each potential employer. An employer is most concerned with the specific value brought to their unique situation and bottom line. This requires a more intimate knowledge of how cost and value behave.

With the increased focus on serving persons with more profound disabling conditions, rehabilitation professionals have been learning the finer points and implications of job design, work flow, behavioural training, reasonable accommodation and use of technology. Supported employment has accelerated the knowledge and understanding of how to work with real work settings. Many persons with severe and pervasive disability require creative, practical, low-cost rehabilitation engineering solutions in order to function effectively within the community and on the job. Leading practitioners are leveraging this need and turning it into a competitive advantage.

Rehabilitation professionals author task-flow and environmental designs that facilitate high performance at a reasonable cost. Practitioners are quite familiar with the notion of doing more with less. Practitioners are combining the skills and knowledge of the rehabilitation field with the abilities of the person with disability to form a synergistic whole that brings increased value to business and industry. The employer is not only obtaining a good employee but is also receiving additional talents, skills and resources from the rehabilitation firm that can directly facilitate increased revenue or decreased costs. The relationship with employers is being redefined as a strategic alliance and partnership in which win-win solutions are created for all parties. 'Know-how' of the rehabilitation industry is directly transferrable into know-how business needs to increase valued outcomes creatively, efficiently and effectively.

Value stream

A key to the strategic alliance strategy is awareness of how and where value can be added and how this is translated into measurable financial gains that can be communicated to the employer. The source of this information begins by analysing the value stream of a business. A value stream is a collection of discrete activities performed by a company that involves designing, producing, marketing, delivering and supporting products or services (Porter, 1980). These activities serve as the building blocks for creating value for the buyer of the product. Buyers include internal and external customers. Improving elements of the value stream serves as a source of organizational advantage for the business and opportunities for the rehabilitation practitioner.

Value activities are divided into core and support functions. Core activities include:

1 Incoming processes, the tasks of receiving, storing and disseminating, such as material handling, warehousing and inventory control.
2 Production process, making input into product form, such as assembly, printing, typing, machining and cooking.
3 Transfer processes, moving the product down stream in the internal value stream or externally to a buyer, such as material handling, order processing and delivery.
4 Marketing and sales processes, facilitating product awareness, promotion and exchange, such as selling, advertising, price quoting, educating and distribution channel development and management.
5 Service processes, ensuring post-sale satisfaction such as installation, repair, training, parts supply and product adjustments.

(Lynch and Werner, 1994; Porter, 1980)

Support activities include:

1 Procurement, the process of dealing with vendors, qualifying purchases and using information systems for ordering and tracking issues related to cost, quality, life cycle and performance of purchased goods.
2 Technology, the fundamental 'know-how', procedures and equipment which influence the production process and product.
3 Human resource management, the recruiting, hiring, training, developing, retention, compensation and motivation of workers.
4 Leadership, management and administration, the overall company supervision, coordination, planning, finance, accounting,

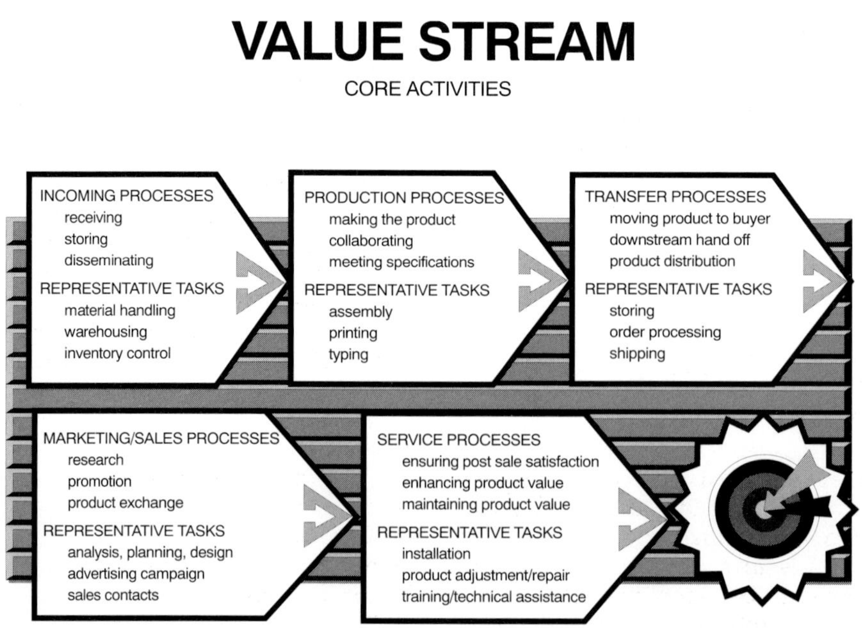

Figure 8.23 Value stream, core activities.

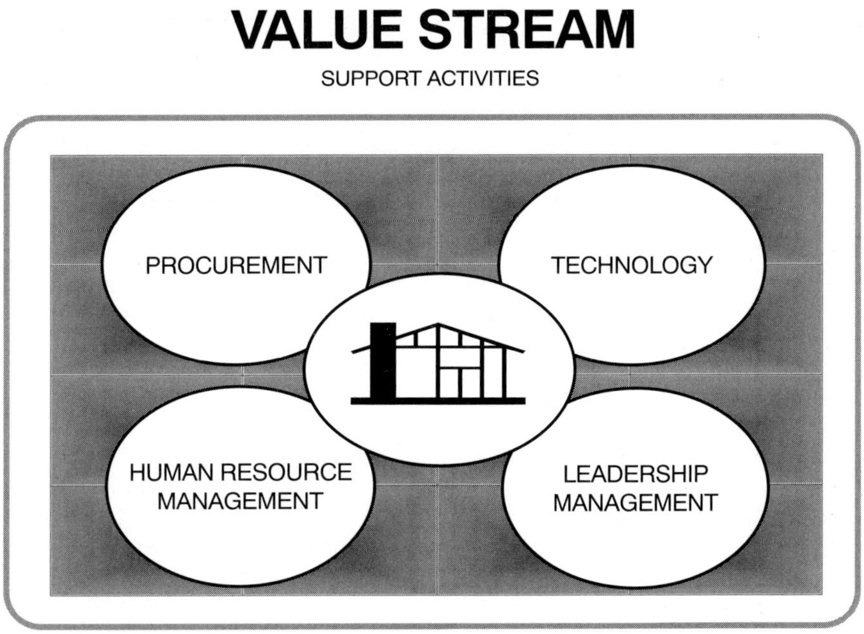

Figure 8.24 Value stream, support activities.

legal, quality control and quality enhancement processes.
(Porter, 1980).

The value stream is a system of interdependent relationships that reflect company history, strategies, assumptions and culture. Enhancing performance of a firm involves optimization and coordination of value-stream activities. Systematic exploration of the value stream reveals opportunities for increasing revenue, reducing costs, avoiding costs and offsetting costs. This opens the door for the practitioner to frame the placement of a client in a job as added value by demonstrating worth in economic terms.

Identifying value-adding opportunities

It is safe to assume that nothing is perfect. There is always room for improvement. There is always variance from an ideal state of affairs. Business is in a continuous quest to reduce the variance between the actual level of operating performance and the idealized vision of how operations could perform. Studying the socio-technical system of a company, within the context of its whole system architecture, pinpoints value-adding opportunities created by variance. The whole-system architecture of a company is the overall structure, alignment and dynamics of elements that influence organizational performance. The socio-technical system is an analytical perspective that focuses on the relationship of the environment with the technical and social systems within a company (Miller, 1994).

The environment represents the expectations, requirements and input of various groups or forces that define or influence the work of the organization. There are two core environments, strategic and operational. The strategic environment is concerned with the external context of the organization. It is represented by elements such as:

- economy
- customer segments
- industry
- technology
- financial stakeholders
- competition
- labour supply
- government

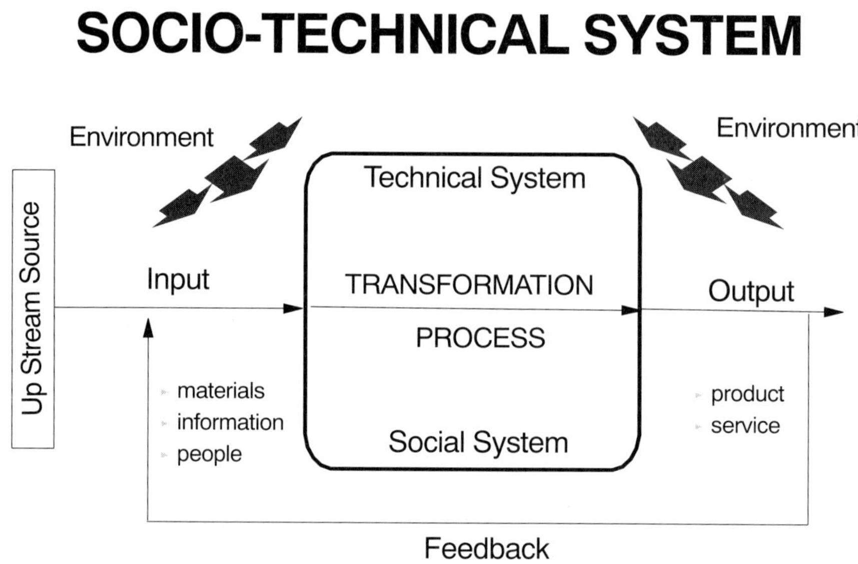

Figure 8.25 Socio-technical system.

- social, political, special interest trends
- supplies.

The operational environment is reflected in elements such as:

- management and administration
- internal, external customers
- marketing and sales
- technology
- finance
- management
- information systems
- human resources
- purchasing
- production processes
- business teams.

The technical system focuses on the processes involved in transforming the incoming materials or information into a final product or service. It is represented by procedures, instructions, techniques, tools, equipment, machines and physical space. The social system is concerned with how people work together to operate, coordinate, and maintain the technical system. Worker characteristics, needs, capabilities, relationships, decision-making procedures, team work, problem-solving protocols, roles and organizational culture mirror key elements (Lytle, 1991; Meyers, 1992; Miller, 1994).

Both the technical and social systems engage in linear and non-linear work. Linear work is represented by sequential production steps that follow an orderly progression and are predictable, measurable, logic based, generally focused on a short time span. Manufacturing is a prime example. Non-linear work is associated with asequential, disorderly, uncertain, fuzzy, intuitive thinking processes involved in continuous trade-offs that frequently span over a long time horizon. Human resource development, improving commitment, building motivation, creating an open system, and increasing worker satisfaction are examples. Non-linear work is involved in knowledge generation, knowledge transfer and knowledge utilization. Knowledge is the most important technology in non-linear work (Lytle, 1991).

The search for value-adding opportunity is a search for variance within the socio-technical system. Variance is that aspect of the socio-technical system that deviates from standards or specifications. Variance results in interference with performance in such areas as quality, quantity, cost and timeliness. Representative causes of variance include:

- the nature of raw materials
- the nature and design of work processes, procedures and techniques

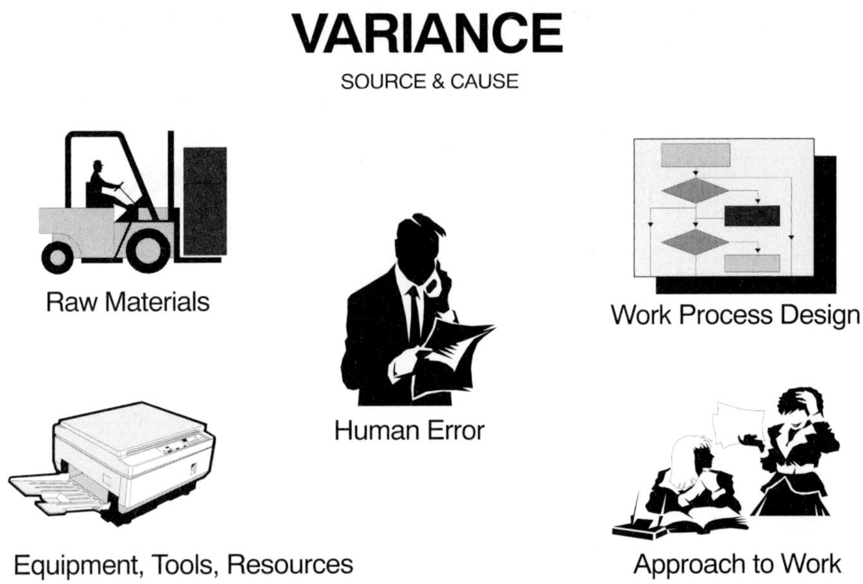

Figure 8.26 Variance.

- human error
- the approach and manner in which workers perform duties
- equipment, tools and resources.

Variances can stand alone or can be inherited from external sources within and outside of the company. They are revealed by searching for:

- frequent mistakes
- handoff points
- rework orders
- customer complaints
- information from inspectors, supervisors and workers
- information from trouble shooters and customer service personnel
- production cycle times
- waste.
  (Lytle, 1991)

Warning and control-cue mechanisms are used to alert a system that it is in variance with intended performance. These reactive mechanisms reveal potential opportunities to improve performance and add value. A value-adding intervention develops ways to prevent, reduce or eliminate the undesirable variance. Preventative and proactive value-adding services reduce, avoid or offset costs.

There are at least six types of mistake-detecting cues that indicate a variance exists:

1 warnings
2 gagging
3 non-response
4 self-correct
5 dialogue
6 impact projections
  (Chase and Stewart, 1995)

Warnings (i.e. beep, flashing light) indicate that a mistake has been made because performance is moving outside of acceptable ranges. The socio-technical system continues with normal activity until such time a corrective action is taken. The warning does not stop the system. *Gagging* (i.e. general protection fault error in software) is a warning cue that brings the system to a halt until the variance is corrected. After the correction is made, the system has to be restarted. *Non-response* warning cues (i.e. soda machine coin recognition, pin number for automatic bank teller machines) do not respond to the variance. They do not allow the system to accept input unless it is within an acceptable performance range. *Self-correct cues* (i.e. spell check in word-processing software) signal a significant variance is occurring and suggest a corresponding correct response. *Dialogue cues* (i.e. financial reports, project reports) set in motion a discussion between relevant participants in order to reach an agreement regarding objectives and the means to achieve desired outcomes. *Impact projection cues* (i.e. navigational software used in a space shuttle) focus on providing extrapolated information regarding future outcomes if the system continues in the variance state.

Variances are symptoms of root causes. Underlying every variance is a rule-, skill- or knowledge-based cause. Under each of these causes is a set of assumptions that serve as the source of the variance. Variances can be machine based and human based. With machines, variances can be caused by:

- being broken
- lack of input
- jammed with input
- improper input
- improper calibration
- worn-out parts
(Chase and Stewart, 1995)

Human error is reflected in task variances, customer treatment variances, and tangible variances (Chase and Stewart, 1995; Hupp *et al.*, 1995; Kobayashi, 1988; Lynch and Werner, 1994; Melan, 1995). Tasks variances exist when:

- tasks are performed incorrectly
- doing a task that was not requested
- doing a task in the wrong order
- doing a task too slowly.

Customer treatment variances occur when:

- not acknowledging the customer
- not listening to the customer
- not reacting appropriately to the customer.

Tangible variances are related to breakdowns in the:

- physical environment
- ergonomic supports
- concrete and adequate resources to manage the tasks of the socio-technical processes.

The physical environment and ergonomic supports are concerned with factors such as noise, odours, light, temperature, lifting, bending, sitting, walking, vibrations and cleanliness. Concrete and adequate resources are concerned with having the right tools in a sufficient quantity to meet the challenge of the tasks. Depending on the task, tools may range from items such as machines and calculators, to pens, paper and personnel.

Variances have a cascading effect on a socio-technical system (Lytle, 1994; Meyers, 1992; Miller, 1994). A minor error in the initial stages of a work process may result in a major variance later in the production process. For example, an incorrect food order is written down by a food server. This results in the chef preparing the wrong meal. The food server delivers the incorrect meal to the customer which is then rejected. The meal results in waste. A new meal is reordered to correct the mistake. The restaurant reworks the order. The labour and material costs double and result in a net loss for the sale. It also results in loosing the opportunity to have a repeat customer. The customer tells a friend and the friend tells five more friends. This results in seven potential customers avoiding the future use of the restaurant. While the original customer was waiting for the correct meal, three other customers notice the mistake and resulting aggravation. The incident tarnishes the image of the restaurant for the customers. They decide to not order dessert (driving down the average sale) in order to leave while they are ahead. However, there is a delay in obtaining their checks because the food server is sidetracked by correcting the order for the original customer. The frustration of waiting turns three more customers away from future patronage. These customers, in turn, discourage future customers away through their networks. The average customer purchased three meals per year with the restaurant. There is a total loss of 28 customers that equates to an average of 84 diners per year. The average diner generates $25 per sale. Reworked meals result in a net loss of $10. The initial mistake results in costing the restaurant not only the $10 to rework the order but also $2180 in future sales over the next year. The food server is let go because this has been a recurring problem. The average cost to recruit, advertise, screen, select and train is $1200. The initial mistake ends up costing the restaurant nearly $3400. An average of three food servers leave each year for a variety of reasons that are not necessarily linked to employee difficulties. During the learning curve, new food servers generate less sales and at a lower amount per sale. This lasts for an average of six weeks. With the addition of the natural attrition of food servers, a total of $8000 to $10 000 per year is taken from the bottom line.

Having this type of information enables a practitioner to discuss the benefits of value-added service. It positions the rehabilitation professional as a business partner. Using the above example, a practitioner can offer a service that can prevent, reduce or eliminate the variance. Instead of asking for a job, a practitioner can offer a profit improvement proposal that will save the employer at least $8000 to $10 000 per year thus allowing management to concentrate on overall quality improvement and expanding the customer base.

For purposes of discussion, assume a practitioner approaches the restaurant manager, from the above example, looking for a bookkeeper position that pays $16 000 per year. Competition for the opening is tough. Because time was taken to learn about the business, the practitioner can demonstrate that by hiring the qualified candidate she represents, additional benefits can be offered to resolve the collateral issues of order-taking errors, turnover of food servers and improving the quality of customer service. The practitioner can demonstrate an understanding of how costs behave with the specific restaurant. A profit improvement proposal can be submitted by the practitioner that offers a package of services at no additional charge to the employer when the client is hired. The additional services include:

1 Designing a system to eliminate or reduce errors in the order-taking process.
2 Developing orientation and training modules to bring employees up to full performance more rapidly.
3 Developing ways to retain valued servers to reduce turnover and orientation training costs.
4 Continuous education in customer service issues such as dealing with difficult customers and increasing the volume of each sale order.

The profit improvement proposal represents an added value to the employer that is not matched by other persons competing for the bookkeeper position. The practitioner is able to demonstrate to the employer that the original cost of $16 000 per year for the bookkeeper position has, in essence, been reduced $8000 to $10 000 per year by preventing and reducing costs in other areas of the operation. This represents a potential savings of 50 per cent to 62.5 per cent in salary expenses within the first year alone. Over a two-year period, the potential savings would be almost equivalent to a full year's salary. With this approach, professionalism, business savvy and added value are the images created in the mind of the employer when referring to the rehabilitation firm. The practitioner is not asking the employer to choose a less-qualified applicant because of the valued-added proposal. The practitioner is offering to provide an excellent candidate who is qualified to compete for the position. By hiring the candidate, additional value can be brought to the company to strengthen its bottom line.

Multiple opportunities exist for adding value to any company by finding ways to:

1 Expand revenue.
2 Maximize working capital.
3 Reduce purchase costs of raw material.
4 Reduce production costs.
5 Reduce administrative overhead costs.
6 Improve the quality of products or services, in areas such as performance and reliability.
7 Standardize products and services.
8 Improve scheduling and planning.
9 Make better use of idle time.
10 Make better use of wasted space.
11 Make better use of existing capacity.
12 Reduce downtime and overtime.
13 Increase the volume of throughout.
14 Redesign and improve the flow of work, tasks and jobs.
15 Reduce inventory.
16 Speed the disposal of slow-moving inventory.
17 Improve responsiveness to customers.
18 Improve information handling.
19 Reduce processing errors.
20 Reduce lost production time due to illness, accidents, personal reasons, complaints and grievances.
21 Improve performance of individual work units.
22 Improve integration and coordination between work units.
23 Establish, strengthen and improve quality enhancement practices.

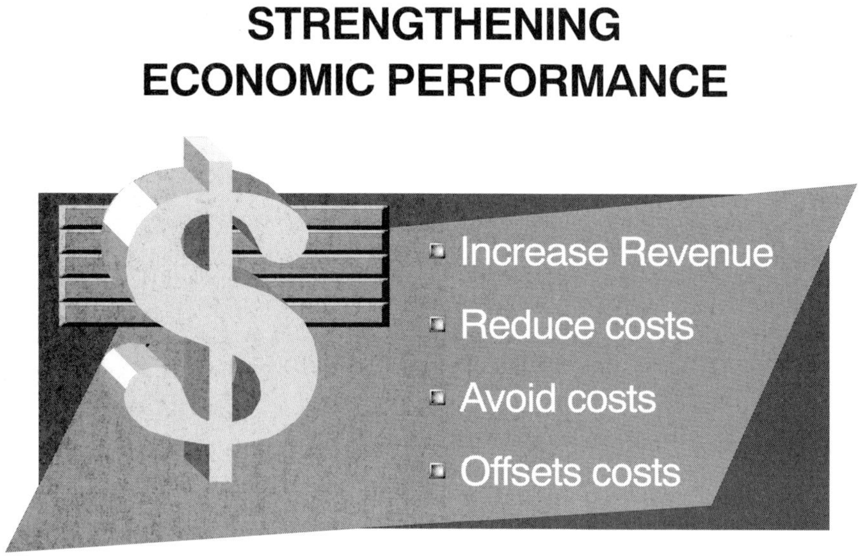
STRENGTHENING
ECONOMIC PERFORMANCE
Increase Revenue
Reduce costs
Avoid costs
Offsets costs

Figure 8.27 Strengthening economic performance.

24 Increase employee ownership, involvement and motivation in the production process and outcome goals.
(Judson, 1990; Kobayashi, 1988; Nagel, 1991)

These areas are representative and not all inclusive.

There are no separate problems. As improvement is administered in one part of the value stream, opportunities emerge throughout other primary and secondary activities of the production process.

A tool that is helpful in targeting value-adding opportunities is process analysis (Lynch and Werner, 1994; Lytle, 1991; Melan, 1995; Meyers, 1992; Miller, 1994). The process analysis maps:

1 Major stages (core work process) of production.
2 Related activities and tasks that take place within the core process.
3 Key individuals, teams or departments that are involved with each core process.

A core process takes input and transforms it into output that is handed off to the next value-adding core process or end customer. Telephone call processing is an example. The core work processes are:

1 Answer phone.
2 Request name of person being called, the name of the caller and the purpose of the call.
3 Call the appropriate extension or pager.
4 Inform person of caller and purpose of the call.
5 Connect caller to the appropriate party or take a message.
6 Disconnect from the call.

The output of one core process needs to meet certain specifications in order to be accepted as input for another core process or customer. When the output of one process does not meet specifications, it sets in motion a series of subsequent errors that compound the problem. Within each of the core processes are subroutines that take place to achieve the outcome goal of the step. Within each subroutine are a series of tasks that are done to complete the superordinate routine. Each of these routines are subject to revision in order to facilitate efficiency and effectiveness. This can translate into dollar-and-cents savings. Opportunities for value-adding are revealed when each core process is explored to identify key variances that most frequently occur and the probable root causes. The impact of the variances can be identified and quantified for the current and subsequent processes downstream. Most solutions can be discovered without moving into the infinite detail of subroutines.

A root-cause analysis is conducted to reveal 'points of entry solutions' that can translate into value-adding services. Root-cause analysis traces the symptom back to underlying issues. The basic process is to identify the symptom, describe the rule of operation that generates the symptom and uncover the underlying assumptions that create the rule. For example, high turnover may be a symptom. The rule may be the profile specifications used to hire applicants for the position. The root cause may be related to management's assumptions regarding the critical success factors required to meet customer expectations.

The following case example illustrates the process of identifying value-adding opportunities:

A rehabilitation practitioner was searching for a clerical-related position on behalf of one of her clients. She was given a lead that a local financial services company may be in the market for hiring. The lead had been provided by the local chamber of commerce. The practitioner was told that the company specialized in providing financial statements for small to medium-size businesses in the local community. The company had been started seven years ago by a former financial officer of a large corporate group in the metropolitan area. She saw the emerging trend of downsizing as many local businesses began restructuring and outsourcing operations. This trend spelled opportunity for her. For years she had wanted to have her own business. Through her professional networking relationships, she had developed an excellent reputation for her technical skills. She never ran a whole company but felt confident that her technical skills in finance outweighed any lack of general management experience. When she left her corporate job, she immediately picked up eight accounts and added 26 more over the following four years. Business was very strong in the beginning.

The owner agreed to meet with the practitioner to explore how both parties might be able to work together. However, the owner let the practitioner know that she was not looking to hire. Her real concerns were to cut costs due to her declining business base. From the initial meeting, the practitioner learned that the last three years had not been as successful as the owner anticipated. She had gradually lost accounts to the point where her current customer list was down to 25 companies from a one-time high of 34. Over the last eight months she had lost six accounts, gained two new accounts and may be losing four more by the end of the fiscal year. The practitioner learned that the average service contract was $24 000 per year per company with a typical monthly invoice of $2000. Annual revenues were in the $700 000 range. The owner felt that the decline in her business was due to the availability of less expensive competitors and some difficulties she was having keeping up with existing accounts.

The practitioner asked if she could observe operations to learn more detail about the company and to determine if there was any potential of being helpful in improving the company's performance. Although the primary mission of the practitioner was to secure a job for her client, she chose not to push in that direction this early in the relationship. The owner agreed and the practitioner scheduled a day to return.

Identification of opportunities for value-added service began with preparation for the job site visit. Discussions with the chamber of commerce revealed that the local economy was growing. The average size of each business was small to medium. This would probably remain the same over the foreseeable future. This meant that the need for financial services from an outside source was projected to remain strong. The practitioner was referred to three small- to medium-size companies by the executive director of the chamber. The executive director actually called on behalf of the practitioner in order to ease entry. The purpose of the visits to the companies was to learn what was important to the company managers and owners regarding financial services from outside firms. This informational interviewing gave the practitioner a quick background briefing on customer expectations. During the interviews she requested the names of financial services companies they thought did an excellent job and why. From the interviews, she was able to construct a profile of excellence from a customer's point of view.

The executive director of the chamber was kind enough also to call a neighbouring chamber outside the local geographic market, twenty miles away, to obtain the names of three financial service companies the practitioner could visit. The chamber executive in the distant community helped arrange interviews. The distant community was chosen to avoid putting the practitioner and the local chamber in an awkward position with the local financial services companies. The practitioner was going to be asking detailed questions regarding how effective operations should be organized, managed and positioned in the market. Both the practitioner and chamber executive did not want the local financial services companies to feel they were giving away company knowledge to competitors just around the corner. Both wanted to avoid any perceptions of conflict of interests.

At the interviews, the practitioner observed everything from the physical environment, how she was greeted and treated by company personnel, to how work was organized, processed and managed. She asked a series of questions regarding the industry, the major challenges it faced, and the essentials each manager felt were necessary for running a superior service. The informational interview was framed as gathering background information so that she would be able to provide career guidance for her client, to learn more about the industry and potentially to secure work with a local company back home. The practitioner was forthright regarding how the information was going to be used to facilitate a job opportunity for her client while providing value-added services to the company.

Following the background interviews and research, the practitioner felt confident she had a solid basic understanding of the business and what it took to be successful. In business terms, she did 'benchmarking' to determine best in-class operating procedures for the industry niche (Camp, 1989). The next step was for the practitioner to conduct the onsite review of the potential employment site.

As the practitioner drove and parked her car on the way to the financial services company she observed that the local business community was filled with small 'mom and pop' companies. The business community appeared vibrant and growing as indicated by the numbers provided by the chamber of commerce. Upon entering the building, the practitioner began developing a working hypothesis regarding the needs of the business, value-adding opportunities, and the basic job match potential for her client. The path to the entrance doorway was lightly cluttered with food wrappers, trash, and cigarette butts. There was a public trash can in the front of the building and an apartment building next to the business. The debris was by no means overwhelming. Yet it left a negative impression. She had noticed the same problem when she visited before. The practitioner immediately began to ask herself why the business would allow their front walkway to remain unattractive. She thought perhaps this was a symptom of a bigger issue facing the company.

When she reported to the receptionist's desk in the lobby she had to wait in line for several uncomfortable minutes. The wait was experienced as longer than it should be. She noticed the others standing in line were agitated. The receptionist was swamped with answering and routing phone calls, posting outgoing mail, light typing and photocopying. The receptionist appeared frazzled and pulled in too many directions at once to be successful with any one duty. One person waiting gave up and left in disgust. The practitioner added this observation to her working hypothesis. Both observations suggested the company had problems with keeping up with basic routine chores. The receptionist was managing too many divergent duties at once. It was difficult to tell what were the real priorities for the role. The practitioner wondered why the owner would allow the reception area to be uninviting and aggravating for visitors. She thought perhaps the owner may have difficulty in planning, scheduling and setting priorities. The initial impressions suggested the company was operating moment to moment instead of having a larger game plan. It was as if the company was so busy counting trees that it forgot about the forest. The receptionist role did not appear well thought out. It appeared the owner had not anticipated the impact on the business of the dirty walkway and a chaotic reception area. This suggested that perhaps the owner did not know how to market or position her company in the market because its image was not being managed well with the basics of greeting customers.

The receptionist finally attended to the practitioner. However, the best he could do was to say take the elevator up the top floor before he was interrupted again by two phone calls and a mail run. The practitioner knew where to go from her first visit but she felt that this was a sloppy way to greet and direct visitors. It did not appear that the receptionist was performing poorly due to lack of skills, talent or ability. In spite of all the pressure, the receptionist worked hard to smile and be pleasant. It looked as if the work system surrounding him interfered with successful performance. The practitioner was curious why the system operated as it did. If the reception process turned off just one existing customer, it meant a potential loss of $24 000. If the reception process turned off one potential new customer, it meant another $24 000 loss. The probability that this had already occurred seemed reasonable to assume.

When the practitioner arrived at the owner's office, she was greeted and directed to work with the administrative assistant. The assistant took the practitioner on an overview tour. The practitioner observed that staff appeared to be in good spirits and working together as a team. Everyone did appear overburdened, with pile upon pile of financial data and reports on their desks. From all the warm welcomes and introductions, the practitioner developed a sense that the work culture was leaning toward a support orientation. Discussions and further observations verified her assumption. Everyone seemed to be reaching out and helping each other. The emotional climate felt positive. There appeared to be strong cohesion and morale despite the obvious chaos of being swamped. Individual discussions with workers indicated they held the owner in high regard. This in part, helped staff deal with the disorganized work environment. This was a positive sign for the practitioner. She felt her client would thrive in the support orientation culture. There appeared to be a basic job match with the culture.

As the practitioner observed operations and discussed issues with staff she noted areas for improvement that could benefit from value-added services. The organizational culture appeared fundamentally positive and supportive but needed to move toward the characteristics found within role orientation cultures. The company needed standardization of the work-flow process. A basic process analysis was conducted that followed the flow of a work order through the system. It revealed that current procedures and routines were not formalized. Many documents were passed on to the next step in the work-flow process that were incomplete or not accurate. Internal mistake proofing did not exist in a formal procedure. This resulted in rework and delays. No hard data existed on the level of incidence. The consensus of people interviewed suggested that at least 30 per cent of the work had to be sent back or corrected. Each rework order or correction process took an average of one hour when counting the initial review and the subsequent review to make corrections. This hour cost the company $40 in direct costs and bad will with the customer because of delays. The internal reworking cost the company $800 per week with an annual impact of $41 600 in wasted labour. The organizational culture promoted forgiving people over getting the job done correctly. It was well intentioned but resulted in significant losses to the company.

There wasn't a procedures manual that mapped out how the work was to be performed or how the various steps tied together. The organization frequently missed schedule commitments. The firm's ability to deliver existing products and services reliably, predictably, on time and in accordance with promises to customers needed to improve. An average of 25 per cent of their work was returned each month due to errors in compiling financial information accurately. Each report represented an invoice of $2000. It took $1000 to produce a report. Industry standards for production costs were $400. When the work was returned the company had to do over the report at an average cost of $800. This translated into the company losing $800 for 84 reports a year. This represented a direct loss of $67 200 a year and resulted in dissatisfied customers. Over the last year, the company lost $100 000 with existing business that decided to take its account to another firm. Over 60 per cent of financial statements were submitted late each reporting period. From interviewing the local businesses it was learned that timely, accurate financials were crucial in current market conditions. Many companies felt a need to be able to make quick decisions regarding business strategies. Slow submission of the financials interfered with the customer company's ability to function efficiently.

Further observations revealed the company was not automated to the level required to process reports accurately and efficiently. The owner didn't feel she could afford the needed system. It cost $150 000. She did not have sufficient cash flow to support the payments. The owner felt lack of automation was compensated by having existing staff hold multiple responsibilities beyond their basic roles. The practitioner concluded that labour costs were contained on paper but rework and late orders were costing the company at least $208 800 when combining the rework costs and lost accounts. Additional costs were associated with taking a line of credit to meet expenses due to slow-moving accounts' receivable activity. The long delays in issuing reports with invoices impacted on their cash position. As long as reports sat on a desk, they were inventory not cash. This also interfered with the owner's ability to earn interest. Between borrowing and lost interest, the owner felt she lost an additional $25 000 in potential income. In terms of opportunity costs, the owner's current operation was off-putting to customers. Industry standards revealed she had the potential of gaining two accounts a year. Instead, the company was losing business and cutting off access to future business. This represented a minimum loss of $70 000 per year and climbing.

From a total of twelve hours of research, benchmarking, onsite observations, and interviews with staff, middle management and senior management, the practitioner was able to develop a profit improvement proposal that created opportunity for her client and identified an improved bottom-line performance for the company. She presented a proposal to the owner that would result in increasing the profit margin conservatively by $100 000 by investing $480 per week. The practitioner pointed out that there was a real potential to increase profit margins by as much as $300 000. The owner was intrigued and asked her to explain. The practitioner reviewed the flow of operations, pointing out the areas for improvement and translated the improvements into dollars. The source of the information was based on actual information provided by members of the company and the owner. She carefully discussed areas for improvement such as:

- flow of work design
- improved work methods and procedures
- increased standardization
- reduced waste and rework
- improved resource utilization
- improved job design
- improved information handling
- improved process cycle time, movement of inventory, and on-time delivery of accurate reports
- improved information processing technology
- improved customer service.

The owner agreed with the observations.

The practitioner presented the concept of value-added services. She showed how $480 per week would translate into significant financial gains. First she demonstrated that by creating a position, Production Coordinator, work could be centrally scheduled, tracked, expedited and delivered on time. Operations were currently fragmented and pulling in different directions at the same time. The position would facilitate integrated priority setting, optimize production flow, dampen potential conflicts and channel the system to perform at a more robust level of output. Over time, the position could incorporate oversight and coordination of continuous quality improvement activities. For the immediate future, the position would work on rapid flow through, standardization of work processes, establish mistake proofing work procedures and integration of work between departments. The outcome would result in a rapid turnaround on report processing, delivery and payment. Accuracy of reports would increase therefore resulting in less rework. This would substantially curb excessive costs. This in turn would allow existing resources to be directed toward new work instead of rework. This position could be filled with an existing staff at no additional expense. Taking a person off line and assigning them to the Production Coordinator role would not take way the existing workload of the person filling the position. This is where the $480 per week investment was introduced. The practitioner demonstrated that most finance staff were handling clerical duties over and beyond their primary duties of preparing financial statements. Clerical duties are non-billable duties. This additional burden was slowing production, not utilizing the higher level skills of the accountant staff, and interfering with peak performance directly related to producing income for the company. The practitioner proposed creating a new position, Administrative Assistant, with a weekly salary of $480. Clerical and administrative responsibilities could be consolidated into this position, thereby freeing the accountant staff to take over the Production Coordinator's old assignments. The accountant staff felt confident they could produce financial statements more rapidly with fewer errors and at a higher volume if not sidetracked by clerical duties. By freeing the accountant staff to do their prime duties, many of the costs associated with reworking internal and external errors would disappear. This represented a little more than $108 800 per year. Preventing lost accounts through improved performance represented an additional savings of at least $100 000. An improved cash position would be established because of a higher volume of reports submitted each month. This meant quicker turnaround time for accounts receivable. Previous delays in payment due to rework and late submission of reports would be diminished. With improved cash flow, it could be expected that there would be an additional $25 000 in increased revenue. The owner would not have to borrow money for pay roll and pay interest on the loan. Instead she would be able to benefit from interest bearing accounts by keeping a high daily balance. Adding two new accounts would bring in at least $48 000. The return on the weekly investment of $480 would range from $108 800 to $281 800 per year. This additional revenue would open the door for the owner to purchase the management information system she needed to remain viable and competitive.

The added value the practitioner offered, beyond the above recommendations, was to assist in development and design of the:

- Production Coordinator and Administrative Assistant positions
- overall work system to align roles and production processes
- continuous quality enhancement process, at a later date, once production was achieving objectives.

The practitioner was not offering to take responsibility for the above. An offer to participate and assist where appropriate was tendered. The level of effort by the practitioner would represent approximately 32 hours over the course of the first year. An average cost of an organizational consultant was estimated at $1500 per day. Value-added service represented an additional resource worth a minimum of $6000. Two objectives were achieved, a job for the practitioner's client and added value for the employer. Advocacy on behalf of the client was accomplished by creating and adding value to the business. The relationship of the business owner with the person with disability and the rehabilitation firm was framed on a higher plane. It focused on images of worth and economic development. A future vision was painted of value enhancement. The vision pulled rather than pushed the process of job placement.

Consultation and collaboration

Tactical and strategic positions

The value-adding approach to vocational rehabilitation is based on creating 'win-win' solutions for all parties. It requires focusing on the larger system surrounding the client, the job and the employer. Creating employment opportunities requires the practitioner to work with performance dynamics that go beyond the traditional boundaries of counselling, guidance, treatment, education and the medical model. These traditional approaches are not cast away. They serve as a foundation that is transferred into application with a variety of business and workforce performance issues. The emerging challenges facing the rehabilitation industry demand a knowledge base that blends rehabilitation with performance technology and business practices. It is compelling practitioners to become comfortable with consulting and collaborating with business around economic performance issues.

Value-adding services are positioned tactically and strategically (Kelly, 1988). Tactical positioning involves consultation and negotiation. Strategic positioning focuses on account affiliation management, relationship management and resource networking. Consultation activities centre on creating an employer's awareness of underlying performance improvement needs followed by providing assistance to meet needs. Negotiation activities occur when the business is aware of needs and is seeking assistance. The employer is looking for the best deal. The solutions offered by the rehabilitation firm are compared to other options that may be available and substituted for less cost. Account affiliation management works to gain a hold in the business community so that the rehabilitation firm is viewed as the preferred or exclusive supplier of human resource and business performance solutions. Relationship management is concerned with maintaining existing consulting relationships with an eye toward expanding and increasing opportunities for value-adding. Resource networking involves bringing together additional experts to facilitate identification of needs and applicable interventions. This is when the rehabilitation practitioner recommends bringing in other consultants to address a technical aspect of performance and value engineering outside the expertise of the rehabilitation firm. In the case example with the financial services company, the practitioner recommended consulting with a management-information systems group. The company had come highly recommended by the other top financial services companies she had benchmarked.

Consultation roles

The roles of a consultant move along a continuum from directive to non-directive activities. The practitioner adjusts role performance according to the needs of the situation. Beginning with the directive stance and moving toward the non-directive position, the following roles come into play:

1 Advocate, most directive
2 Expert
3 Trainer and Educator
4 Joint Problem Solver
5 Solutions Analyst and Broker
6 Fact Finder

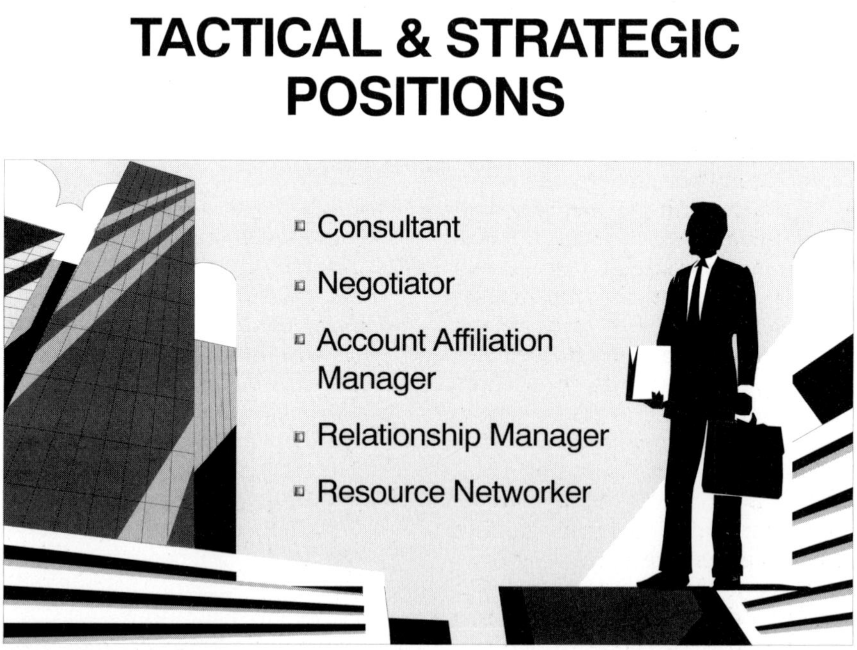
TACTICAL & STRATEGIC POSITIONS
Consultant
Negotiator
Account Affiliation Manager
Relationship Manager
Resource Networker

Figure 8.28 Tactical and strategic positions.

7 Process Counsellor
8 Objective Observer, least directive.
(Lippitt and Lippitt, 1986; Dougherty, 1990).

In the Advocate role, the practitioner promotes an explicit position on a topic, issue or opinion. Activities involve taking charge of a problem solving process, championing a solution and persuading others to support a particular course of action. In the Expert mode, the practitioner provides services based on specialized knowledge and skills. The practitioner serves as a content expert. A tax attorney, expert witness in a trial or travel counsellor are examples. Responsibility for activities and outcomes resides with the client (rehabilitation client or business client). The role of the consultant is to provide authoritative information and advice. In the Trainer and Educator role, the practitioner assesses learning needs, designs learning activities, provides instruction for knowledge and skill building, and evaluates learning outcomes. Teaching conflict resolution, use of a specific software product, operating a machine or briefing on licensing regulations for an industry are examples. Joint Problem Solver role involves the practitioner and the client working together to collaborate on identifying issues that need to be addressed, developing alternative solutions, committing to a plan of action, implementing the plan, evaluating the outcomes and adjusting course as necessary. This is a role that is collaborative by nature. The consultant is an active participant yet remains objective. Even though the consultant works closely in partnership, achieving outcomes is the responsibility of the client. The client and consultant operate as peers. The role of Solutions Analyst and Broker focuses on helping the client identify alternative courses of action, weigh the probable impact of each option, choose a course of action and link the client with appropriate resources to achieve goals. Through a neutral and objective stance the consultant facilitates the client's thinking. The consultant does not pass judgement on options generated or chosen. The Fact Finder role serves as a research assistant who gathers relevant information for the client and stimulates the client's creative and critical thinking. The role of Process Consultant is involved in observing the client's problem solving process, giving feedback statements that reflect the *modus operandi* and raising issues for exploration. For example: 'Let's take a look at how this decision just took place. All of the members of the management team were participating in the discussion except for Mary and Chris. They seemed to shut down. The team went ahead and made a decision but it was the opposite of what everyone publicly said they felt was best. The team then jumped to the next topic. There was no discussion why the sudden change in opinion took place. What do you think is going on? I'd like each of you to share your thoughts. Let's begin with Bill.'

The Objective Observer role stimulates the client's ability to develop insights into the problem to be solved without the consultant revealing any personal beliefs or ideas. The consultant asks a series of questions to open exploration and assist the client to become curious, such as: 'You say that you and your staff are upset with your payroll clerk. For years it has been almost impossible to have a decent interaction with her without an argument erupting. Yet, as the manager, you have chosen to keep her and loose other coworkers instead. Is this an accurate statement? Does this suggest anything to you? What does it tell you? Are you comfortable keeping the situation as it now exists? Why?'.

Consultation process

There are four basic phases in the consultation process:

1 entry
2 diagnosis
3 implementation
4 disengagement.
(Lippitt and Lippitt, 1986; Dougherty, 1990; Manzini, 1988)

The entry phase is the period in which the practitioner explores the organizational needs of the business to determine if there is a possibility of a working relationship. Activities during this phase are concerned with determining whether to go forward or move on to other options. The practitioner screens the situation to determine:

1 Congruence between the preferences and needs of the client with the employer.

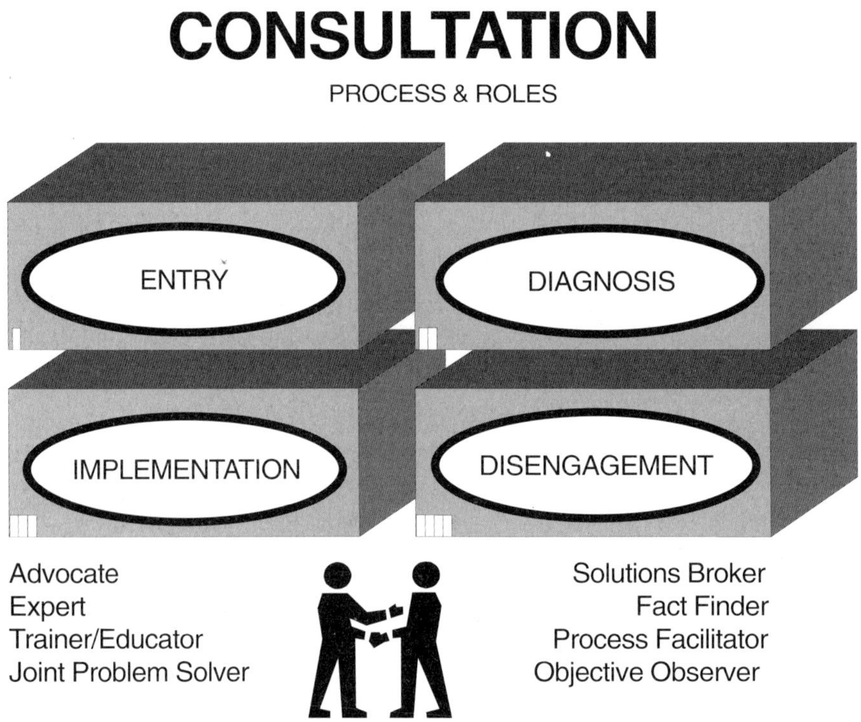

Figure 8.29 Consultation.

2 Congruence between the needs of the business and the value the client and rehabilitation practitioner bring to the relationship.
3 Congruence between the practitioner and the employer.
4 The amount, availability and commitment of required resources.
5 Employer's perceived need for establishing a working relationship.
6 Clarity of mutual gains and expectations.
7 Agreement on the mutual roles and responsibilities of the client, business and practitioner.
(Dougherty, 1990; Lippitt and Lippitt, 1986)

If satisfactory answers are obtained regarding these issues, then the possibility of moving the process forward exists.

During the entry phase, the business typically opens dialogue with the practitioner around the many unknowns. Employers want to know the purpose of the consultation, a picture of the consulting process and results expected, an understanding of the practitioner's plan to achieve outcomes, and an understanding of everyone's part in the series of actions proposed.

Most people are typically hesitant and conservative when faced with an unknown. Particularly an unknown that could potentially change the way business is conducted. Most people tend to approach the unknown with concerns around loss rather than gain. People do not resist change. They resist loss and grieving. Basic instincts take over. When faced with uncertainty and the unknown, it is natural for anxiety to increase. When anxiety goes up, IQ goes down. The mode of behaviour moves into flight, fight, freeze, fumble or forward. People may run from the unknown, push it away and try to minimize it, become paralysed, hedge or decide to explore how to grow and develop opportunity.

One of the practitioner's challenges, during the entry phase, is to overcome the employer's natural tendency to say no before saying yes. This begins by establishing credibility. Credibility can be earned, transferred or gained through reputation. Credibility is earned by having a previous success with the employer. It can be transferred when a third-

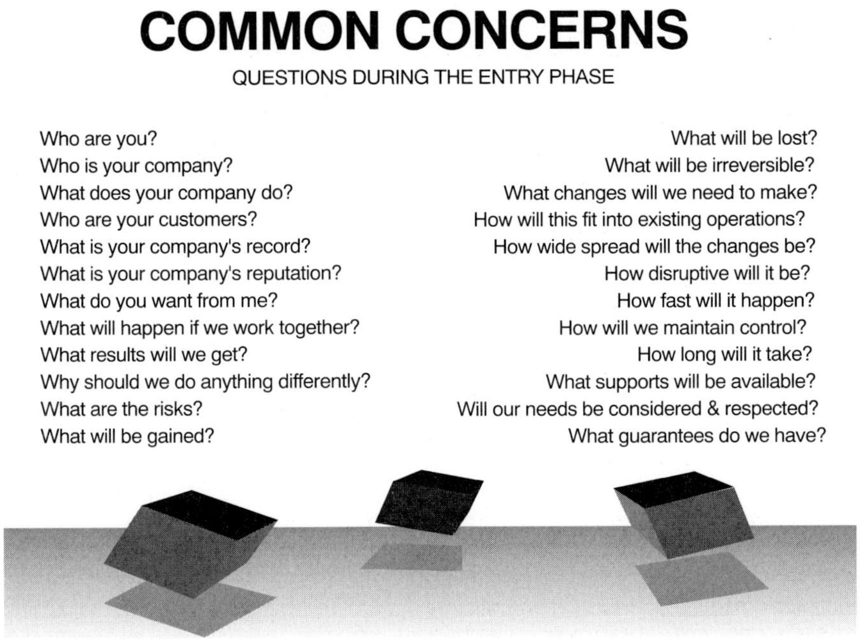

Figure 8.30 Common concerns.

party reference vouches for the practitioner. It can be established by reputation when a practitioner is associated with a rehabilitation firm held in high esteem. Earned credibility is by far the strongest source. Solid product and service knowledge, a clear understanding of employer needs, honouring commitments, following relationship protocols established by the employer, and achieving bottom-line results, all contribute to establishing a credible image. Credibility is built by asking precise, relevant questions and by active listening. Superficial statements and a 'know-it-all' approach do not work. They do not convey a sense the practitioner has the best interest of the employer in mind. The practitioner is viewed more as a peddler than a win-win partner.

An employer will not move forward in the consulting process unless basic conditions exist as represented in the formula.

$$D \times V \times FS > R \qquad \text{(Jacobs, 1994).}$$

The business must be dissatisfied (D) with the current or projected status of the company. Dissatisfaction may be driven by an approach or an avoidance motivation. As an approach motivation, the employer wants to build on the positive foundation of the existing operations and become even better. Issues such as reducing cycle time, strengthening staff skills or opening a new product line all point toward growth and further development of a healthy organization. As an avoidance motivation, the business is trying to move away from trouble. Issues such as deteriorating staff morale, high turnover, frequent error rates, damaged customer relations or declining market share are driving the business to consider outside help to bring health back to the organization. Once the employer feels the motivation to consider consultation services, there needs to be a compelling vision (V) of a better future. The employer needs a vivid image of the organization and the net results it will be producing. Before allowing the vision to pull the business toward the future, the employer wants to have a sense of the game plan to get from point A to point B. The first steps (FS) need to be mapped out to identify how the process will be set in motion. The plan of action needs to be concrete and reasonable before the company will buy into the effort required. When the dissatisfaction (D), vision (V) and first steps (FS) have been satisfied, then the employer is ready to set aside resistance (R) to becoming involved.

Underlying the formula are a set of ten conditions that must be addressed to the satisfaction of the employer in order to advance interest in hiring the person with disability and accepting the services of the practitioner. Lack of advancement is related to not satisfying one or more of the following prerequisite conditions:

1 Need, the prospect recognizes a need exists.
2 Responsibility, the prospect feels personal ownership and responsibility to fill the need or share in the responsibility to fill the need.
3 Authority, the prospect has authority to fill the need or participate with the proper authority to fill the need.
4 Discomfort, the prospect believes that dissatisfaction with the company's state of affairs will continue if the proposals put forth by the practitioner are not accepted.
5 Priority, the prospect believes the company need is a priority and can therefore justify allocation of resources to meet the need.
6 Satisfy, the prospect believes the solutions proposed by the practitioner will satisfy the need of the company.
7 Capability, the client or practitioner are credible and have the capability to satisfy the need.
8 Optimal Solution, the solution proposed by the practitioner is the best to the exclusion of others.
9 Price, the prospect believes the price to pay for the solution is a good return on the investment based on cost to obtain and use over time.
10 Viable Plan, the prospect views the plan of action proposed by the practitioner as workable.

(Sales Training America, 1994)

There are tangible and intangible motivators that facilitate the prospect's desire to work with a rehabilitation firm. At a basic level, the prospect and practitioner are engaged in an exchange process. The exchange is accomplished through use of a range of valued currencies. The practitioner needs to determine which type of currencies are germane to the prospect. From this understanding, the practitioner frames the presentation of proposals in terms that are relevant to the prospect. The valued related currencies can be categorized as:

- task
- position
- inspiration
- relationship
- personal.

(Cohen and Bradford, 1990)

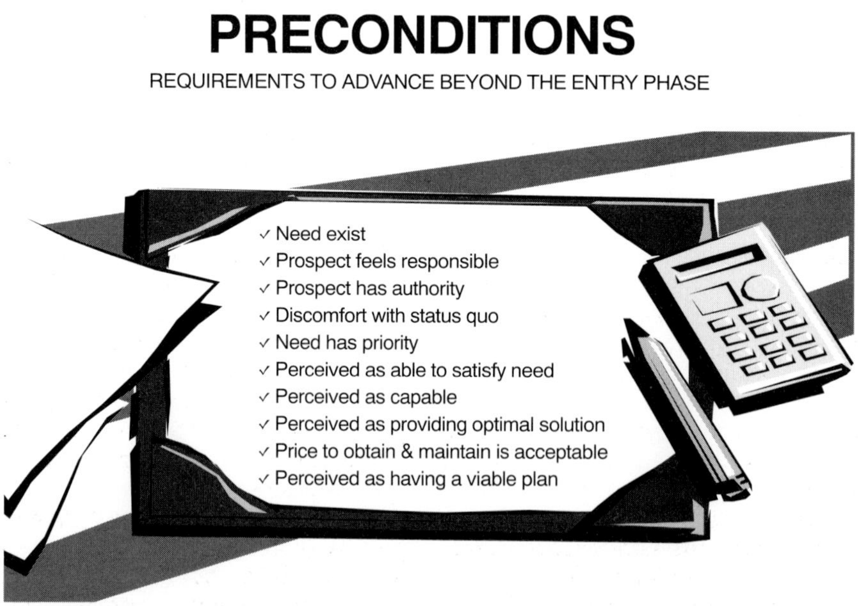

Figure 8.31 Preconditions.

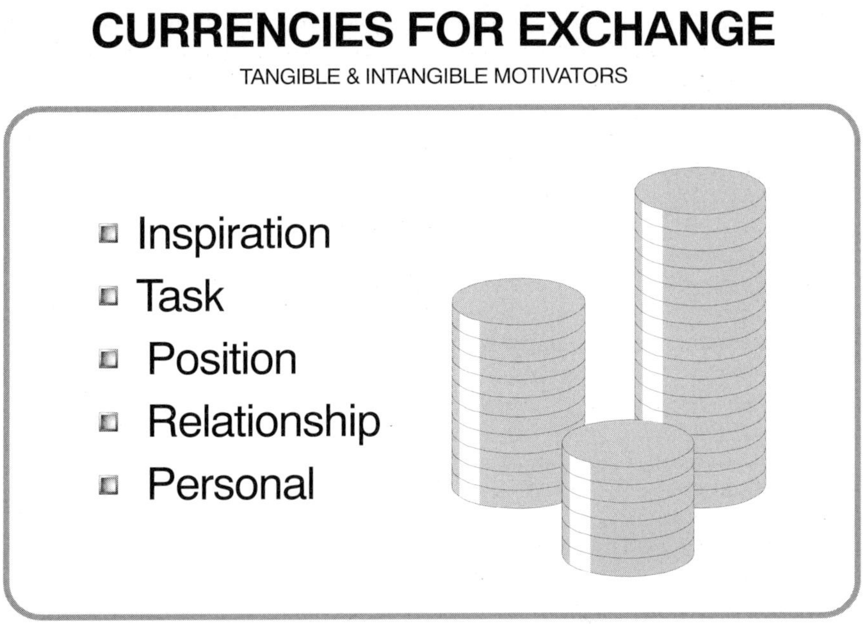

Figure 8.32 Currencies for exchange.

Task-related currencies focus on providing the prospect with new resources, technical assistance, task support, improved system performance, information, challenge or learning. Task-related currencies may include tax credits, on-the-job training payments to cover initial start-up costs, personnel, help with existing projects or unwanted tasks, performance training, access to technical knowledge, and value-added services such as team building, work-flow design or planning. For example, a conference centre located outside of a major metropolitan area experienced difficulty in recruiting and maintaining entry-level positions in the laundry room, guest-room cleaning, building maintenance and food service. The centre was not located on a public transportation route. It was not economically feasible for potential employees to buy cars or pay for private transportation to come to work for the wages offered. A rehabilitation firm proposed a solution that removed the barriers experienced by the conference centre. The rehabilitation firm offered to provide multiple candidates for employment in the various positions. With the candidates came guaranteed transportation to and from work through the transportation system of the provider, at no cost to the centre. In addition, the rehabilitation firm assisted in recruitment and transportation of non-disabled persons from the same geographic area served by the agency, thereby opening the door to a broad array of potential employees. The non-disabled workers paid the rehabilitation firm a reasonable amount for transportation and received a personalized service. The rehabilitation firm also offered to provide an onsite supervisor and job trainer, at no cost, as long as at least eight clients were hired throughout the complex. The employment specialist would provide technical assistance to the work supervisors in order to ensure the successful performance of the clients. The rehabilitation firm offered to arrange for on-the-job training money, through the state vocational rehabilitation agency, to cover part of the client wages for the first three months of employment. This would bring in thousands of dollars to cover operating expenses. The proposal offered task-related currencies to the employer in exchange for employment opportunities.

Position-related currencies provide the prospect with recognition, visibility, access to an inner circle of power, professional contacts, and reputation enhancement. Through the use of position-related currencies, the practitioner exchanges opportunities for the prospect to achieve a higher professional standing. For example, a prospect who was district manager for a claims department of a major insurance carrier wanted to become known as a civic leader in order to improve his chances for promotion to regional manager. A practitioner was seeking clerical employment for one of his clients. During the course of discussion regarding employment, the manager mentioned his interest in becoming a leader in the local community. The practitioner suggested to the manager that he could arrange a meeting with the local president of the chamber of commerce who served as chair on the board of directors of the rehabilitation firm. He mentioned his board was looking for a strong business leader to champion employment opportunities for disadvantaged persons and serve as a spokes person for the agency. The practitioner stressed the stature of board membership with his firm in the local community. He explained that each year a feature story was done by the newspaper entitled 'Rising Star'. The article was an in-depth report on the leadership qualities of a community board member. This is followed by a reception held in the person's honour. To be selected for this prestigious recognition, the person had to demonstrate first-hand experience promoting the welfare of others. The practitioner stated he would be more than pleased to help the manager once the employment opportunity was made available and proved to be successful.

Inspiration-related currencies focus on providing an opportunity for the prospect to participate and serve in an activity that is viewed as important to society, the company or the work unit. The activity is held in high moral esteem and represents excellence. A regional human-resource manager for a national food chain had a longing to move into more spiritual work, either by becoming a minister or by actively doing something for the greater good of the metropolitan area. When approached regarding employment opportunities, the practitioner directed the discussion toward the broader meaning of moving persons with severe disability into the mainstream of community life. It was framed in the context of creating opportunities for full citizenship and as a way to restore a person's civil rights. They discussed how the world for persons with severe and profound disability had in many ways turned into an apartheid-type relationship with the larger society, separate and not equal. Supported employment had proven itself as a worthy tool to remedy the unjust situation. The manager talked to the practitioner to determine how supported employment could become a central theme and initiative for the chain of stores that came under his jurisdiction.

Relationship-related currencies are concerned with a prospect feeling subjectively understood, accepted and part of an interpersonal bond with others. The practitioner's role is to facilitate the opportunity for personal support so that the prospect has a sense of membership, connection and friendship with people. For example, a practitioner made it a standing practice to invite the owners of several small businesses to attend business management seminars with the rehabilitation firm's senior management staff. This fostered a feeling of community and intimacy the small-shop owners felt lacking in their day-to-day business life. This led to employment opportunities directly from the participants and indirectly through personal sponsorship of the firm to other business connections. The small-business owners looked out for the rehabilitation firm.

Personal-related currencies focus on exchanges linked to expressions of a prospect's gratitude and influence. The currencies are used by a practitioner to affirm values, self-esteem, identity and power of the prospect over important tasks. For example, a prominent business leader's daughter was injured in an automobile accident when she was 16. It resulted in a traumatic brain injury. A rehabilitation hospital worked with the daughter for two years. They assigned an occupational therapist and a vocational rehabilitation counsellor to assist the daughter in learning how to restore functioning, hold a job, and begin a career. At 18 the daughter was prepared to transition from high school to the adult world. The mayor of the city asked the business leader to chair an employment initiative for youth in transition from school to work. The business leader was more than eager to demonstrate her appreciation for what rehabilitation services had done to help her daughter. The business leader made personal contacts with the top one hundred employers in the city on behalf of the school system. She orchestrated a major media event to boost the initiative and established an annual scholarship for transitioning youth.

After screening, defining mutual benefits, establishing credibility, and overcoming initial resistance, the consultant negotiates a preliminary contract that outlines the basic parameters of the consultation process. Areas in the contract cover:

1 goals and outcomes
2 work products
3 time frame
4 mutual responsibilities
5 services to be provided
6 methods to be used
7 boundaries and limitations of the consultation
8 protocols for relating to the employer, such as contact person, chain of command to be followed, internal sponsorship, access to sources of data and people, approval check points, confidentiality
9 reporting requirements
10 escape clauses indicating the mechanism for terminating the process by either party.

The contract can be oral or written. There is a benefit in drafting a simple written statement. It keeps mutual expectations and responsibilities clear, and demonstrates professionalism. The degree of formality is dependent on the relationship between parties and the complexity of the consultation.

Once the consultation process is agreed upon, the consultant physically and psychologically enters the system. The leader within the organization plays a key role in smoothing the transition and paving the way for the consultant to be well received. The leader:

1 gives the membership advance notice
2 describes the reason, purpose and use of findings
3 outlines the consultation process
4 indicates the role members are expected to play
5 states the degree of confidentiality that will exist with each member's input
6 stresses the importance of each person's perceptions, thoughts, feelings, ideas, and candour.

When physically within the system, the consultant works on gaining psychological acceptance by members of the organization. Acceptance is achieved when the consultant is viewed as being predictable, reliable and trustworthy. The consultant facilitates acceptance by being genuine, empathic, straightforward, polite, truthful, realistic, consistent, avoids implying ulterior motives or taking sides, avoids placing others in an uncomfortable light in front of coworkers, keeps confidences where appropriate, shows respect and deference to members, projects an accepting and non-judgemental attitude, asks relevant questions instead of giving personal opinions, and is willing to explore conflictual or sensitive issues without implying blame or fear.

Upon completion of the entry phase tasks, the consultant moves into the diagnostic phase. Major tasks include:

1 formulating the method and type of data to gather
2 gathering the data
3 analysing the data
4 formulating a working hypothesis regarding key issues and root causes
5 verifying and developing a consensus regarding key issues and root causes
6 establishing remediation goals.
(Dougherty, 1990; Lippitt and Lippitt, 1986; Manzini, 1988)

The method of data gathering characteristically involves direct observations, interviews and document reviews. It is not uncommon for staff to reveal, very directly, the key issues, problems and solutions that need to be addressed. As discussed previously, focusing on variance data sources and process analysis provides valuable insights.

This is a time when there are bruised feelings and defensiveness. The consultant's role is to provide emotional support so that the parties can face issues directly. A way to ease the process is for the consultant to establish basic principles everyone agrees to follow. One such basic principle is concerned with the concept of blame. The consultant stresses the purpose of the analysis is not to fix blame but to seek clarity and direction to improve performance. Another guideline includes an agreement to present feedback in a manner that supports a person's self-confidence and self-esteem. Private counsel is provided to management on how to role model facing critical feedback. No matter how positive a work culture, workers will always be dissatisfied with management and feel things are worse than management wants to admit. Sharing this information with management, before the feedback is presented, normalizes the defensiveness that is bound to be experienced. It draws upon management to rise to the occasion to demonstrate leadership when facing potentially unpleasant feedback. The process is further eased by cascading the reporting. First, the consultant briefs the senior management followed by middle management and then the entire body at once. This minimizes the potential of placing management in an embarrassing light where they may feel ambushed. It also allows management to shape how the information will be presented. Not to avoid any truths, but in a way that management does not feel out of control.

Setting goals occurs when there is consensus regarding the key issues and root causes. The tasks associated with this step involve facilitating creative and analytical thinking so that members of the organization can discover new possibilities to improve performance. During this time the consultant works to open thinking to discover alternative scenarios and avoid erroneous extrapolation. The task then shifts to narrowing thinking to identify end states to be achieved based on a future vision of how the organization will function. The goals are set in accordance with criteria that they must be:

1 behavioural, clear, concrete, specific, operational
2 measurable and verifiable
3 stretching yet realistic and capable of being accomplished with available resources
4 worthwhile, adding value, doing more with less more efficiently and effectively
5 compatible with organizational and consultant values
6 accomplishable within a reasonable time frame.

The consultant supports the consultees in working through challenges of goal setting by minimizing unhealthy stress or anxiety that may interfere with envisioning new scenarios, and by facilitating the consensus building processes. Discussions take place regarding issues such as:

- risk taking
- failure as a learning experience
- conflict resolution
- choosing quality and excellence over expediency
- personal and shared commitment to achieve objectives
- mutual support
- team work
- progress measurement and feedback
- mid-course corrections
- the importance of achieving bottom-line results.

During the implementation phase, the consultant facilitates the process of choosing an intervention, formulating a plan, implementing the plan, and evaluating the plan (Dougherty, 1990; Lippitt and Lippitt, 1986; Manzini, 1988). Implementation strategies are successful when there is:

1 A clear vision of a desired future state.
2 A clear and accurate definition of the business.
3 A clear and accurate definition of strategic business units.
4 Proper preparation of line managers.
5 A balance between quantitative and qualitative goals.
6 A proper and balanced focus on external, environmental issues and internal operations considerations.
7 A realistic and candid self-assessment.
8 Sufficient action detailing.
9 Effective participation across functions and key stakeholders.
10 Healthy management of conflict.
11 Congruence of controls and systems with the strategic direction and values.
12 An ability to move from strategic visioning and planning to strategic management. (Judson, 1990)

Before moving forward it is imperative that there is a shared vision of the destination both at the organizational and personal levels. Without the shared vision people will pull in different directions thereby immobilizing the process and creating unnecessary conflict. The shared vision needs to be as concrete as possible. Prior to establishing a shared vision, it is important to define the business mission and purpose properly. It has often been commented by leaders in the rehabilitation field that, from an outsider's point of view, it appears that day activity centres for persons with severe disability were in the ceramic business. The focus had narrowed so much that staff's main objective turned into managing the production of ceramic art instead of preparing the person for a life in the community. Management and staff lost sight of the broader intended mission of the industry, organization, work unit and roles.

Implementation of a plan of action will fail if front-line supervisors are not properly prepared. In the late 1960s and early 1970's, a New England state hired a prison commissioner who set a major frame-breaking reform initiative in motion. A variety of issues resulted in its demise. One of the key factors was a lack of training and support for the front-line prison guards and management. They were left without a clear sense of their new role. Nor were they clear on the overall initiative and its relationship with their existing understanding of the purpose of prison. The initiative went flat and the prison commissioner was relieved of his duties.

Excessive focus on financial and production numbers initially appears to create a winning situation. Operations become very focused and concrete results are produced. This is true for the short run but fails over time. It gives a false sense of success. Myopic focus on numbers constrains performance and dramatically reduces a person's time horizon. The emphasis moves from actions that invest in the future to decisions and behaviours that represent harvesting in the present. The controls, rewards and systems become designed around immediate gain with little regard to long-term strategy. This may lead to misplaced attention on optimizing internal operations to the detriment of broader more profound strategic positioning issues in the environment. It is critical that measures of success are congruent with the strategic direction stated in the implementation plan. All too frequently new measures of success are added while old measures still remain. On the contrary, an organization can spend too much time on scanning the environment and planning. This leads to difficulty in translating grand designs into practical realities. Implementation will fail if the strategic thrusts and goals are not translated into a coordinated set of action steps, assignments, accountably, time frames, milestones and concrete results.

Forward movement needs to be based on a realistic self-assessment of the present strengths and weaknesses as they relate to strategic positioning. False analysis leads to improper diagnosis of needs, mistaken goal setting and off-based implementation planning. The organization ends up working on the wrong issues. Time, effort and resources go to waste. Waste is also generated when the planning fails to take into account key stakeholders across multiple functions. Without synthesizing the variety of views each stakeholder brings to the table, an implementation plan will hit many dead-ends as it reveals needs that were not proactively addressed. Upstream participation and discussion with key stakeholders combined with explicit action detailing are time-consuming activities that ensure efficient and effective implementation downstream. Well begun is half done.

Conflict is unpleasant. It is a part of organizational life that must be recognized and leveraged positively. Management plays a significant role in facilitating the resolution of conflict in healthy ways by ensuring that open and fair treatment is given to all parties. When issues are not dealt with honestly, openly and fairly, the situation becomes political. Power over others replaces collaboration and win-win strategies. A sense of scarcity overtakes people's emotions. This does not mean that all parties get an equal distribution of resources, attention or other forms of privilege. It does mean that management is forthright regarding the decision-making process.

Conflict resolution training and operational forums to which members can turn to resolve issues are useful. An interdepartmental collaboration and coordinating committee is an example. Although it is important to focus on differences and diversity, it is equally important to focus on common ground. Frequently the conflicts of divergent positions can be translated into gains for both parties by searching for the essence of what each party wants or needs. Once the essence is understood, then a creative solution may come forth to meet underlying needs in ways not conceived before the dialogue was opened. In other words, a party may get what is wanted but in a way not anticipated. For example, a worker may request a raise to cover child-care costs but there is no money available to meet the need in the traditional manner. One solution may be to pay the person the same for fewer hours of work. This would allow the person to spend more time with his children without incurring the cost of child-care during those days. He is able to retain his revenue position while decreasing his expenses. He has a net gain.

In essence, the degree of success in implementing an action plan is tied to seven basic issues:

1 understanding
2 commitment
3 resources
4 ability
5 accountability
6 tracking
7 mid-course corrections.

Achievement of results is enhanced when there is a clear understanding of the external and internal customer needs. The more people comprehend the reasons for the change, the desired outcomes, the work-plan strategy and each person's required behavioural performance, the higher the probability goals will be reached. Understanding, however, is not enough. There needs to be credible objectives and strategies that employees and key stakeholders can own. Without ownership any plan is condemned to failure. Adequate resources need to be identified and made available to make the journey and maintain the success. People and systems need to have the ability to meet the challenges put forth. People need to keep promises and be held accountable for deliverable, measurable results. A culture of taking personal responsibility is required. If performance outcomes are expected, then they need to be inspected. That which is given attention grows. Staff closely observe the real focus of management in order to take cues regarding the real agenda that is expected to be followed. Through ongoing comparison of actual versus planned outcomes, modifications can be made to get back on track before compounding problems. Measurement not only tracks errors but is also used to catch people doing things right. Objectives, goals and strategies need to be constantly re-evaluated to determine relevancy in face of changing realities.

The disengagement phase is the point at which the consultant and the targeted organization:

1 evaluate the consultation process
2 plan post-consultation issues
3 fade involvement
4 ensure long-term support mechanisms are in place to sustain success
5 terminate the assignment
6 engage in post-consultation follow along, if required.
(Dougherty, 1990; Lippitt and Lippitt, 1986; Manzini, 1988)

The purpose of the evaluation is to step back and evaluate the overall success of the project. The basic question of whether or not the project achieved what it set out to accomplish is discussed. It serves as a quality review and learning mechanism to determine customer satisfaction, outline areas where the process could be improved, and reflect on what was discovered. Each party reviews what was learned about the organization, human resources, market forces, planning, goal setting, implementation, and quality improvement needs that still need to be addressed. Assumptions made at the beginning of the process are compared to the reality of what was encountered along the way.

Fading involvement begins the day the consultation begins. The objective is for the organization to be adaptive and self-sustaining. The role of the consultant each step along the way is to facilitate implementation, development and ownership. By the end of the project the consultant should be viewed as a peer colleague who is available to provide future help and follow along support. Yet the work to sustain the improvements belongs to the members of the organization. Before fading, the consultant ensures the conditions are in place to provide a positive and lasting future for the client.

Final comments

Rapid discontinuous change is surrounding every industry. Business is faced with market fragmentation, mass customization, and shrinking product life cycles. It is a time of fundamental uncertainty. Industries across the board are redefining their purpose and direction. Motion is everywhere. Company resources are under continual realignment. New forms of organizational structure are emerging that cross traditional boundaries. Companies are forming strategic alliances and networks that result in virtual corporation structures. The waves of change are accelerating. Business is moving from an information wave to a productivity wave. The driving forces demand 'doing more with less'. The phrase 'once and for all' is an obsolete notion. Everyone is surrounded with contradictory information. Ambiguity is fast becoming a way of life. Business leaders are confronted with the fact that they can no longer afford to drive their companies through the rear view mirror. It is a time that demands breakthrough thinking and the unleashing of creative capacities. Unification of divergent parts of various systems under a common purpose is opening doors to the future. Flexibility, agility and creativity are hallmarks for survival. It is a time when the anchor of the past is being replaced by the pull of the future.

Permanent structural relationships within organizations are being replaced with loose couplings with resources from outside. Networks and alliances are forming the core logic of organizational design. Companies are 'desperately seeking synergy'. Maximum flexibility is required that allows for putting together and taking apart resource requirements as they change. Access to energy and resources outside the firm is paramount. Networking and strategic alliances facilitate a firm's ability to improve timing, develop rapid access to markets, lower costs, increase service, improve quality, and be open to growth or development opportunities.

The field of vocational rehabilitation is not immune to these dynamics. In fact it is intimately tied to the business environment. The objective of vocational rehabilitation is employment. Jobs are located within business. While business is learning to 'do more with less', social services are learning to 'do less with less'. The general tax paying public, in the United States, is no longer willing to invest in social programmes that do not show more immediate, practical returns. The key to success is by beginning at the end. If the objective is employment, then starting with a real job delivers the results more directly. From recent experiences with supported employment, this axiom has reaped rewards previously considered unobtainable.

To ensure employment opportunities for persons with severe disability, vocational rehabilitation practitioners need to expand the range of skills to incorporate organizational, performance and business consultation. Practitioners will need to become more familiar with value and process engineering. Services need to be reframed as adding economic value to business by improving revenue opportunities, reducing costs, avoiding costs or offsetting costs. The relationship with business needs to be viewed as a strategic alliance and partnership. As many other industries seek to network with other companies to meet business objectives, vocational rehabilitation practitioners are well positioned to follow suit.

Economic value can be demonstrated to business by analysing the socio-technical work processes. Searching for ways to streamline or reconfigure operations creates value for the company and opportunity for employment. Providing ongoing consultation in organizational and human resource development areas positions the practitioner as providing value-added services that positively exceed customer expectations and translate into access to jobs and maintenance of previous placements.

Enhancing cognitive performance for persons with intellectual impairment is more efficiently achieved through contextual learning. The functional issues and elements of the work environment are factored into what is taught, including becoming a member of the company culture. There is less time spent on non-relevant training and support. Building and using naturally occurring supports within the work setting reduces alienation and separation of the person with severe disability. It strengthens the company's ability to provide the long-term support that may be needed. With reduced internal resources in the rehabilitation firm, the practitioner needs to find creative ways to arrange for someone else to do as many of the duties traditionally man-

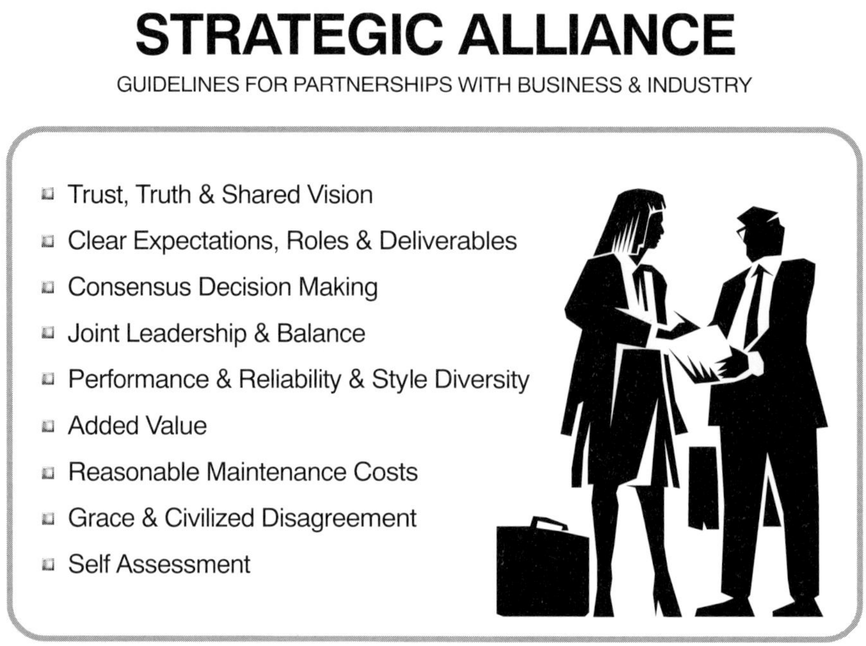
STRATEGIC ALLIANCE
GUIDELINES FOR PARTNERSHIPS WITH BUSINESS & INDUSTRY
Trust, Truth & Shared Vision
Clear Expectations, Roles & Deliverables
Consensus Decision Making
Joint Leadership & Balance
Performance & Reliability & Style Diversity
Added Value
Reasonable Maintenance Costs
Grace & Civilized Disagreement
Self Assessment

Figure 8.33 Strategic alliance.

aged by the disability professionals. Building the capacity of the employer or generic community resources will be a major focus for the practitioner.

Strategic alliances and partnerships directly with business meet the needs of the client, business and the rehabilitation firm. Rehabilitation practitioners have a wealth of knowledge and skills that can translate into value-adding services to an employer. Psycho-educational aspects of training, learning and motivating are skills and resources many businesses need to remain competitive. By helping a business identify critical success factors for enhancing performance, the practitioner becomes a valued resource. With the addition of business knowledge and skills, the practitioner becomes a valuable partner and resource. Not all businesses are candidates for forming a strategic alliance and partnership. Careful weighting of the required investment for the desired outcome needs to be considered. Ingredients of a healthy partnership need to be nurtured for long-term success.

The most effective advocacy for vocational rehabilitation services and the client is to create and add value for business and the community.

References

Albin, J. M. (1992). *Quality Improvement in Employment and Other Human Services*. Baltimore: Paul H. Brookes Publishing Co.

Ashkenas, R., Ulrich, D., Jick, T. and Kerr, S. (1995). *The Boundaryless Organization*. San Francisco: Jossey-Bass Publishers.

Band, W. A. (1991). *Creating Value For Customers: Designing and Implementing a Total Corporate Strategy*. Canada: John Wiley & Sons, Inc.

Bell, C. R. (1994). *Customers As Partners*. San Francisco: Berrett-Koehler Publishers.

Bellak, L. and Small, L. (1978). *Emergency Psychotherapy and Brief Psychotherapy*, 2nd edn. Larchmont, NY: Library of Congress Cataloging in Publication Data.

Camp, R. C. (1989). *Benchmarking: The Search for Industry Best Practices that Lead to Superior Performance*. Milwaukee: Quality Press.

Chase, R. B. and Stewart, D. M. (1995). *Mistake-Proofing*. Portland: Productivity Press, Inc.

Cohen, A. R. and Bradford, D. L. (1990). *Influence without Authority*. New York: John Wiley & Sons.

DeRose, L. (1989). *Value Selling: The Strategy for Reaching the Industrial Customer, Satisfying Customer Requirements, Competing in Cost-Conscious Markets*. New York: AMACOM.

Dougherty, A. M. (1990). *Consultation: Practice and Perspectives*. Pacific Grove, CA: Brooks/Cole Publishing Co.

Fabian, E. S., Luecking, R. G. and Tilson Jr., G. P. (1994). *A Working Relationship: The Job Development Specialist's Guide to Successful Partnerships with Business*. Baltimore: Paul H. Brookes Publishing Co.

Feuerstein, R. (1979). *The Dynamic Assessment of Retarded Performers: The Learning Potential Assessment Device, Theory, Instruments, and Techniques*. Baltimore: University Park Press.

Frost, P. J., Moore, L. F., Louis, M. R., Lundberg, C. C. and Martin, J. (1985). *Organizational Culture*. Beverly Hills, CA: Sage Publications, Inc.

Gilbert, T. F. (1978). *Human Competence*. New York: McGraw-Hill, Inc.

Goldstein, J. (1994). *The Unshackled Organization*. Portland: Productivity Press, Inc.

Heinssen, R. K. and Glass, C. R. (1990). Social skills, social anxiety, and cognitive factors in schizophrenia. In *Handbook of Social and Evaluation Anxiety* (H. Leitenberg, ed.) pp. 325–55, Plenum Publishing Corporation.

Hupp, T., Polak, C. and Westgaard, O. (1995). *Designing Work Groups, Jobs, and Work Flow*. San Francisco: Jossey-Bass, Inc. Publishers.

Jacobs, R. W. (1994). *Real Time Strategic Change*. San Francisco: Berrett-Koehler Publishers.

Janis, I. L. (1982). *Counseling On Personal Decisions: Theory and Research on Short Term Helping Relationships*. New Haven, CT: Yale University Press.

Judson, A. (1990). *Making Strategy Happen*. Cambridge, MA: Basil Blackwell, Inc.

Kegan, R. (1982). *The Evolving Self*. Cambridge, MA: Harvard University Press.

Kelly, P. J. (1988). *Situational Selling: Six Keys to Mastering the Complex Business Sale*. New York: AMACOM.

Kilmann, R. H. (1989). *Managing Beyond The Quick Fix: A Completely Integrated Program for Creating and Maintaining Organizational Success*. San Francisco: Jossey-Bass Publishers.

Knefelkamp, L. and Cornfeld, J. L. (1978, October). Combing student stage and style in design of learning environments using Holland Topologies and Perry's Stages. Paper presented at the University of Maryland, College of Education. College Park, MD.

Kobayashi, I. (1988). *20 Keys to Workplace Improvement*. Portland: Productivity Press, Inc.

Langs, R. (1982). *Psychotherapy*. New York: Jason Aronson, Inc.

Lawton, R. L. (1993). *Creating a Customer-Centered Culture*. Milwaukee: ASQC Quality Press.

Lekak, M. D. (1976). *Neuropsychological Assessment*, 2nd edn. Oxford: Oxford University Press, Inc.

Lewis, J. D. (1990). *Partnerships For Profit: Structuring and Managing Strategic Alliances*. New York: The Free Press, A Division of Macmillan, Inc.

Lippitt, G. and Lippitt, R. (1986). *The Consulting Process In Action*, 2nd edn. San Diego: University Associates, Inc.

Lovett, H. (1985). *Cognitive Counseling and Persons with Special Needs: Adapting Behavioral Approaches to the Social Context*. New York: Praeger Publishers.

Lynch, R. F. and Werner, T. J. (1994). *Reengineering Business Processes and People Systems*. Atlanta: QualTeam, Inc.

Lytle, W. O. (1991). *Socio-Technical Systems Analysis and Design Guide*. Plainfield, NJ: Block-Petrella-Weisbord, Inc.

Manzini, A. O. (1988). *Organizational Diagnosis: A Practical Approach to Company Problem Solving and Growth*. New York: AMACOM.

Melan, E. H. (1995). *Process Management: A System Approach to Total Quality*. Portland: Productivity Press, Inc.

Meyers, C. H. (1992). *Improving Whole Systems*. NJ: Block Petrella Weisbord, Inc.

Miller, L. M. (1994). *Whole System Architecture*. Atlanta, GA: Miller Howard Consulting Group, Inc.

Mirsky, A. F. (1987). Behavioral and psychophysiological markers of disordered attention. *Environmental Health Perspectives*; **74**, 191–9.

Morton, M. S. S. (1991). *The Corporation of the 1990s: Information Technology and Organizational Transformation*. Oxford: Oxford University Press.

Nagel, K. (1991). *The 6 Keys To Company Success*. Great Britain: Fitzwilliam Publishing Limited.

Nilson, T. H. (1992). *Valued-Added Marketing*. London: McGraw-Hill Book Company.

Porter, M. E. (1980). *Competitive Strategy*. New York: The Free Press, A Division of Macmillan Publishing Co., Inc.

Quinn, R. E. (1990). *Beyond Rational Management*. San Francisco: Jossey-Bass Inc., Publishers.

Rickards, T. (1974). *Problem-Solving Through Creative Analysis*. Great Britain: Gower Press Limited.

Risher, H. and Fay, C. (1995). *The Performance Imperative: Strategies For Enhancing Workforce Effectiveness*. San Francisco: Jossey-Bass, Inc.

Robinson, D. G. and Robinson, J. C. (1995). *Performance Consulting*. San Francisco: Berrett-Koehler Publishers, Inc.

Rummler, G. A., Brache, A. P. (1995). *Improving Performance*. San Francisco: Jossey-Bass Publishers, Inc.

Sales Training America (1994). *Criteria Driven Value Selling*. Woodlands, TX: Sales Training America.

Shea, G. F. (1994). *Mentoring*. New York: AMA Membership Publications Division.

Sims Jr., H. P., Gioia, D. A. *et al.* (1986). *The Thinking Organization*. San Francisco: Jossey-Bass Inc. Publishers.

Smith, P. and Kearny, L. (1994). *Creating Workplaces Where People Can Think*. San Francisco: Jossey-Bass Publishers.

Swanson, R. A. (1994). *Analysis for Improving Performance*. San Francisco: Berrett-Koehler Publishers, Inc.

Wolf, M. D. and Ernest, S. (1988). *Treating The Self*. New York: The Guilford Press.

9

Work Programmes to Enhance Motor and Neuromusculoskeletal Performance Components

Ev Innes

Learning Objectives

At the end of this chapter the reader should be able to:

1. Identify the major forms of workplace-based and clinic-based approaches to enhancing neuromusculoskeletal and motor performance components.
2. Identify the key components of each form of return-to-work programme and indicators of appropriate use.
3. Define work fitness and the key aspects which must be addressed to improve neuromusculoskeletal and motor performance function.
4. Design a basic clinic-based and workplace-based rehabilitation programme.

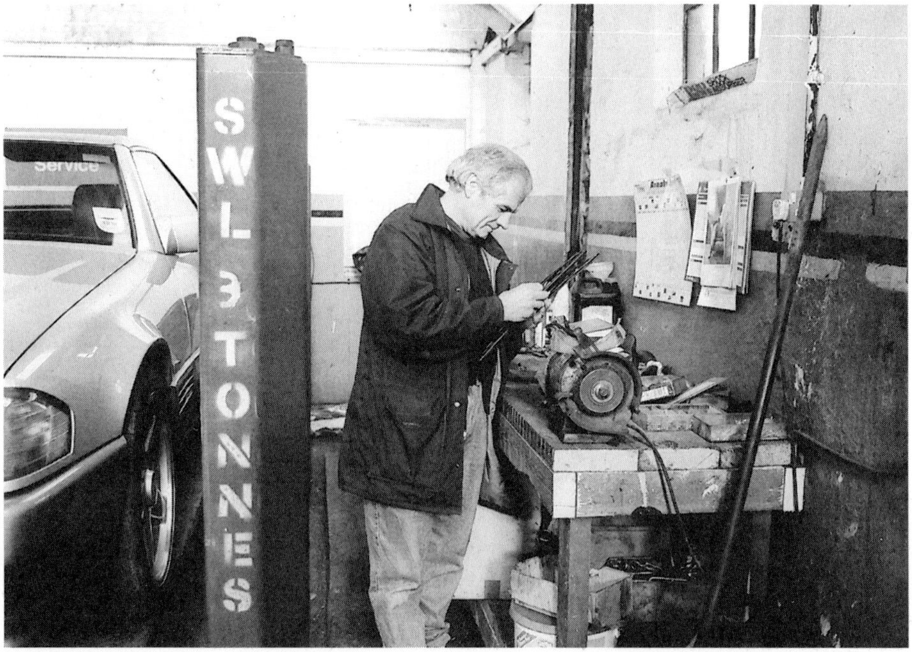

Abstract

A continuum of return-to-work programmes ranging from work hardening through work conditioning, to workplace-based is presented. Work hardening and work conditioning are clinic-based programmes focused on improvement of neuromusculoskeletal and motor performance component function, while workplace-based rehabilitation is focused on improvement in overall job performance. Aspects of work fitness are identified and described with particular emphasis on areas to improve neuromusculoskeletal and motor performance. The concept of suitable duties is presented and explained. Case studies exemplify both clinic and workplace based programmes and how they are interrelated.

Introduction

This chapter presents the three major approaches to return-to-work programmes (work hardening, work conditioning and workplace-based rehabilitation) for individuals with neuromusculoskeletal and motor impairment. These programmes are based on the concept of work fitness and the elements which comprise it. In order to appreciate the components of the return-to-work programmes presented, it is necessary to be familiar with the elements of work fitness and how each of these may be individually addressed.

All areas of occupational performance require the physical performance, or 'doing', of an activity or task to carry out the occupations that fulfil our role repertories. The neuromusculoskeletal and motor performance component areas translate what a person perceives, recalls and plans into action or physical performance (Ranka and Chapparo, 1995).

Rehabilitation should address all the roles an individual fulfils, rather than only the worker role (Bammer *et al.*, 1994). This implies that not only the work requirement and environment are considered, but also other aspects of an individual's lifestyle, such as

Key words and definitions in this chapter

Clinic-based rehabilitation: Rehabilitation that occurs in a facility removed from the actual workplace.

Motor performance component: Consists of gross coordination, crossing the midline, laterality, bilateral integration, motor control, praxis, fine coordination/dexterity, visual–motor integration and oral–motor control.

Neuromusculoskeletal performance component: Consists of reflex, range of motion, muscle tone, strength, endurance, postural control, postural alignment and soft tissue integrity.

Occupational rehabilitation: 'The restoration of . . . injured worker[s] to the fullest physical, psychological, social, vocational and economic usefulness of which they are capable, consistent with pre-injury status. It is a managed process aimed at maintaining injured or ill workers in or returning them to suitable employment. It involves early intervention with appropriate, adequate and timely services based on assessment of the injured worker's needs' (WorkCover Authority of NSW, 1993, p. 9).

Suitable duties: Duties identified in the workplace which match the individual's capacities, avoid risk of further injury and have regard for the injured worker's abilities and limitations, pre-injury employment, age, education, skills, work experience, place of residence, rehabilitation plan and any other relevant aspects.

Work fitness: The capacity to meet successfully the present and potential challenges of work requirements with vigour, and to demonstrate the traits and capacities associated with low risk of premature development of occupational injuries and diseases.

Workplace-based rehabilitation: Rehabilitation of individuals, usually those with a work-related injury, in the workplace.

home, leisure and social life. 'The arbitrary isolation of a single aspect of a person's life and focus on the worker role alone, has the effect of devaluing and failing to acknowledge the impact and interplay that occurs between the various roles and activities performed by individuals within their own environments' (Innes, 1995: 151).

Work and productive activities, however, play an important part in the lives of individuals. They are viewed as being central to the self-identification of adults in Western societies. The work we perform, particularly paid employment, is how we describe and define ourselves to others. It is the response made to the usual question, 'What do you do?'

An inability to perform the worker role, therefore, greatly interferes with overall occupational performance. Many work-related injuries and disabilities affect the neuromusculoskeletal and motor performance component areas. Other disorders, although not workplace related, also result in neuromusculoskeletal and motor impairment, making it difficult to perform the activities and tasks required to achieve satisfactory work performance.

Neuromusculoskeletal and motor performance components

The neuromusculoskeletal performance component encompasses reflex, range of motion, muscle tone, strength, endurance, postural control, postural alignment and soft tissue integrity (American Occupational Therapy Association, 1994). The motor performance component includes gross coordination, crossing the midline, laterality, bilateral integration, motor control, praxis, fine coordination/dexterity, visual–motor integration and oral–motor control (American Occupational Therapy Association, 1994).

The neuromusculoskeletal and motor performance components most commonly affected by work-related problems are those of strength, range of motion, endurance (both cardiorespiratory and muscle endurance), postural alignment and fine coordination/dexterity. Together with these aspects of physical dysfunction, there is also the problem of pain, both acute and chronic, associated with a neuromusculoskeletal or motor impairment. Pain is particularly debilitating when it becomes chronic in nature.

The physical demands of work as defined by the US Department of Labor (1991) include strength, climbing, balancing, stooping, kneeling, crouching, crawling, reaching, handling, fingering, feeling, talking, hearing, tasting/smelling, near acuity, far acuity, depth perception, accommodation, colour vision and field of vision.

When neuromusculoskeletal and motor components are considered in the context of work, it is usually these physical demands of work that are addressed, particularly strength through to feeling.

The impact of neuromusculoskeletal and motor performance component deficits on work

Within the workplace the most common types of injuries and disorders which affect an individual's capacity to perform usual productivity tasks are those that impact on the neuromusculoskeletal and motor performance components. These types of impairments include sprains, strains, crush injuries, lacerations, burns, fractures and dislocation-type injuries to various parts of the body. Overuse injuries, or cumulative trauma disorders, affecting the back, neck and upper limbs are also common. Conditions which result in a reduced energy capacity such as cardiac and respiratory disorders and deconditioning due to prolonged inactivity also affect an individual's capacity to perform necessary work activities and tasks. The movements and postures or positions required in some jobs can contribute to the development of work-related disorders.

The basic components of occupations in which impairment of the neuromusculoskeletal and motor components results in difficulty performing job tasks include:

- Maintaining prolonged static postures and positions. This includes standing, sitting, stooping, twisting (of the neck and trunk); maintaining upper extremity positions such as being in a 'key ready' position for keyboard operators; working at inappropriate heights requiring excessive shoulder abduction, wrist extension, etc.

- Performing repetitive movements for extended periods of time, or fast bursts of repetitive movements performed infrequently without the opportunity to adequately warm-up. This may include work with little variety or opportunity to change tasks, or piecework, where workers are paid on the number of items produced, rather than the time worked;
- Heavy work requiring strength and/or endurance, or having to cope with a sudden unexpected load. This encompasses more than just lifting, and includes such things as pushing or pulling and other aspects of manual handling. It also includes work with high energy expenditure.
- Working in extreme ranges of motion while also applying force.
- Working in confined or restricted conditions which do not enable the individual to be in a 'good' working position.
- Periods of very heavy workload, such as at the end of the financial year, before a public holiday, at the end of the month, and so on, resulting in overload.
- Stressful environments within the workplace and at home. This may be physical, cognitive or psychosocial stressors such as conflict with the supervisor or other workers, or family conflict or stress.

Link with other performance components and their impact on work

Contrary to expectations, in the case of neuromusculoskeletal and motor injuries, the severity of a person's injury is not related to the likelihood of that individual returning to work (Lusted, 1993; Strautins and Hall, 1989). That is, the assumption that the more severe the injury the less likely a person is to return to work is not supported by the literature for the majority of injuries which affect the neuromusculoskeletal and motor components. This indicates that there are other factors which influence a person's capacity and ability to return to work successfully. It is not possible, therefore, to make assumptions about return-to-work potential on the basis of the injury or impairment of the neuromusculoskeletal and motor components alone. There are multiple factors which influence a person's ability to return to work.

This finding has implications for the type of programmes which are developed to assist injured workers to return safely to work and productive employment. This situation also demonstrates the interrelatedness of all performance components on overall occupational performance. Job satisfaction, for example, has been found to be a predictive factor in the development of back pain and successful return-to-work following an injury (Bigos *et al.*, 1991; Hurri, 1989; Linton and Warg, 1993).

Work programmes designed to improve neuromusculoskeletal and motor performance component problems should also include aspects which address other performance components, such as psychosocial, cognitive and sensory. This is the case particularly when chronic pain also affects performance.

Person–activity–environment fit

The person–activity–environment fit is a crucial concept in the development of work programmes. It is necessary to identify the match and/or mismatch which exists between the person, the job performed and environment or context in which it is performed.

Identification of person–activity–environment match and/or mismatch can be achieved by:

- Assessing the person's capacity and abilities using an appropriate selection of work assessments (see Chapter 6).
- Performing a worksite visit and a job analysis of the person's job, or a range of jobs, to which the person may return and the environment in which they are performed.

- Identifying the match and/or mismatch between the person, the job and the environment.

This determination of match and mismatch between the person, the job and the environment assists in identifying appropriate intervention approaches and strategies and treatment modalities which may be used. For example, when there is a match between the individual's capabilities and specific job and environmental requirements it is possible to determine suitable duties for the person to perform. This ensures that the client is able to return to work as soon as possible. Further upgrading at work in terms of time, duties, effort, weight and so on can then occur at the workplace.

In cases where a mismatch between a person's capabilities and the job requirements occurs, it is possible to determine the nature of the problem and identify possible intervention strategies. These may include job or environmental modifications, or targeting neuromusculoskeletal or motor component areas requiring improvement within the individual. It may be possible for this to occur at the workplace without the client leaving the job. It may be necessary for the client to attend a health practitioner for specific treatment (e.g. physiotherapy) but continue at work. If the mismatch between the individual's capabilities and job requirements is too severe, then there is the need to consider other options, such as centre-based programmes.

Work fitness

Physical fitness has been defined by various authors as:

> the capacity to meet successfully the present and potential physical challenges of life. (Lamb, 1984, cited in Minor, 1991: 200)

> a state characterized by (a) an ability to perform daily activities with vigour, and (b) demonstration of traits and capacities that are associated with low risk of premature development of hypokinetic diseases (i.e. those associated with physical inactivity). (American College of Sports Medicine, 1991: 35)

If these definitions are considered in the context of work, then work fitness can be defined as the capacity to meet successfully the present and potential challenges of work requirements with vigour, and to demonstrate the traits and capacities associated with low risk of premature development of occupational injuries and diseases.

This definition of work fitness considers not only the current demands required of the job at hand, but also the prevention of future injury by lowering the risk of developing occupational injuries or diseases through improving the status of the elements which make up work fitness. Unlike physical fitness, which consists of cardiorespiratory endurance, muscle strength and endurance, flexibility and body composition, work fitness includes capacity in all performance component areas required to function successfully in all the roles an individual fulfils, including work. In the context of this chapter, however, only the neuromusculoskeletal and motor components of work fitness will be considered.

By considering the concept of work fitness in a way similar to fitness for athletic performance, it is also possible to consider the treatment of work injuries in a similar way to sporting injuries. The worker is then considered as an industrial athlete. This is based on the assumption that all jobs require a level of work fitness to enable the worker to perform the job requirements successfully. In the same way that athletes train and are coached to obtain their maximum performance in a particular sport, so workers train and are coached for their specific occupations.

The treatment approach adopted for sporting injuries is based on very early identification of the problem, early and appropriate intervention and continuation of appropriate levels of activity, possibly with an adjusted training programme. This ongoing commitment to appropriate activity and training is also applicable when an athlete returns to competition following a break. The athelete gradually increases the level of performance in a graded manner. This concept of a graded return to usual levels and types of activity is also applicable to the industrial athlete in the workplace. Work programmes offered to enhance the neuromusculoskeletal and motor components can incorporate this concept by including the expectation that injured workers will train and upgrade to a level which is consistent with their job requirements.

Consider Steve who is a science teacher, weekend competitive soccer player and rock climber. He slipped down some wet stairs at work injuring his right knee. He received appropriate treatment immediately following his injury and was also referred for ongoing treatment to enable him to return to his usual activities. Steve stopped playing soccer and rock climbing and had difficulties when standing for extended periods of time, ascending and descending stairs and crouching to reach low cupboards. Under the supervision of his therapist, Steve returned to soccer training when the acute phase of his injury had subsided. He walked instead of ran around the oval, performed stretches and strengthening exercises specifically designed for him when the rest of the team were also doing these activities and remained a part of the team by assisting the coach and manager. Steve returned to work a couple of days after the injury and was able to continue with only minor modifications. Over two months Steve gradually increased his training regime, was playing soccer for short periods of time, began attending the indoor climbing centre and had no difficulties at work.

This example demonstrates the similarities between sporting and workplace injuries and how they both benefit from speedy intervention, appropriate grading and continuation of usual activities.

General aspects of fitness

Fitness must also be considered in the context of the activity to be performed. A marathon runner may be considered extremely fit in terms of long-distance running but not fit for weightlifting or gymnastics. In the same way, a worker may be fit to be a courier but not able to cope with the demands of a word processor. When considering whether a person is fit, it is always necessary to ask: 'Fit for what?' This is important for identifying match and mismatch between performance and work requirements and for designing appropriate intervention programmes.

Åstrand and Rodahl (1986: 422) emphasize that an 'analysis of the demands that a particular athletic event places on the body should form the basis for the training program, taking into consideration whatever deficiencies there may be in the athlete's resources or capabilities to meet these demands.' This concept should also be applied to the workplace. Work programmes for neuromusculoskeletal and motor deficits, therefore, should be based on the specific work requirements identified in a thorough job analysis. These job tasks and activities become the basis of the programme for the individual, with neuromusculoskeletal and motor deficits targeted through engagement in relevant and specific job tasks and activities. This concept forms the basis of all return-to-work programmes.

Elements of fitness

The neuromusculoskeletal and motor components of fitness are considered to be cardiorespiratory endurance, muscle strength, muscle endurance and flexibility or range of motion. Various approaches to improve fitness are used depending on the component of fitness which is to be targeted. Training techniques which improve cardiorespiratory endurance will not necessarily improve flexibility or muscle strength. Weight training may improve muscle strength and muscle endurance, but may have no impact on cardiorespiratory endurance. It is essential, therefore, that work programmes target the appropriate and relevant elements of fitness, and should be structured to meet the specific job requirements.

Cardiorespiratory endurance

Improvement in all aspects of fitness is reliant on a level of training or workload which is sufficient to produce a noticeable training effect. This is usually referred to as the overload principle and implies that the individual should work at a level above that which can be normally carried out comfortably (Egger and Champion, 1990).

The FITT formula is usually applied when developing programmes to improve cardiorespiratory endurance (Egger and Champion, 1990). The acronym stands for Frequency, Intensity, Time (or duration) and Type of

FITT formula

Frequency: The person should engage in the programme 3 to 4 times weekly to have a training effect. These sessions should be spread evenly throughout the week, rather than occurring on consecutive days, or having more than 1 training session per day.

Intensity: Sedentary people need to train at an intensity which results in the individual being slightly out of breath (Åstrand and Rodahl, 1986). Training should raise the heart rate to 60–85 per cent of maximal heart rate. When first beginning, the intensity should be at a lower level and gradually increase as cardiorespiratory endurance improves. Take factors such as general health, level of activity, weight and blood pressure into consideration when determining an appropriate level of intensity. Maximal heart rate decreases with age, but is not related to gender (American College of Sports Medicine, 1991; Minor, 1991). It can be calculated in a number of ways (American College of Sports Medicine, 1991) all of which should be viewed as guidelines only when determining the appropriate level of intensity.

Time: To have an impact on cardiorespiratory endurance it is necessary to keep the heart rate at the appropriate level of intensity for 20 to 40 minutes. This does not include warm-up activity and cool-down periods. Warm-up and cool-down periods of 5 to 10 minutes each are very important to ensure that there is decreased risk of injury. Some clients may have received their injuries through engaging in strenuous activity without an adequate warm-up.

Type: To have an impact on cardiorespiratory endurance the activity performed should be aerobic and performed on a continuous basis rather than in a stop/start nature. Activities commonly used in these types of programs for individuals with neuromusculoskeletal injuries include brisk walking, swimming and cycling. Jogging and high-impact aerobics are avoided due to the potential risk of injury in this group of clients.

activity. As with any fitness programme, if an individual is deconditioned due to illness, injury or sedentary lifestyle, it may be necessary to ensure that it is medically safe to commence.

Steve, who was moderately fit and active before his injury, was involved in a cardiorespiratory training programme on Tuesday and Thursday evenings and Sunday afternoons. He enjoyed swimming on Sundays at the local pool and cycling during the evenings. When cycling Steve began slowly on the local cycle track which was relatively flat. Following his 5–10 minute warm-up he increased speed and cycled through areas which had hills and inclines for about half an hour and then slowed down to cycle home. At home he finished off with some stretches which he had been taught.

For some individuals who have been inactive for lengthy periods and are severely deconditioned it may be necessary to have a 'pre-aerobic' programme. This type of programme would emphasize increasing tolerance to activity rather than increasing cardiorespiratory fitness. The frequency and type of activity would be the same, however, the intensity and duration would be at lower levels for shorter periods of time. These would gradually be increased until they reached a level which will improve cardiorespiratory endurance.

Glenn injured his shoulder twelve months previously and stopped playing tennis and volleyball. He has a sedentary job as a tollbooth attendant and was severely deconditioned, becoming breathless when climbing a flight of stairs, or walking 50 metres. Due to his deconditioning, Glenn was not able to engage safely in cardiorespiratory training immediately and required a 'pre-aerobic' programme to increase his activity tolerance before commencing fitness training. Glenn's programme involved walking every day during his lunch hour in a park across the road from work. He began by walking for 5 minutes at a comfortable pace. This was gradually increased in time to 10, 15 and then 20 minutes. The intensity also increased until Glenn was walking at a pace where he was slightly breathless, but could comfortably continue with the activity. At this stage he was able to commence a cardiorespiratory training programme.

Activities to improve cardiorespiratory endurance may be incorporated into work conditioning or work hardening programmes. Due to the nature of the programme and the need to maintain heart rate within the target range, it would not be appropriate to conduct cardiorespiratory endurance training in the workplace as part of work duties. However, it may be possible to engage in them before or after work, or during an extended break, such as lunch.

Monitoring

An important aspect of any programme is the need for monitoring the client. To encourage involvement in the programme, self-monitoring by the client is suggested. This may be through monitoring heart rate to ensure it is within the target range, or through the use of Rate of Perceived Exertion (RPE) scales (see Table 9.1). When using these scales, exercise should be within the range of 12 to 16 ('somewhat hard' to 'hard') when using the 15-point scale (6 to 20) (American College of Sports Medicine, 1991; Wilmore and Costill, 1994). If the 10-point scale is used, ratings should be between 4 and 6.

Muscle endurance

Do not confuse muscle endurance with cardiorespiratory endurance. A keyboard operator may have a high level of muscle endurance in the wrist extensors and long finger flexors and extensors to key quickly and for prolonged periods of time. This person, however, may have poor cardiorespiratory endurance due to the all day sedentary nature of the work performed. Muscle endurance is the capacity of a muscle or muscle group to continue contracting efficiently over a prolonged period of time (Egger and Champion, 1990) or the ability to sustain a submaximal contraction (Minor, 1991). This is considered as either dynamic contraction, where movement occurs, or static contraction, where no movement occurs.

Dynamic endurance and strength are developed by isotonic and isokinetic contractions, while static endurance and strength are developed by isometric contractions. Often both dynamic and static endurance and strength are required in different muscle groups at the same time in order to perform an activity. For example, dynamic endurance and strength are required when repeatedly lifting an object, and static endurance and strength are required to carry the object to the required location. Static endurance and strength are also required to sustain postures and balance (Minor, 1991).

Table 9.1 Borg's Rate of Percieved Exertion scales

Rating	*15 point scale – A*	*15 point scale – B*	*Rating*	*10 point scale*
6		No exertion at all	0	Nothing at all
7	Very, very light	Extremely light	0.5	Very, very weak
8			1	Very weak
9	Very light	Very light	2	Weak (light)
10			3	Moderate
11	Fairly light	Light	4	Somewhat strong
12			5	Strong (heavy)
13	Somewhat hard	Somewhat hard	6	
14			7	Very strong
15	Hard	Hard (heavy)	8	
16			9	
17	Very hard	Very hard	10	Very, very strong
18				
19	Very, very hard	Extremely hard		
20		Maximal exertion	–	Maximal

(Borg Scales of Perceived Exertion, in Wilmore and Costill, 1994, p. 524) Permission requested from *Human Kinetics*.

Muscle endurance is an important factor in the development of many neuromusculoskeletal injuries in the workplace. Injuries associated with repetitive movements include occupational overuse syndromes or cumulative trauma disorders, back injuries, carpal tunnel syndrome, de Quervain's disease, tenosynovitis, epicondylitis and so on.

Muscle endurance for specific muscles or muscle groups can be improved by repetitive isotonic contractions (15 to 30 repetitions, performed for 2 to 3 sets) with a low intensity or resistance (15+ RM or repetition maximum), performed at a medium pace, with minimal rest periods between sets (Egger and Champion, 1990).

Neuromusculoskeletal injuries may occur if postures are maintained for prolonged periods of time. Static muscular work has been identified as the major postural health hazard (Luopajarvi, 1990). This static contraction of muscles for an extended time is also an important aspect of muscle endurance in the performance of work tasks.

Static contraction

When considering muscle endurance, the stronger the force of the contraction the shorter the endurance time. This may not be surprising, however it has been found that regardless of the force of static contraction, people begin to report fatigue when approximately 15 per cent of the total endurance time has elapsed (Jonsson, 1984). After approximately 33 per cent of the endurance time, people would prefer to rest, and after approximately half the endurance time, people would stop working due to muscle exhaustion (Jonsson, 1984). The fatigue is a product of reduced blood flow to the muscles and the speed of fatigue is dependent on the level of force or exertion applied by the muscles (Chaffin and Andersson, 1991).

Muscle endurance is increased by the provision of small rest breaks. Some studies have found that the endurance limit for maintenance of a static contraction for an 'unlimited' period of time is 8 per cent of maximal voluntary contraction (MVC), with 5 per cent being recommended for continual static work (Chaffin and Andersson, 1991). Jonsson (1984: 67) recommends that to avoid the effects of muscular fatigue during prolonged periods of work (i.e. for an hour or more):

1 The static load should not exceed 2–5 per cent of the maximal voluntary contraction (MVC) during continuous work.
2 The average force of contraction should not exceed 10–14 per cent of MVC in long-lasting intermittent or dynamic work (e.g. typing or keying).
3 Maximum peaks should not exceed 50–70 per cent of MVC so that full fatigue within less than one minute is avoided.

There are also estimates related to the duration of rest periods during work. According to Jonsson (1984: 73) for a rest period to be of benefit it may be necessary to:

1 Have a micropause (e.g. a pause between two contractions) of at least 2 seconds.
2 Rest for at least 2 minutes between two work periods when a third of the endurance time had been used.
3 Rest for at least 5 minutes after a work period which has continued to marked muscular fatigue (e.g. 55 per cent of the endurance time).
4 Rest for at least 60 minutes after a work situation which has continued to full muscular exhaustion.

Muscle strength

Muscle strength is the ability of a muscle or group of muscles to produce a maximum force in one contraction. Within the workplace, muscle strength is required in many areas, particularly those related to manual handling. This may be lifting, pushing, pulling and carrying. Muscle strength and endurance are closely linked, and muscle strengthening programmes also affect muscle endurance.

As with other areas of fitness, strengthening programmes are most effective if they target the specific work or activity requirements. Strengthening muscles using the same type of contraction, speed of contraction and position or joint angle as is required in the specific work task will be the most effective (Minor, 1991). Motivation is also increased when the activity is of direct benefit to the individual. This is of relevance when designing work hardening programmes and selecting appropriate work simulation activities. Strengthening is also possible in workplace-based programmes where upgrading the work requirements can readily occur as the individual continues performing the specific work tasks which are suitable.

In order to increase dynamic strength, people should begin with 8 to 12 repetitions performed for 2 to 3 sets using 8–12 RM (repetition maximum) at a slow-to-medium pace with 2 to 3 minutes rest between sets (Egger and Champion, 1990). As improvement occurs this can be gradually upgraded to 2 to 6 repetitions for 3 to 6 sets using 2–6 RM at a slow-to-medium speed with 3 to 5 minutes rest between sets. Isometric training in isolation from dynamic training is rarely practised today; rather, it is incorporated with other forms of muscle strengthening (Egger and Champion, 1990).

When designing muscle strengthening programmes be aware that eccentric contractions (where the muscle develops tension when lengthening – such as in the biceps when lowering an object) may produce muscle soreness in untrained persons (Åstrand and Rodahl, 1986). This has relevance in work hardening programmes, particularly the lifting components, or when descending stairs and ladders. The quadriceps muscles of the things require concentric contraction to extend the knees when lifting an object from a low position, such as from the floor, and eccentric contraction to lower the weight to the floor. Individuals may have difficulty or soreness the following day if they are unused to this level of activity and are also required to perform eccentric contractions against resistance, such as when lowering a weight.

Flexibility (range of motion)

Flexibility of joints ensures adequate range of motion required for normal movement. Limited flexibility can affect activities of daily living as well as work activities. Of particular concern is adequate flexibility of the lower back and posterior thigh region. Limited flexibility of this area has been associated with increased risk for the development of low back pain (Åstrand and Rodahl, 1986). Immobility, such as maintaining static postures and positions for prolonged periods of time, can adversely affect flexibility leading to stiffness and reduced range of motion.

Stretching exercises can assist in maintaining and improving joint range of motion. These may be 'pause gymnastics' performed in the workplace to maintain range, or a more detailed stretching regime integrated within the warm-up and cool-down phases of an overall exercise programme. 'Pause gymnastics' are stretches and exercises performed for short periods of time (2–5 minutes) throughout the day to take a 'pause' from work, change postures and stretch muscles which have been in constrained positions. Åstrand and Rodahl (1986) provide the following guidelines for flexibility exercises:

- They should be performed slowly with a gradual increase in range, but should not cause extreme pain.
- Movement should be slow and dynamic, followed by a static stretch sustained for 10 to 30 seconds.
- Sets should consist of 3 to 5 repetitions of each exercise performed at least 3 times per week.

Return-to-work programmes

Having identified various components of neuromusculoskeletal and motor dysfunction relevant to work, and the requirements of work fitness, we must also identify suitable strategies and interventions which facilitate clients' return to work. Terms such as occupational rehabilitation, work hardening, work conditioning and workplace-based rehabilitation may all be familiar, but what are these approaches and when is it appropriate to use them?

Perhaps one way is to view these strategies on a continuum, rather than as mutually exclusive strategies.

Occupational rehabilitation

Occupational rehabilitation is defined as:

> the restoration of ... injured worker[s] to the fullest physical, psychological, social, vocational and economic usefulness of which they are capable, consistent with pre-injury status. It is a managed process aimed at maintaining injured or ill workers in or returning them to suitable

> employment. It involves early intervention with appropriate, adequate and timely services based on assessment of the injured worker's needs. (WorkCover Authority of NSW, 1993: 9)

While 'occupational rehabilitation' identifies strongly with work and employment, there is also a component which addresses quality of life issues and the ability of the individual to function not only in the workplace, but also at home and within the community (CCH Occupational Health and Safety Editors, 1990). There are a number of principles which underpin successful occupational rehabilitation which are relevant no matter whether the approach to rehabilitation is work hardening, work conditioning or workplace-based:

- Rehabilitation should occur at the workplace except where appropriate intervention for the injured worker's disability cannot be supplied by the workplace rehabilitation systems (CCH Occupational Health and Safety Editors, 1990).
- Intervention should recognize work as therapy, be function-oriented and avoid rest, inactivity and passive therapies (other than those required during the acute phase of care) (CCH Occupational Health and Safety Editors, 1990).
- Early intervention results in the maximum gains from rehabilitation (CCH Occupational Health and Safety Editors, 1990, **29**; WorkCover Authority of NSW, 1993, **340**).
- A multidisciplinary approach to occupational rehabilitation is necessary due to the range of factors encompassed by each injured worker's disability (CCH Occupational Health and Safety Editors, 1990; Innes, 1995).
- There is a shared responsibility and commitment by all parties to the rehabilitation of the injured worker. This includes not only the worker and the rehabilitation provider, but also the employer, unions, insurance companies, doctors and other health providers (CCH Occupational Health and Safety Editors, 1990; Innes, 1995; WorkCover Authority of NSW, 1993).
- Absences due to work-related injuries incur both 'hidden' and actual costs to the worker and the employer (Ganora and Wright, 1987; WorkCover Authority of NSW, 1993).
- Rehabilitation provision is an essential component in ensuring the health and productivity of the workforce (WorkCover Authority of NSW, 1993).

Clinic-based programmes: work hardening

Some have suggested that an injured worker who is only capable of performing 'a job specifically tailored to his or her needs, for example two hours per day, self-paced, in an ergonomically and biomechanically redesigned workstation' (Ogden-Niemeyer and Jacobs, 1989: 22) is in 'sheltered employment' due to the goodwill of his or her employer. However, it is work hardening programmes which occur away from the place of employment which should be considered as sheltered employment. Programmes which take place in the workplace are open employment. This does not suggest, however, that it is always appropriate or possible to develop and implement workplace-based programmes for all injured workers.

Clinic-based programmes, such as work hardening, may be the preferred option for individuals who:

- Identify with a patient or sick role rather than a worker role. These individuals have inappropriate worker behaviours to meet the requirements and expectations of the workplace.
- Have levels of work fitness which are inadequate for any suitable duties in the workplace and cannot be accommodated through job or environmental modifications.
- Have specific limitations in critical job demands which would risk further injury or compromise the safety of themselves or others if they were in the workplace.
- Require close and frequent supervision to ensure safety regarding techniques and the use of equipment (Bidencope, 1994).
- Have symptoms, such as pain, which are not adequately controlled or managed to enable functioning within the workplace.
- Are unable to determine accurately safe end-points of their physical capacities and either severely under- or overestimate their abilities.

The development of chronic pain syndromes, loss of self-esteem, depression and anxiety, over and above the initial physical injury, indicate the need for work hardening programmes. Many individuals who have sustained neuromusculoskeletal injuries, such as back injuries and occupational overuse syndromes or cumulative trauma disorders, may have pain. This may be of an acute or chronic nature and may be the most limiting aspect of their disability.

There may also be factors which prohibit an injured worker returning to the workplace other than individual limitations and reduced capacity. These factors include:

- A lack of suitable duties available in the workplace, but the individual is capable of upgrading and improving function (Bidencope, 1994).
- An inability to return to work until fully work fit, with no opportunity of upgrading in the workplace.
- No job or workplace to return to and the worker requires maintenance or improvement in work fitness before a work trial or work retraining programme is commenced (Bidencope, 1994).
- No job or workplace to return to but work fitness levels require maintenance or upgrading on a short-term basis while job seeking (Bidencope, 1994).
- Political, social or legislative limitations or restrictions which do not make it possible or feasible to implement workplace-based programmes.

Work hardening programmes place emphasis on improvement in all performance component areas through the use of real or simulated work activities and other conditioning tasks. This can be seen in the following definition by the Commission on Accreditation of Rehabilitation Facilities (1989: 69):

> Work hardening programs, which are interdisciplinary in nature, use conditioning tasks that are graded to progressively improve the biomechanical, neuromuscular, cardiovascular/metabolic and psychosocial functions of the individual in conjunction with real or simulated work activities. Work hardening provides a transition between acute care and return to work while addressing the issues of productivity, safety, physical tolerances, and worker behaviours. Work hardening is a highly structured, goal oriented, individualised treatment program designed to maximise the individual's ability to return to work.

Many descriptions of work hardening programmes state they are based on the Stage Model of Industrial Rehabilitation (Matheson *et al.*, 1985). These include Ellexson (1989), Matheson and Ogden-Niemeyer (1987), Matheson (1988) and Ogden-Niemeyer (1989). Others may not identify this model, but use similar terminology when describing the basis of the programme (Demers, 1992). In this model an individual can be referred for work hardening

Table 9.2 Stage Model of Industrial Rehabilitation

Stage	*Description*
1	**Pathology** Identification of the injury or disease process (e.g. L4/L5 disc protrusion).
2	**Impairment** Measurable consequence of pathology taken as a disruption of physical or mental integrity (e.g. decreased range of motion of trunk flextion).
3	**Functional limitation** The inability to perform general tasks which are found in a variety of roles (e.g. lifting 10 kg from floor to waist level; sitting for 2 hours).
4	**Disability** The social consequence of the injured worker's functional limitations, or how impairment affects role performance (e.g. ability to work as a long-distance truck driver).
5	**Feasibility for competitive employment** The acceptability of the injured worker as an employee to an employer (i.e. the physical and behavioural match between the worker's tolerance and the job demands, with emphasis on safety, productivity and interpersonal behaviour).
6	**Employability** The ability to become employed within a particular labour market.
7	**Vocational handicap** The ability actually to perform the tasks required of a specific job at an acceptable level of performance with safety.
8	**Earning capacity** It is measured in terms of work-generated income over the worker's lifetime.

Source: Author [Adapted from Matheson (1988), and Ogden-Niemeyer and Jacobs (1989)].

at any stage from impairment (stage 2) through to vocational handicap (stage 7) (Ogden-Niemeyer and Jacobs, 1989).

Work hardening programmes may be provided for up to 8 hours per day, 5 days per week, for up to 8 weeks in length (Lechner, 1994). These tend to be upper limits rather than averages, with many programmes being completed within shorter time frames. For example, work hardening programmes in Wisconsin, USA were completed in four weeks for 71 per cent of clients, 86 per cent of clients completed programmes within six weeks and 95 per cent within eight weeks (King, 1993).

A survey of 192 work hardening and work adjustment programmes throughout the United States was conducted in 1991 to determine the types of services offered (Wyrick *et al.*, 1991). They found that the most consistently provided services were:

- Graded work simulation and exercise to increase employability (91%).
- Baseline assessment of functional limitations (91%).
- Assessment between the match of an individual's capabilities and critical job demands (90%).
- Client education for the prevention of injury (90%).

For individuals with chronic pain and psychosocial dysfunction subsequent to their physical injury the focus of a work hardening programme is to increase activity tolerance and reinforce principles of body mechanics, while also demonstrating that an individual is capable of performing productive activities. This may be achieved through therapeutic projects (e.g. woodwork, pottery, etc.) or realistic job simulations in conjunction with a more regulated and specific physical demands component which addresses, in detail, limiting physical factors, such as lifting, carrying, pushing, pulling, walking and so on. For example, Lucy had sustained a whiplash injury to her neck and had worn a soft neck collar for eighteen months. She had chronic pain and had only been able to cope with her immediate self-care needs. She had not worked on a process-line or been involved in any home duties since her injury. While in work hardening Lucy chose to make a macramé planter hanger. This required her to perform repetitive, gross, dynamic movements of her arms, remove the soft collar and maintain good head and neck alignment. Lucy was able to continue this activity for an hour at a time. She was also involved in an upgrading of her walking tolerance and lifting and carrying capacity. Lucy successfully completed the project and gave the planter hanger to her daughter who had taken on all the home duties following Lucy's accident.

These programmes do not attempt to relieve pain. They do, however, attempt to demonstrate to individuals that it is possible to engage in functional activities and work-related tasks at appropriate and increasing levels of frequency, duration and intensity that do not result in unacceptable and debilitating increases of pain or dysfunction. Lucy, for example, reported no decreases (or increase) in her neck pain when she was involved in macramé. She did, however, express pleasure and surprise at having completed a gift to give to her daughter.

An integral component of all work hardening programmes is education. Client education entails not only the obvious aspects of biomechanical precautions and injury prevention associated with neuromusculoskeletal and motor disorders, such as back injuries or overuse injuries, but also aspects such as the relationship between stress and pain, the importance of general fitness to overall health and the use of relaxation techniques when engaged in functional activities.

The focus of the activity tolerance/work simulation component is to develop a basic ability to function in a work context. Expectations related to worker behaviours, such as attendance, appropriate dress and behaviour, are built into the programme. The types of activities or work simulations in which the client is engaged vary between individuals. The selection of appropriate activities is based on the individual's background experience and work history, personal preferences and suitability of the activity with respect to the client's medical history.

One of the key aspects of the activity tolerance/work simulation component is the development of tolerances to a variety of work positions relevant to the job. Many occupations require individuals to work in a wide variety of postures for prolonged periods of time. While acknowledging the basic principles related to improving general physical fitness, it is also necessary to develop an ability to perform specific job requirements. This may be the ability to remain standing for up to an hour at a time, sitting for up to 1+ hours, or maintaining any number of unusual postures due to the nature of the work and the work environment (e.g. working overhead, or in a confined space).

The specific physical demands component is based on identified critical demands of an individual's job. These critical demands may include lifting, carrying, climbing, walking and so on. Routines or circuits may be developed, or tasks incorporated into a work simulation activity. Frequency, intensity and duration are gradually increased as the client improves. These circuits can be equated with the weight and training circuits seen in gymnasiums and fitness centres. This would also assist in creating the image of the industrial athlete engaged in an individually prescribed programme designed to improve work fitness.

As with all treatment programmes, SMART (Specific, Measurable, Achievable, Realistic and Time-bounded) treatment goals should be set. For example, a goal for Jim, who works in a warehouse and has a low-back injury, may be that he will be able to lift and lower 10 kg between knee and shoulder height, five consecutive times, three times per day, within two weeks. Goals must be related to work requirements, as this one is for Jim who needs to load and unload pallets of materials.

As the individual improves and begins to meet the critical work demands identified from a job analysis, the programme becomes workplace-based. The individual returns to work on a graded basis in terms of job requirements and time. The workplace-based programme may continue in conjunction with a work hardening programme until it is appropriate to continue upgrading in the workplace only.

Clinic-based: work conditioning

A more specifically targeted type of programme is work conditioning, which aims to improve an injured worker's physical or neuromusculoskeletal functioning resulting in a return to work. It uses physical conditioning and functional activities related to work (Lechner, 1994) and may be similar to the specific physical demands component of a work hardening programme.

Work conditioning is defined as 'a program with an emphasis on physical conditioning that addresses the issues of strength, endurance, flexibility, motor control, and cardiopulmonary function' (Lechner, 1994: 472).

Work conditioning programmes are suitable for individuals who:

- Have identified themselves as having a worker role.
- Have identified neuromusculoskeletal physical and functional deficits that interfere with work (Lechner, 1994: 472) and cannot be accommodated through job or environmental modifications.
- Have specific physical limitations in critical job demands which would risk further injury or compromise the safety of themselves or others if they were in the workplace.

These programmes tend to involve only one discipline, while work hardening programmes are interdisciplinary. They may be offered up to four hours per day, five days per week for up to eight weeks in length (Lechner, 1994). Many of the recommendations made earlier regarding specific neuromusculoskeletal work fitness aspects and specific physical demands components of work hardening would be appropriately incorporated into work conditioning programmes. Building in the concept of the industrial athlete, circuit training could incorporate specific work-related features such as lifting a 10 kg box five times from floor to waist height, or pushing a trolley with 25 kg up and down a ramp three times. As with work hardening programmes, work conditioning programmes may be continued in a transition from clinic-based to workplace-based rehabilitation.

Workplace-based programmes

The underlying principle of workplace-based rehabilitation is that 'the workplace, and not a medical institution or the home, may be the most appropriate and effective place to rehabilitate the majority of injured workers' (WorkCover Authority of NSW, 1993: 8). It is assumed that all parties involved in the workplace, including the worker, worker's family, employer, coworkers, union, insurer, rehabilitation provider and other health professionals, benefit socially and economically from an individual's safe and speedy return to work following a work-related injury or illness (Innes, 1995).

Not all injured workers will require rehabilitative services. However, early assessment of the need for rehabilitation is necessary (WorkCover Authority of NSW, 1993). For example, it has been estimated that in New South Wales, Australia only 6 per cent of injured workers actually require referral to rehabilitation services (Yates, 1992) and for most of those individuals rehabilitation could occur at the workplace.

Workplace-based rehabilitation programmes are suitable for individuals who:

- Have identified themselves as having a worker role and exhibit worker behaviours appropriate to the workplace.
- Are able to perform safely the basic critical demands of identified suitable duties.
- Are able to be upgraded in terms of duties and time at the workplace (Bidencope, 1994).
- Do not pose a danger to themselves or others due to functional limitations.
- Are able to manage or control symptoms, such as pain, appropriately in the workplace.

Guidelines for the establishment of workplace-based rehabilitation programmes have been developed and consist of a number of essential elements (WorkCover Authority of NSW, 1993). These elements include demonstrated commitments to:

- Prevention of occupational injuries and illness – this incorporates the occupational health and safety legislation into the workers' compensation legislation.
- Early commencement of occupational rehabilitation to minimize time off work and ensure that the worker role is maintained.
- Ensuring that a return to work as soon as possible is a normal expectation in the workplace from top level management to factory floor workers.
- Provision of suitable duties/employment where practicable, for an injured worker as an integral part of the rehabilitation process.
- Consultation with workers and, where applicable, any industrial union of employees representing those workers.
- Participation in a rehabilitation programme will not, of itself, prejudice an injured worker.

Multiple factors obviously influence the effectiveness of workplace-based rehabilitation programmes. The key factors appear to be early and appropriate referral for rehabilitation services, ready access to the work site enabling onsite supervision and support, ongoing support in the workplace from the rehabilitation coordinator and demonstrated commitment on the part of management.

Rather than take extended periods of time off work because they are unable to cope with a full-time workload, or because some of the duties of their job are inappropriate, workers are facilitated to remain at work. This is achieved through the development of individualized rehabilitation programmes where workers perform appropriate or suitable duties and attend for the period of time which best suits their post-injury abilities. The rehabilitation programme is gradually upgraded by increasing time at work and the reintroduction of pre-injury duties. Where this is not possible or feasible, long-term plans regarding the retraining or permanent redeployment of the injured worker are developed.

Workplace-based rehabilitation may take a number of forms. Clients may return to work in a number of capacities which are gradually upgraded. These are return to work with the same employer, performing:

- The same duties for the same hours.
- The same duties for reduced hours.
- Modified duties for the same hours.
- Modified duties for reduced hours.
- New/alternate duties for the same hours.
- New/alternate duties for reduced hours.
- Or any of the above alternatives with a different employer.

If injured workers are unable to return to their original job, then they may be redeployed within the organization and undergo retraining. There is also the option of work trials, where clients are unable to return to their original employer or may have had their employment terminated and undergo a work trial of approximately twelve weeks with another employer. This last alternative is an excellent option when the person may have received treatment, such as a work hardening programme, is work ready, but has no job to return to. All the benefits gained in work hardening may be lost if the momentum is not retained and the person returned to work, in this case on a work trial.

Preferred heirarchy of suitable duties

- Same job modified
- Same area, similar job
- Same area, different job
- Different area, similar job
- Different area, different job
- Different workplace.

Suitable duties

Suitable duties are designed specifically for an injured worker to enable a safe and speedy return to work. They are carefully designed and selected to match the individual's capacities and avoid risk of further injury, therefore enabling ongoing recovery. Important features of suitable duties are the nature and value of the work performed (Innes, 1995). 'A return to work will not be successful if the suitable duties do not ensure the dignity and job satisfaction of the injured employee' (CCH Occupational Health and Safety Editors, 1990: 150). Suitable duties have regard for the injured worker's abilities, pre-injury employment, age, education, skills, work experience, place of residence, medical restrictions, rehabilitation plan and any other relevant aspects (CCH Occupational Health and Safety Editors, 1990). They do not include work which is demeaning or of a token nature considering the individual's experience, skills and previous employment. For example, a worker who was a leading hand (in charge of a group of workers) was returned to work as a 'billy boy' (general hand assisting other workers when requested, making morning tea, etc). This was unsuitable as the employer did not consider the worker's reaction to this new position (CCH Occupational Health and Safety Editors, 1990). Suitable duties should be seen as a temporary step on the way to achievement of the final goal of returning to work in the same capacity as pre-injury if possible.

When designing or selecting suitable duties it is desirable to provide duties which are as close as possible to the injured worker's pre-injury position (CCH Occupational Health and Safety Editors, 1990).

As with all aspects of the rehabilitation programme the determination of suitable duties should involve negotiation between the injured worker, employer, supervisors and co-workers, rehabilitation provider, treating medical practitioner and relevant unions. The duties which have been negotiated and how they will be upgraded should also be documented.

Case studies

Work hardening and workplace-based programme

Greg is a 36-year-old man who is employed as a labourer in an ink factory. He is married and has three children aged 9, 6 and 2 years. Greg injured his back at work eighteen months ago when a 400 kg vat of ink he was pushing jammed a wheel in a crack in the concrete floor, severely jarring his back. He has been off work since. The injury resulted in an L4/5 disc prolapse and Greg underwent surgery (discectomy) six months after the injury. He reports minimal pain reduction following the surgery and has been abusing prescribed analgesic medications, which also provide only minimal short-term effects. He is not aware of any other ways of controlling his pain.

Greg has not attempted a return to work and currently spends his time laying on the couch at home watching television or reading, walking around his garden, driving his wife to the shopping centre and his children to athletics training and school. He is independent in self-care, although he performs tasks slowly and has some difficulty reaching his feet. He is not aware of any alternative ways of performing these tasks. Greg formerly enjoyed riding his Harley Davidson motor bike, tending his vegetable and herb garden, going on family outings and being involved in his children's athletics club. He has not engaged in any of these activities since his injury. Greg has not been sleeping well, is irritable, depressed and anxious, believing that he will never work again, although he says he would like to go back to work.

Greg understands his injury but is not aware of correct back-care techniques. He has also identified that there is a relationship between his pain levels and stress. Greg has the following physical tolerances:

- Sitting: 5–10 minutes
- Standing (static): 5 minutes standing (dynamic): 10 minutes
- Walking: 100 metres on a flat surface
- Climbing: a flight of stairs (approx. 10 steps) using a rail
- Lifting: unable to squat; lifts <5 kg at waist height unable to lift above chest height
- Pushing/pulling: not attempted.

Greg was referred to the clinic-based work hardening programme, and, following a medical examination and review of his medication, he attended occupational therapy, physiotherapy and psychology. Intervention focused on back-care education which continued throughout the programme and had input from all team members, and upgrading of work tolerances with the goal of return to work on suitable duties.

Greg was involved in progressive relaxation and meditation sessions to manage his pain and control his anxiety. He carried his relaxation techniques over into functional activities and used EMG biofeedback to monitor his levels of muscle contraction during activities. This assisted in monitoring correct posture and techniques as well as monitoring tension levels.

Greg also learned appropriate back exercises and identified that ice packs gave him temporary pain relief. He commenced in the woodwork shop assisting with the manufacture of footstools and angled writing tables and performing tasks such as painting, light sanding, some hammering and using a power drill. He alternated between sitting and standing for gradually increasing periods of time (up to a total of three hours with breaks) when performing woodwork. As he progressed, more resistive activities, such as sawing, planing and using coarser grades of sandpaper, were introduced. Specific work demands were gradually introduced as Greg's activity tolerance improved. This included lifting, commencing with objects weighing 500 and progressing to 10 kg, lifted between knee and shoulder height. He also began a fitness programme targeting specifically cardiorespiratory endurance and flexibility. Swimming and walking were identified as aerobic activities which Greg could pursue near his home and with his family. He commenced at a pre-aerobic level due to his severe deconditioning and physical limitations. Greg commenced with walking 100 m on a flat service and walking across the swimming pool twice. He progressed to walking 2 km and swimming 500 m.

A work visit was conducted to identify suitable duties to which Greg could return. These included assisting the quality control manager with some clerical duties such as filing, telephoning and delivering test results to various units around the factory. He could also assist with sampling and consideration was given to retraining so that Greg could assist in analysing some samples. All these duties were within the tolerances Greg had achieved during the programme.

When Greg could comfortably complete four to five hours per day in the rehabilitation unit after a six week programme, he returned to work for three hours per day, two days per week (Tuesday and Thursday). He also had to travel for 30 minutes each way from his home to work. Greg continued attending the rehabilitation unit on the days he did not go to work, continuing with his programme and enabling team members to monitor his progress and adapt aspects to deal with his immediate needs.

Time at work was gradually upgraded from two to three to four and finally five days a week. He remained at three hours per day until he was working four days per week and then began increasing his hours at work. Greg never returned to his original job, but was able to manage on new duties in a different area with the same employer. He also returned to gardening using long-handled tools and becoming more involved in family outings and his children's athletics club.

Workplace-based programme

Gemma is a 23-year-old woman employed as an administrative assistant in a large government department. This work involves mainly clerical tasks such as word processing and other keyboard activities, filing, photocopying and so on. She lives with her partner in an inner-city apartment. Gemma developed wrist and thumb pain in her dominant right hand two months ago following four weeks of intensive work which had to be completed before the end of the financial year. This required Gemma to spend up to seven hours per day inputting data into the computer. Gemma attempted to remain at work but was unable to continue with her normal duties due to the pain and was given a week off work by her doctor.

Gemma is fully independent in self care and can manage most home duties but has difficulty with vacuuming, sweeping, ironing, hanging out heavy items of laundry (e.g., towels and sheets), chopping and grating hard foods and carrying heavy loads of washing or shopping. She is able to attain all grips but has difficulty if they are maintained for extended periods of time or if applying force, such as squeezing clothes pegs open. Gemma enjoys playing the flute, ballroom dancing and watching foreign language films. She hasn't played her flute for about 6 weeks, and while she still goes ballroom dancing she is concerned that someone may bump into her. Gemma wants to return to work as soon as possible as she is concerned that other people are having to carry her workload. She has worked for the same government department since leaving school at 18 and is considered to be a 'good worker'.

Gemma's supervisor was concerned that Gemma may have a recurrence of her pain on her return to work. A work visit was performed with Gemma present several days prior to her return. Problems with her workstation were identified and some immediate adjustments made. Gemma was not aware of how to correctly adjust her work station, nor was she familiar with correct postures to use during her work tasks.

Following discussions between Gemma, her supervisor, the workplace rehabilitation coordinator and the rehabilitation provider, temporary alternative duties were identified. The department had several projects which required completion. Several of these projects required discussions with relevant people within the department, telephoning suppliers and manufacturers of equipment, negotiating with contractors, some word processing, writing and filing. Due to Gemma's previously demonstrated competence it was agreed that she would be responsible for one of these projects. All word processing, writing and filing could be performed at times during the day when Gemma felt comfortable. There was no time pressure involved regarding when these tasks were to be completed. Gemma was also given a programme of pause gymnastics to be completed every one to two hours. Her workstation was correctly adjusted and Gemma was made aware of how she could arrange her work space more conveniently. She was provided with a document holder, footstool, wrist rest and shoulder rest for the telephone.

Gemma returned to work full time performing alternative duties in her original work unit. She found these duties did not exacerbate her pain. Due to the localized nature of her pain, she was given a wrist support orthosis incorporating the thumb which she wore only when performing heavier tasks which previously caused pain. Gemma continued with her pause gymnastics and began walking after work with her partner. At the natural completion of the project Gemma returned to her previous duties, ensuring that she did not perform keyboard activities for more than four hours per day, with a maximum of one hour at any one time. This limitation was implemented throughout the organization following several other similar situations with other workers. Gemma developed new skills while working on the project which she was able to use later to demonstrate her competence and proficiency when applying for a promotion. Gemma's return to playing the flute was slow and tentative, however, she was successful and incorporated her pause gymnastics and warm-up exercises into her routine.

Summary

Clinic-based and workplace-based programmes can be seen as a continuum of return-to-work programmes which facilitate the re-establishment or continuation of the worker role for individuals who have sustained neuromusculoskeletal or motor performance dysfunction. While the focus of the programmes is to improve physical performance, work fitness in its broadest sense can be improved through these structured programmes. The concept of the industrial athlete enables the intervention approach to resemble that of a sporting athlete, receiving appropriate coaching and an individualized training schedule which meets the capacities and limitations of the injured worker.

The use of suitable duties within the workplace enables the continuation of the rehabilitation programme in the workplace, with gradual upgrading of duties and time enabling injured workers to regain a positive productivity role which is consistent with their overall lifestyle and role repertoire.

Acknowledgements

The author would like to thank Dr Maureen Fitzgerald and Anne Hillman for their helpful comments and editing on the text of this chapter.

Multiple choice questions

1 Which of the following is NOT a principle of occupational rehabilitation?
   (a) Use a multidisciplinary approach to occupational rehabilitation due to the range of factors encompassed by each injured worker's disability.
   (b) Encourage early intervention to obtain maximum gains from rehabilitation.
   (c) Rehabilitation should occur at the workplace except where appropriate intervention for the injured worker's disability cannot be supplied by the workplace rehabilitation systems.
   (d) Intervention should recognize work as therapy, be function-oriented and use rest, inactivity and passive therapies as an integral part of rehabilitation.

2 Which of the following is NOT an indication for a workplace-based rehabilitation programme?
   (a) Identification with a patient or sick role.
   (b) Able to perform safely basic critical demands of identified suitable duties.
   (c) Able to manage symptoms, such as pain, appropriately in the workplace.
   (d) Do not pose a danger to themselves or others due to functional loss.

3 Grace has reduced cardiorespiratory fitness following the fracturing of several metatarsals in her left foot when a heavy box was dropped on her foot. Which of the following would be an appropriate programme for her?
   (a) Playing an hour of doubles tennis on Mondays, Wednesdays and Friday. Grace reports she rarely gets out of breath because it is mainly a social game and nobody is very good, so they stop a lot to pick up the ball.
   (b) Playing 9 holes of golf with a couple of friends on Wednesday and Sunday afternoons. This usually takes about 45 minutes and they stroll around the golf course with their golf buggies. Grace reports this is very pleasant and relaxing.
   (c) Swimming for 30 minutes at a continuous pace on Tuesdays, Thursdays and Saturdays. Grace reports she is 'puffing, but I can still talk' at the end of this.
   (d) Walking to the local shops to buy bread and milk a couple of times a week. It usually takes Grace about 5 to 10 minutes each way.

4 Heino is a maintenance mechanic in a pharmaceutical company. His dominant right hand was crushed when the machinery that Heino was working on was switched on by a co-worker. This resulted in amputation of his index and middle fingers at the PIP joints, and at the IP level of his thumb. The injury was four months ago and Heino has had good healing over the wounds but is very hypersensitive over the scarred areas. He has difficulty holding tools in his right hand and is afraid of moving machinery. Which return-to-work approach would be most suitable initially?

(a) A workplace-based programme returning on suitable alternate duties, such as checking incoming and outgoing orders, which is in a different area of the factory, starting on four hours per day.
(b) A work hardening programme incorporating relaxation and anxiety management techniques, desensitization and reintroduction of various hand tools, commencing for four hours per day.
(c) A work conditioning programme to improve his hand strength and range starting at 2 hours per day.
(d) A workplace-based programme returning on suitable modified duties, such as assisting the other maintenance mechanic by collecting appropriate tools, cleaning them, etc., in his usual work area of the factory, starting on four hours per day.

5 Consider the case study of Greg who injured his back at work. Which of the following situations was the most likely contributor to the development of his work-related injury?
(a) Maintaining a prolonged static posture or position.
(b) Working in extreme ranges of motion while applying force.
(c) Working in confined or restricted conditions.
(d) Performing heavy work requiring strength or endurance.

For answers to multiple choice questions see p. 309.

References

American College of Sports Medicine (1991). *Guidelines for Exercise Testing and Prescription*, 4th edn. Philadelphia: Lea & Fabiger.

American Occupational Therapy Association (1994). *Uniform Terminology for Occupational Therapy, Application to Practice*: 3rd edn. Rockville, MD.

Åstrand, P. and Rodahl, K. (1986). Textbook of Work Physiology: Physiological Bases of Exercise, 3rd edn. Singapore: McGraw-Hill.

Bammer, G., Calcino, P., Chadwick-Masters, J., Pollini, C. and Rainforth, J. (1994). The experience of rehabilitation from RSI: What determines success? *Journal of Occupational Health and Safety – Australia and New Zealand*, **10**(4), 353–8.

Bidencope, M. (1994). An evaluation of work hardening and workplace-based rehabilitation programs. Unpublished Masters treatise, The University of Sydney.

Bigos, S. J. *et al.* (1991). A prospective study of work perceptions and psychosocial factors affecting the report of back injury. *Spine*, **16**(1), 1–6.

Borg, G. (1982). Psychophysical bases of perceived exertion. *Medicine and Science in Sports and Exercise.* **14**(5), 377–81.

CCH Occupational Health and Safety Editors (1990). *Workplace Rehabilitation Manual.* Sydney: CCH Australia.

Chaffin, D. B. and Andersson, G. B. J. (1991). *Occupational Biomechanics*, 2nd edn. New York: John Wiley & Sons.

Commission on Accreditation of Rehabilitation Facilities (1989). *Standards Manual for Organizations Serving People with Disabilities*. Tucson, Arizona: Author.

Demers, L. M. (1992). *Work hardening: A practical guide.* Boston: Andover Medical Publishers.

Egger, G. and Champion, N. (ed.) (1990). *The Fitness Leader's Handbook*, 3rd edn. Sydney: Kangaroo Press.

Ellexson, M. (1989). Work hardening. In *Work in Progress: Occupational therapy in work programs* (S. Hertfelder and C. Gwin, eds) pp. 67–126, Rockville, Maryland: American Occupational Therapy Association.

Ganora, A. and Wright, G. (1987). Occupational rehabilitation: Costs and benefits. *Journal of Occupational Health and Safety – Australia and New Zealand*, **3**(4), 331–7.

Hurri, H. (1989). The Swedish back school in chronic low back pain. Part II. Factors predicting the outcome. *Scandinavian Journal of Rehabilitation Medicine*, **21**(1), 41–4.

Innes, E. (1995). Workplace-based occupational rehabilitation in New South Wales, Australia. *Work*, **5**(2), 147–52.

Jonsson, B. (1984). Muscular fatigue and endurance: Basic research and ergonomic applications. In Neural and Mechanical Control of Movement (M. Kumamoto, ed.) pp. 64–76, Kyoto: Yamaguchi Shoten.

King, P. M. (1993). Outcome analysis of work-hardening programs. *American Journal of Occupational Therapy*, **47**(7), 595–603.

Lechner, D. E. (1994). Work hardening and work conditioning interventions: Do they affect disability? *Physical Therapy*, **74**(5), 471–93.

Linton, S. J. and Warg, L. E. (1993). Attributions (beliefs) and job satisfaction associated with back pain in an industrial setting. Perceptual and *Motor Skills*, **76**(1), 51–62.

Luopajarvi, T. (1990). Ergonomic analysis of workplace and postural load. In *Ergonomics: The Physiotherapist in the Workplace* (M. I. Bullock, ed.) pp. 51–78, London: Churchill Livingstone.

Lusted, M. (1993). Predicting return to work after rehabilitation for low back injury. *Australian Journal of Physiotherapy*, **39**(3), 203–10.

Matheson, L. N. (1988). Integrated work hardening in vocational rehabilitation: An emerging model. *Vocational Evaluation and Work Adjustment Bulletin*, **21**, 71–6.

Matheson, L. N. Ogden, L. D., Violette, K. and Schultz, K. (1985). Work hardening: Occupational therapy in industrial rehabilitation. *American Journal of Occupational Therapy*, **39**(5), 314–21.

Matheson, L. N. and Ogden-Niemeyer, L. (1987). *Work Capacity Evaluation: Systematic approach to industrial rehabilitation*, Rev. edn. Anaheim, CA: ERIC.

Minor, M. (1991). Physiological dimensions of performance. In *Occupational Therapy: Overcoming human performance deficits* (C. Christiansen and C. Baum, eds.) pp. 198–229, Thorofare, N.J.: Slack.

Ogden-Niemeyer, L. and Jacobs, K. (1989). *Work Hardening: State of the art*. Thorofare, New Jersey: Slack Inc.

Ranka, J. and Chapparo, C. (1995). Assessing information processing deficits through observations of function: The PRPP system. Paper presented at the Quest for Quality: 12th World Congress of the International Federation of Physical Medicine and Rehabilitation, Sydney, Australia.

Strautins, P. and Hall, W. (1989). Does early referral to an on-site rehabilitation program predict an early return to work? *Journal of Occupational Health and Safety – Australia and New Zealand*, **5**(2), 137–43.

US Department of Labor, Employment and Training (1991). *The Revised Handbook for Analyzing Jobs*. Indianapolis, IN: JIST Works.

Wilmore, J. H. and Costill, D. L. (1994). *Physiology of Sport and Exercise*. Champaign, IL: Human Kinetics.

WorkCover Authority of NSW (1993). *Rehabilitation Guidelines: Guidelines for workplace-based occupational rehabilitation programs for large and medium sized businesses*, rev. edn. Sydney.

Wyrick, J. M., Ogden-Niemeyer, L., Ellexson, M., Jacobs, K. and Taylor, S. (1991). Occupational therapy work-hardening programs: A demographic study. *American Journal of Occupational Therapy*, **45**(2), 109–12.

Yates S. (1992). Measuring the effectiveness of workplace rehabilitation. *Journal of Occupational Health and Safety – Australia and New Zealand*, **8**(6), 493–6.

Section IV

Practice Tools

10

Challenging Tradition: Measuring Quality as Outcomes for People

James Gardner and Tina Campanella

Learning Objectives

At the end of this chapter, the reader should be able to:

1. Define the difference between an organizational process and outcome measure of quality for individuals with disabilities.
2. Define the impact of organizational suboptimization on people with disabilities.
3. Identify the two distinct roles that professionals assume in promoting outcomes for people.
4. Explain how generic outcomes can be used to structure the work or supported employment setting for an individual with disabilities.

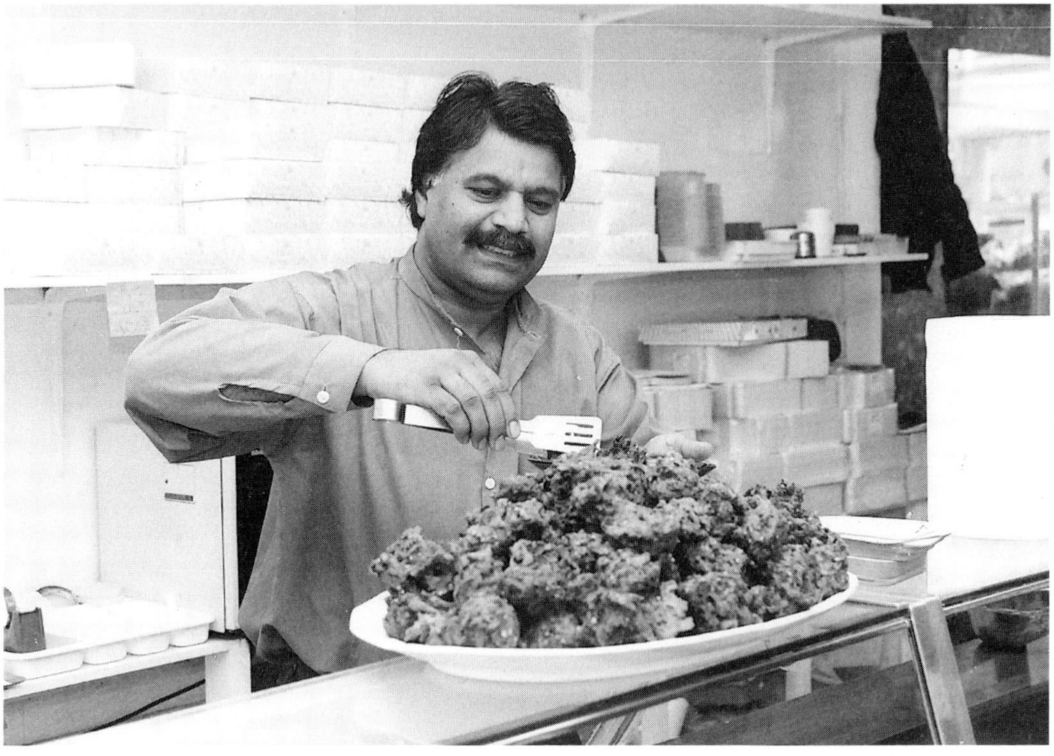

Abstract

The fields of health, rehabilitation and human services have traditionally defined quality in terms of compliance with professional norms, government requirements, or provider consensus. The Accreditation Council redesigned its standards for accreditation on the basis of individual and focus group interviews with people with disabilities. These *Outcome Based Performance Measures* published in 1993 are generic and can be applied to a wide range of disability and service settings. The Accreditation Council in 1995 published a set of outcomes for work and supported employment services. The work and supported employment outcomes define work as a process of intermediate variable that leads to outcomes. The *Outcomes for Work and Supported Employment* are individually defined. *Outcomes for Work and Supported Employment* are used to design the unique set of services and supports that will facilitate outcomes for each person. Outcome measurement forms the basis of The Accreditation Council's international quality enhancement, organizational support and accreditation programme.

Introduction

The fields of health, rehabilitation, education and human services have traditionally defined quality in the context of compliance with professional norms, governmental regulations, or consensus standards. While some evaluation research has focused on quality-of-life criteria and individual benefits, in practice, the measurement of quality generally occurs through the process of programme evaluation. Recently, however, the advocates of total quality management (TQM) and continuous quality improvement (CQI) have questioned the traditional definitions and measures of quality. Researchers and practitioners of enhanced quality in service settings are pointing to the importance of producing valued outcomes for the customer. Proponents of 'reinventing government' are questioning the viability of government programmes that meet the test of compliance with norms and standards but fail to produce outcomes for the people served.

The measurement of quality

The input–process–outcome model provides the beginning structure for defining and evaluating quality. Variations of the model include an antecedent, transaction and outcome classification (Stake, 1972). Inputs are the resources that are allocated to services and supports for people with disabilities. Frequent measures of input are the number of staff, the

Key words and definitions in this chapter

Outcome: Statement of what the individual expects from services and supports.

Organizational process: The methodology for providing services and supports that result in an outcome for an individual.

Accreditation: Independent, third-party assessment of the quality of services and supports provided by an organization

Suboptimization: Becoming more efficient and effective while performing the wrong task.

Interview: The formal and informal process of talking with people with disabilities to identify their prioritized outcomes.

Individualized organizational process: On organizational policy, procedure or practice that is individualized and made applicable for each individual.

Quality as a design variable: The interviews that identify people's prioritized outcomes are used to plan, develop and design services and support that facilitate those outcomes. Quality is achieved through the identification and facilitation of people's outcomes.

size of the budget, and the furnishings, equipment and facilities operated by the organization (Suchman, 1967). Schalock includes an organization's knowledge base as an input, citing assessments, individualized plans, programme objectives and environmental demands (Schalock 1983; 1986).

Organizational process measures define how the organization uses the resources. The process measures frequently determine whether the services and supports were provided in accordance with the programme design. The process measure addresses the question of whether 'the program was implemented as intended' (Rutman, 1977: 62). Process measures also indicate whether the organization complies with required local, state, provincial and federal requirements (Posavac and Carey, 1980). Frequent measures of process are: compliance with requirements concerning assessment, treatment planning, record keeping and reviews, case closure, and compliance with professional norms and codes of conduct.

Organizational outcome measures identify the outcomes produced by the services and supports of the organization (Posavac and Carey, 1980). These organizational outcomes generally focus on such accomplishments as the number of people placed in work settings, the number of assessments completed, or the average wage or hours worked per week. Outcomes in criminal justice programmes are arrests, convictions, or reimprisonment (Rutman, 1977). Outcomes in education might include the impact of instruction on students, teachers and administrators (Stake, 1972). Health programmes measure changes in incidence and prevalence rates, and drug-abuse programmes might measure repeat addiction (Patton, 1978).

In the area of health care, Donabedian (1980) designed a framework for determining quality in health care that incorporated the dimensions of input, process and outcome. Donabedian defined input as the structure and resources of the organization that included financial capital, technology and physical and human resources. Structure encompassed variables that influence the financing and delivery of health care such as public policy and financing. The influence of structure on quality was most apparent in the planning, design and implementation of health-care services.

Donabedian (1980) defined the process of health care as 'the set of activities that go on within and between practitioners and patents.' The activity is evaluated in the context of normative behaviour derived from the science of health care and societal values and ethics. The outcomes of health care are the changes in individual health status that can be traced to the provision of health care. Outcomes might include improvements in social, psychological and physiological performance as well as individual satisfaction, knowledge and behavioural change.

Donebadien identified the process measure as the most direct measure of quality because of the observable normative behaviour on the part of the practitioner. Outcome measures, in contrast, could serve as quality indicators only when the other possible causes for change in health status had been eliminated. In general, quality measurement systems in the field of health, vocational rehabilitation and human services have emphasized the organizational process and, to a lesser extent, the organizational outcomes related to services and supports. State regulations and licensing requirements and federal certification requirements place a heavy emphasis on compliance with specified requirements, and those requirements are often derived from the norms and patterns of the particular professions. The requirements of national accrediting organizations, such as the Commission on Accreditation of Rehabilitation Facilities, the Joint Commission on Accreditation of Health Care Facilities, and the Accreditation Council on Services for People with Disabilities, focused on organizational process compliance.

Causes and consequence

The focus on organizational process and organizational outcomes results from problems in measurement. The first problem is that the desired payoffs of human service programmes may lie in the future. This difficulty of waiting, and knowing when to measure, leads many evaluators to focus on intermediate goals that are defined in terms of organizational process and outcomes (Weiss, 1972). Fuzzy goals and the lack of consensus on the definition of quality also lead to a

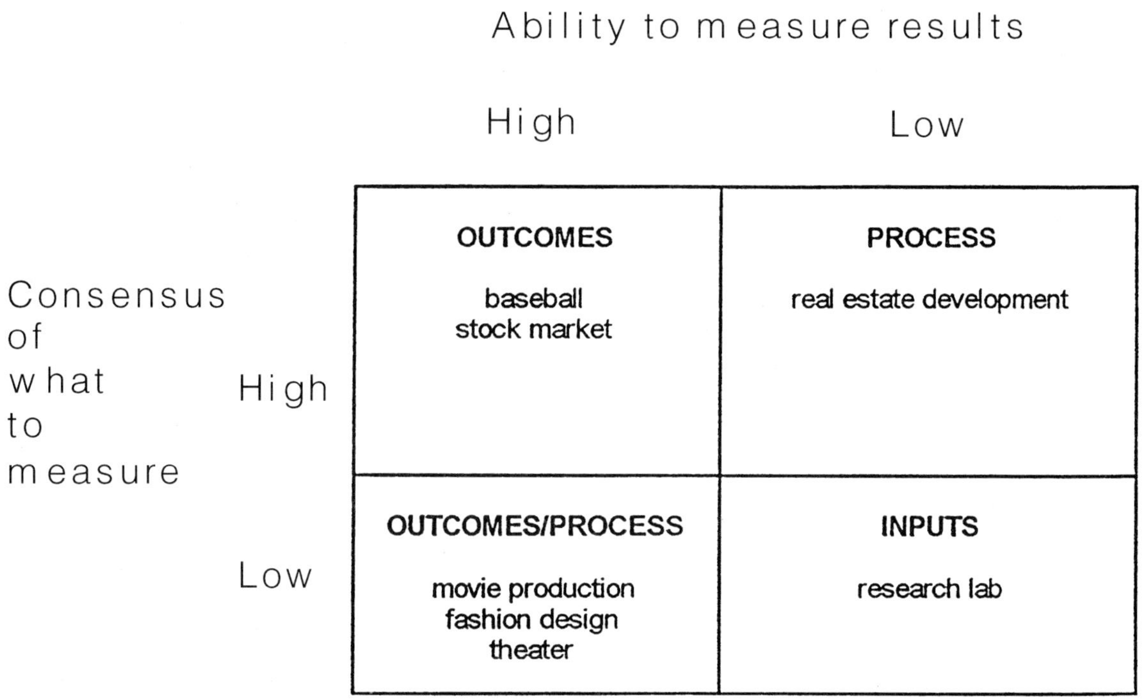

Figure 10.1 Feedback variables. Adapted from Merchant (1982).

preoccupation with organizational process. Merchant (1982) analysed the input–process–outcome model in terms of two variables – goal congruence and measurement capability. As Figure 10.1 indicates, a high level of agreement on what to measure and a high level of capability results in an emphasis on outcomes. A corresponding low consensus on goals and poor measurement methods results in a focus on input measures.

The problems of measurement are compounded by the focus on programmes. Programmes represent the reification of professional and bureaucratic abstractions and classification schemes. This reification enables professionals and bureaucrats to conduct their business. It affords primacy to the organizational process and the programme outcome rather than a discovery and definition of individual status. The tradition of programmes facilitates professional practice toward unambiguous ends. Programme structures provide a stable structural context in which to accomplish ends.

The process of professionalization itself simplifies the complexities and ambiguities of practice. Programmes represent the traditions and conventions of the particular professional subculture. This results in the phenomenon of pigeonholing, or slot assignment, wherein the professional defines the perceived client need in terms of a defined programme and standardized organizational process.

The focus on programme process and programme outcomes furthers the influence of the professional. In the health-care arena, Donabedian (1980) noted the emphasis on process will 'give primacy to the practitioners who are the high priests in charge of its technical mysteries and who also generate and control the information needed to assess it' (118). Berkowitz (1987) has noted the emphasis on 'professionalism' in the vocational rehabilitation programme in the United States and described the conflicts between the professionals who managed the organizational process and the individuals receiving services and supports.

The focus on programmes and organizational process increases the possibilities for suboptimization, when one unit of an organization attempts to optimize its goals at the expense of overall organizational performance (Wheelen and Hunger, 1989). Habilitation and human service programmes suboptimize when they elevate organizational process and outcomes above individual outcomes. These organizations become more efficient and effective at accomplishing the wrong tasks. The workshop becomes more efficient and effective in securing contracts for clients who desire integrated and competitive employment. The day treatment programme becomes more proficient in teaching activity of daily living skills to people who want supported employment.

Global transformations and new definition

Kuhn (1962) defined a paradigm shift as a change in the conceptual framework supporting belief systems. During the past decade, the shifting paradigm has been examined in the fields of management, business, disability, investment, leadership, biology and physics (Ray and Rinzler, 1993; Bradley, 1994; Waldrop, 1992; Wheatley 1994; Zuboff, 1988). The current attention to paradigm shifts, however, was foreshadowed by Daniel Bell's *The Coming of Post-Industrial Society* (1973) and Allan Toffler's *The Third Wave* (1980).

Bell (1973) noted that the increasing competitiveness of the world economy and the proliferating of advanced technologies, such as information processing, communications, biotechnology, advanced materials and superconductivity were resulting in global transformations. He considered the transition from an industrial to post-industrial society as momentous as the previous shift from agrarian to industrial society. For Bell, the pre-eminence of the professional and technical class and the primacy of theoretical knowledge were major characteristics of the new knowledge-based society. The focus on a post-industrial society is not a Western phenomenon. From an Eastern perspective, Sakaiya (1992) describes a knowledge-value society that will emerge in the aftermath of the industrial society. Wheatley (1992) describes the new paradigm in terms of old and new science and organizations. The old science, using machine imagery, focused on understanding parts of the whole. The Newtonian model was characterized by 'materialism and reductionism – a focus on things rather than relationships.' Reality could be disassembled into smaller parts, and the whole could be understood by examining the smaller units. The new science, in contrast, stresses synthesis and holism. The new science 'gives primary value to the relationship that exists among seemingly discrete parts.' Wheatley characterizes organizations not as mechanistic formulations from the industrial/bureaucratic age, but rather as fluid, organic structures in a knowledge-based society. This transformation in organizational structures was also observed by Kanter (1989) who noted that managers are 'watching hierarchy fade away and the clear distinctions of title, task, department, and even corporation, blur' (1992: 84).

The emergence of knowledge-based societies where the provision of services has replaced the manufacture of goods is influencing the definition and measurement of quality. Shewhart, an engineer at Western Electric in the 1920s, first recognized the importance of, and measured, the variability in product dimensions and attributes. Deming, working with Shewhart in the 1930s and 1940, modified and improved quality control methods and techniques. In the aftermath of Japan's defeat in the Second World War, Japanese scientists, engineers and business leaders studied and adopted the quality assurance methods of Deming and Juran. The commitment to quality contributed to the Japanese economic expansion in the 1960s and 1970s. The American rediscovery of Deming and Juran resulted in the popularization of total quality management (TQM) and continuous quality improvement. Manufactures adopted the quality improvement methodologies to increase their competitiveness in an emerging global economic competition (Sashkin and Kiser, 1993).

The popularization of the quality improvement approaches has emphasized the integrated system of tools, techniques and training that results in the continuous improvement of organizational processes. Yet the continuous improvement of organizational processes is only a means toward the end of delivering quality for the customer. As such, Deming, Juran, Crosby and Ishikawa defined quality as the continuous discovery and fulfilment of customer needs and desires (Sashkin and Kiser, 1993).

The gradual shift from an industrial to a service economy is resulting in a greater emphasis on defining the customer's desired outcome prior to engaging in the continuous improvement of organizational process. Indeed, there is little sense in perfecting organizational process if it yields the wrong outcome. Such a situation would result in almost total suboptimization.

In service settings, quality is determined at the point of interaction with the customer. Moreover, as Armand Feigenbaum indicates, 'Quality is what the customer says it is' (Sashkin and Kiser, 1993: 56). Since the desired outcomes may vary from customer to customer and for any individual may change over time, the service provider must pay continuous attention to customer preferences. Successful service organizations are developing a sharper market focus where they first identify customer outcomes and then customize the service accordingly. Albrecht states that 'In the customer value paradigm, the primary focus is on outcomes' (1992: 41). In contrast to the mass marketing of the industrial era, Peppers and Rogers emphasize dialogue and interaction with the customer. They suggest that the crucial question is 'What does this [individual] customer really want?' (1993: 16).

New definitions and transformations in rehabilitation

The literature in the fields of work preparation and habilitation reflects this emerging focus on identifying and facilitating outcomes. Albin (1992) advocates determining quality performance on the basis of the customer's definition of quality. In addition, she urges an ongoing adjustment of quality measures based on changing customer expectations and feedback. McLoughlin, Garner and Callahan equate quality with outcomes as defined by the customer. They argue that 'In the final analysis the outcome selected, the philosophies that guide their selection, and the degree to which the outcomes are achieved by, consumers are the ultimate measures of program effectiveness' (1987: 22). Walls and Tseng, in a review of client outcomes in rehabilitation, declare that the 'mission of rehabilitation must be expressed in terms of demonstrable client outcomes' (1987: 198). The merit of the rehabilitation process, they argue, is found only in the outcome for the client. Similarly, McLoughlin, Garner and Callahan (1987) have pointed to the distinction between rehabilitation structure and outcomes. They define structures as the frameworks or models used to provide vocational training and employment services. As such, outcomes selected by individuals must dictate the service process. The rehabilitation service process is the means to the outcome.

This distinction between the identification of preferred outcomes and the habilitation process that facilitates the outcome alters the relationship between the professional and the individual receiving services and supports. The identification of outcomes becomes an individual responsibility. The role of the professional in outcome identification is to listen and understand the context and reasons for the decision. The professional may provide guidance and counselling, but the choice of the outcome rests with the individual.

Once the individual has identified a set of preferred outcomes, professionals can summon their education, training and experience to facilitate the outcome for the individual. Based on their expertise, they can make recommendations from a variety of possible rehabilitation models and programmes. At this point, the professional plays a proactive role in facilitating outcomes.

In addition to a focus on outcomes, there is a growing recognition that the value of the work experience is individually determined and may extend beyond the traditional indicators of vocational habilitation or work quality. McLoughlin, Garner and Callahan indicate that the quality job is one that 'meets the personalized needs of the worker' (1987: 7).

They argue that the individual (as opposed to the programme designer or evaluator) has the opportunity to define the determinants of the quality job for oneself. Schalock (1988) has discussed quality-of-life indicators in the context of work programmes and indicated that measuring quality of life requires that organizations consider the individual's own perceptions and evaluations of their own life experience. Finally, Matson and Rusch (1986) have indicated how work can enhance quality of life in non-traditional areas, such as friendships, community participation, enhanced social roles, increasing respect and integration.

Redesigning accreditation around outcomes for people

Recognizing the changing definitions of quality in service settings, the Board of Directors of the Accreditation Council began to re-evaluate the role of accreditation in the early 1990s. The changing definitions of quality and the emergence of competing methods of quality enhancement resulted in a reconsideration of the traditional roles and methodologies for a national accreditation organization. The Accreditation Council redefined its mission as quality enhancement and identified its quality enhancement methods as the design and development of standards, the publication of educational materials, the provision of consultation and technical assistance, and the management of a national accreditation programme for organizations providing services and supports to people with disabilities.

The board decided against continued incremental changes to the previous set(s) of accreditation standards last revised in 1990. In contrast, the Accreditation Council engaged in a discontinuous change process by setting the old standards and methodologies aside and starting over. The design criteria for these new standards established by the board of directors were reflected in three primary descriptors. The new measures were to be:

1 Concise.
2 Generic (be applicable to a wide variety of disabilities, service and settings).
3 Person-centered outcomes.

Instead of soliciting professional opinion concerning quality in services, the Accreditation Council asked people with disabilities what outcomes were most important in their life. Staff of the Accreditation Council conducted individual and focus-group meetings with people experiencing a wide range of disabilities throughout the State of Illinois during 1992–1993. The Accreditation Council staff also held meetings with families, advocates and providers of service. The purpose of these meetings was to identify the primary outcomes of supports and services from the perspective of people with disabilities.

The action research interview process resulted in a list of thirty outcome measures. The thirty outcomes and a quality review methodology based on interviews with people receiving services and supports were pilot tested four times in the States of Illinois and Maryland. The revised set of thirty outcomes was then field tested at ten sites in the United States and Canada in 1992–1993. Measures of inter-rater reliability, construct validity, and correlation between outcomes and individualized process were compiled by researchers at Johns Hopkins University, Baltimore, Maryland. The outcomes were finalized with the publication of the *Outcome Based Performance Measures in 1993* (Accreditation Council, 1993) (see Fig. 10.2).

The principle purpose in developing a set of person-focused performance measures was to measure organizational responsiveness to people rather than compliance with organizational process. As such, the person-focused performance measures are used to structure interviews and discussions with people that result in the identification of individual priority outcomes.

The *Outcome Based Performance Measures* (Accreditation Council, 1993) are first used as a resource guide for learning about people. The *Outcome Based Performance Measures* manual provides questions and probes that can be used in discussions with people to identify the priority outcomes in their lives. The manual provides instructions and methods for talking with staff, family and friends to discover preferences of people with significant cognitive limitations, psychiatric dysfunction or communication challenges. Each outcome must be defined for the person served before the presence of the outcome can be measured.

PERSONAL GOALS	1.	People choose personal goals.
	2.	People realize personal goals.
CHOICE	3.	People choose where and with whom they live.
	4.	People choose where they work.
	5.	People decide how to use their free time.
	6.	People choose services.
	7.	People choose their daily routine.
SOCIAL INCLUSION	8.	People participate in the life of the community.
	9.	People interact with other members of the community.
	10.	People perform different social roles.
RELATIONSHIPS	11.	People have friends.
	12.	People remain connected to natural support networks.
	13.	People have intimate relationships.
RIGHTS	14.	People exercise rights.
	15.	People are afforded due process if rights are limited.
	16.	People are free from abuse and neglect.
DIGNITY AND RESPECT	17.	People are respected.
	18.	People have time, space and opportunity for privacy.
	19.	People have and keep personal possessions.
	20.	People decide when to share personal information.
HEALTH	21.	People have health care services.
	22.	People have the best possible health.
ENVIRONMENT	23.	People are safe.
	24.	People use their environments.
	25.	People live in integrated environments.
SECURITY	26.	People have economic resources.
	27.	People have insurance to protect their resources.
	28.	People experience continuity and security.
SATISFACTION	29.	People are satisfied with services.
	30.	People are satisfied with their personal life situations.

Figure 10.2 Outcome based performance measures for people.

While the initial focus of the *Outcome Based Performance Measures* is on priority outcomes for the person, the application process also requires the user to identify the individualized organizational processes that facilitate, or can facilitate, outcomes for the person. Organizational process is considered important, but only when it is clearly connected to outcomes for the person. Outcome measurement challenges organizational processes that are not clearly connected to outcomes for people.

The outcomes were developed and field tested across a wide range of disability and service delivery disciplines and methodologies. The results of the focus group interviews and field tests indicated that these generic outcomes are the same for all people with disabilities. They pertain to people with mental retardation, brain injury, physical disability or chronic psychiatric disorder. The differences between and among people with different disabilities lies not in outcomes, but in the unique processes that facilitate the outcomes. Thus, people with different disabilities may need a medical, therapeutic, educational, or rehabilitation process or programme to achieve the same outcome.

The *Outcome Based Performance Measures* also challenge professional roles. The first role of the professional is to support and assist the individual in identifying his or her priority outcomes. Professionals play a support role in the identification of outcomes. The person with the disability, and not the professional, controls the definition of outcome. Once the priority outcomes are identified, the professional uses his or her training, experience and expertise to facilitate the outcomes. The service provider implements the necessary rehabilitation services and structures to facilitate the attainment of outcomes for the individual.

Outcomes do not require or prescribe specific services for people. Rather, as a tool, outcomes function as a framework for identifying priorities for each person served. Outcomes assist the provider to develop an understanding of how each person prioritizes issues and activities in his or her life. This understanding enables professionals to make decisions about which service and support practices will be most relevant to each person.

Outcomes for assessing quality in work and employment

Upon publication of the *Outcome Based Performance Measures* (1993), considerable debate arose around the question of whether the Measures pertained to the world of work, or whether a subset of the thirty, or an alternative set of outcomes were necessary to assess the quality in work settings. Providers of employment and work training requested outcomes for work and employment.

With an emphasis on outcomes rather than organizational process, and on discovering how work and employment contribute to quality of life, the Accreditation Council initiated a process to investigate outcomes for people receiving employment and work supports that paralleled the development of the original outcomes. People with disabilities, their families, guardians, advocates and support personnel were interviewed in individual and group meetings to gather information about prioritized personal outcomes related to employment. This process yielded a list of items such as money, security, respect and social interaction, that were used to draft outcomes for people related to employment services.

The first set of outcomes drafted for use in employment settings was divided into two sections. Twenty-two outcomes were linked to benefits from employment. A list of eight supplemental outcomes were also identified as important, but indirectly linked to work and employment related concerns. Figures 10.3 and 10.4 identify the initial two categories of outcomes. Field tests were conducted at four organizations providing employment supports to test the applicability and relevance of the draft outcomes.

The four field-test sites served people with a range of disabilities. Collectively, the sites provided a range of employment services including sheltered work, developmental training, on-the-job training, supported and competitive employment. The twenty people who participated in the field test included people with both mild and severe disabilities in areas of cognitive, physical and emotional functioning. Field-test participants ranged in age from 24 to 59 and had a variety of prior work experiences. Each person was directly

1. People choose personal outcomes.
2. People realize personal outcomes.
3. People have friends.
4 People are respected.
5. People decide when to share personal information.
6. People are safe.
7. People use their environments.
8. People work in integrated environments.
9. People choose where they work.
10. People choose services.
11. People choose their daily routine.
12. People exercise rights.
13. People are afforded due process if rights are limited.
14. People are free from abuse and neglect.
15. People are satisfied with supports and services.
16. People are satisfied with their personal life situations.
17. People interact with other members of the community.
18. People perform different social roles.
19. People have the best possible health.
20. People have economic resources.
21. People have insurance to protect their resources.
22. People experience continuity and security.

Figure 10.3 Draft outcome measures for employment.

1. **People choose where and with whom they live.**
2. **People decide how they use their free time.**
3. **People participate in the life of the community.**
4. **People remain connected to natural support networks.**
5. **People have intimate relationships.**
6. **People have time, space and opportunity for privacy.**
7. **People have and keep personal possessions.**
8. **People have health care services.**

Figure 10.4 Draft outcome measures for employment – supplemental outcomes.

interviewed and visits were made to both work and home.

Both the direct and supplemental outcomes were applied for all people in the employment settings. The Accreditation Council was able to determine the presence of outcomes and individualized organizational processes through talking with people served, the people who knew them best and support staff. The only difficulty in the implementation process was finding adequate time to interact with staff providing direct support to people at work. These individuals had the greatest amount of information about people participating in the interviews, but had the least time for interviews due to the demands of their job responsibilities.

The data collected at each site presented a highly individualized profile of each organization's strengths and weaknesses. Figures 10.5 and 10.6 indicate the outcomes and individualized organizational process that were present for the five people in the interview sample at each of the four field-test sites. Although some outcomes were present for a larger number of people in the sample, with the exception of economic resources, these outcomes were not the ones most frequently associated with work. The outcomes related to access and use of physical environments, personal integration, abuse and neglect, optimal health and economic resources were found to be present for over 85 per cent of the people in the sample.

The outcome measures found to be most closely linked to work and employment preparation were those such as: choice and achievement of personal goals, the location of work and daily routines, attainment of economic resources, safety, security and continuity, confidentiality and personal satisfaction with services and general life circumstances. These outcomes reflect a combination of personal priorities, typical norms in the work environment and rationales for the selection of specific jobs and work environments.

Outcome measures often considered less directly connected to work address issues that involve the social aspects of work environments. For example, work environment and interactions can influence outcomes associated with social inclusion and relationships. Many people find close friends and important social roles through their work. Where and how people work may also influence outcomes associated with dignity and respect, health and environment. In the field test, these outcomes were found to be present for only 50–65 per cent of the people in the sample and the direct support that might have facilitated these outcomes was less frequently provided in the work environment.

Finally, some outcome measures do not have an obvious direct linkage to work or employment activities. These outcomes serve to promote an understanding of the person and his or her life experience. Information about personal issues such as living situa-

OUTCOMES PRESENT

NUMBER IN EACH SAMPLE = 5

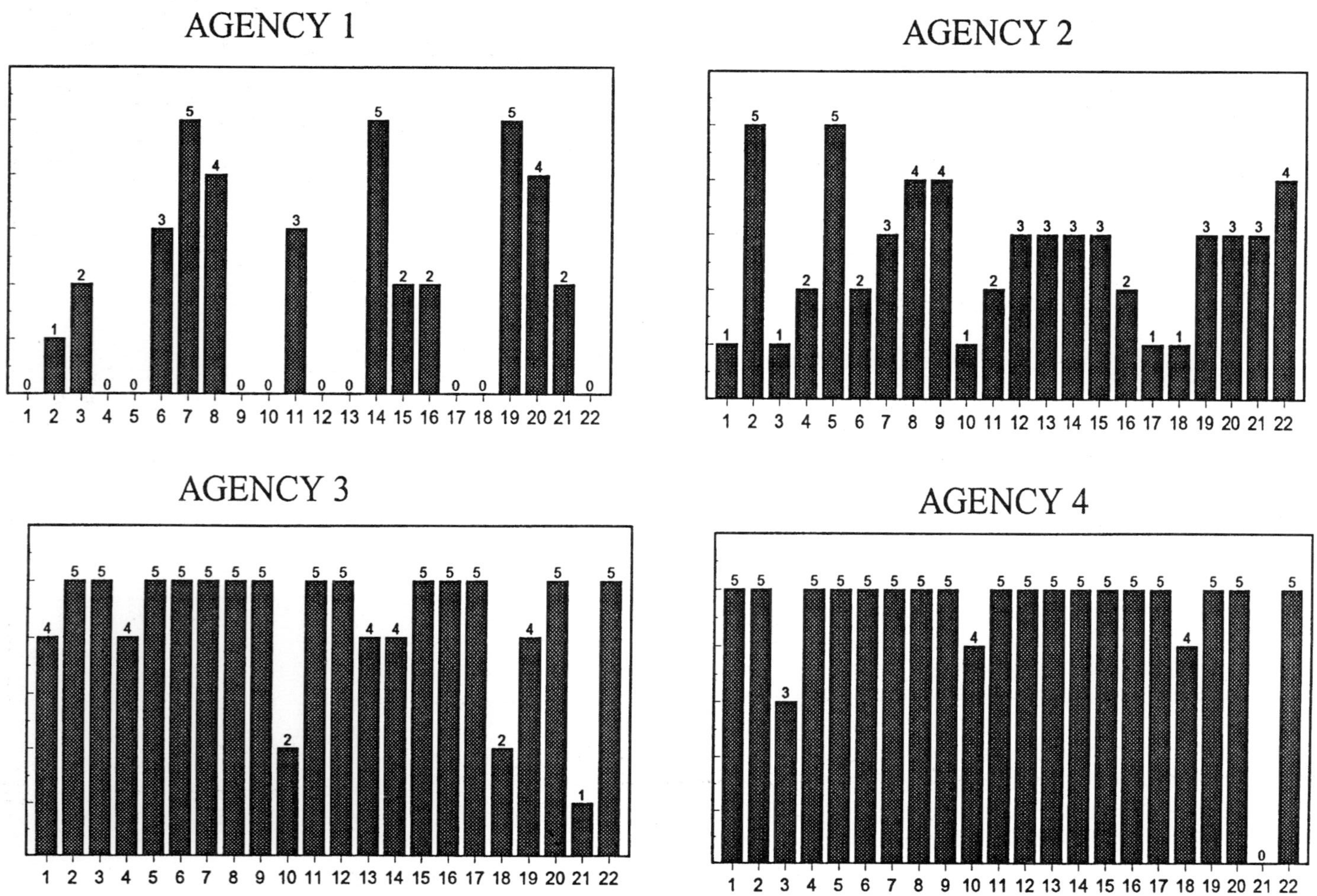

Figure 10.5

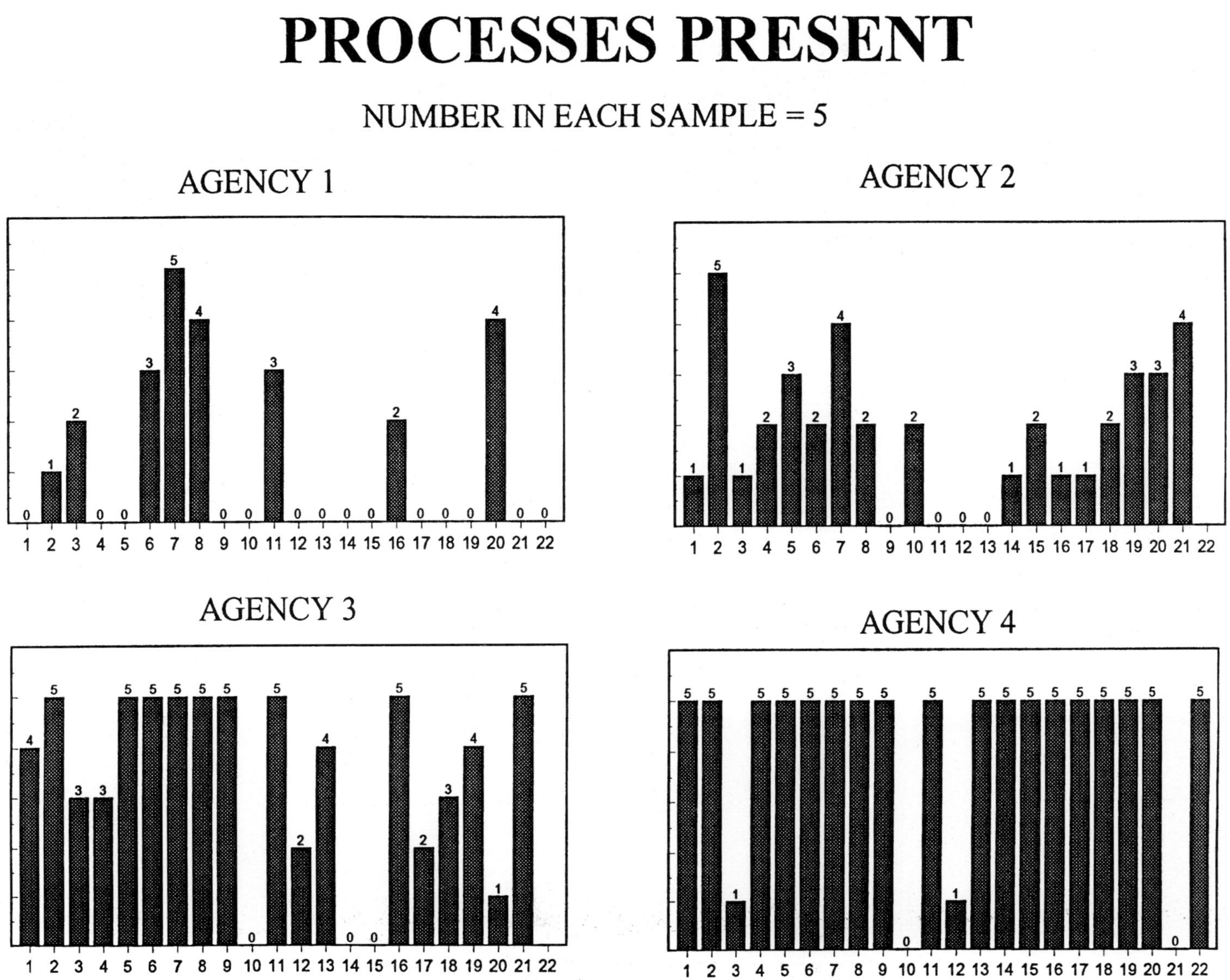
PROCESSES PRESENT
NUMBER IN EACH SAMPLE = 5
AGENCY 1
0 1 2 0 0 3 5 4 0 0 3 0 0 0 0 2 0 0 0 4 0 0
1 2 3 4 5 6 7 8 9 10 11 12 13 14 15 16 17 18 19 20 21 22
AGENCY 2
1 5 1 2 3 2 4 2 0 2 0 0 0 1 2 1 1 2 3 3 4
1 2 3 4 5 6 7 8 9 10 11 12 13 14 15 16 17 18 19 20 21 22
AGENCY 3
4 5 3 3 5 5 5 5 5 0 5 2 4 0 0 5 2 3 4 1 5
1 2 3 4 5 6 7 8 9 10 11 12 13 14 15 16 17 18 19 20 21 22
AGENCY 4
5 5 1 5 5 5 5 5 5 0 5 1 5 5 5 5 5 5 5 5 0 5
1 2 3 4 5 6 7 8 9 10 11 12 13 14 15 16 17 18 19 20 21 22

Figure 10.6

tions, family demands and support, and relationships provide insight about the person. This information may assist staff to understand how factors outside the work environment may support or interfere with work. In addition, although work or employment support services may not facilitate these outcomes, the person's work situation or employment supports should be arranged to minimize interference with the attainment of outcomes in other aspects of the person's life. For example, a work training programme that requires travel of great distances and long hours and results in diminished opportunities for relationships and free time might need to be reconsidered if it is causing difficulty for the person.

The field test experience demonstrated the difficulty of predicting which outcomes would be most important to people with disabilities in guiding the development of their employment supports. Although a majority of people receiving employment services prioritized outcomes such as choice of work and satisfaction with services as important, they selected and defined outcomes from a personal and individual perspective. A person-centered, outcome-based approach does not yield clear and separate work and non-work related priority outcomes.

The rigid separation between narrowly defined work-related outcomes and other 'non-work' outcomes reflects professional behaviour and perspective. Employment and rehabilitation activities are often specialized processes that occur in specific environments (e.g. workshop, clubhouse, clinic) to address specific individual issues (e.g. productivity, social adjustment and motor skills). Feedback from people with disabilities during focus-group interviews and interviews during the four field tests revealed a much greater linkage between work and overall quality of life than reflected by typical employment and rehabilitation programme activities. The preferences and personal expectations for support expressed by people reflected the integration of home, work and other personal issues.

The area of social interaction provides a good example of how personal outcomes functionally connect to the work environment. While intimate and friendship relationships are not typically considered relevant to the work environment, individual perceptions and needs related to intimacy and friendship had significant impact on work success for some people in the field tests. The lack of personal relationships and opportunity for social interaction outside the work environment caused some people to search for those outcomes through social contacts with co-workers. In contrast, other people needed support to learn appropriate interactions with co-workers because of limited prior experience with social interaction in general or because of specific disabilities. The relevance of, and need for, support in the area of social interaction was determined by the person, his or her skills, experience and personal context, not by the type or intensity of work.

The field tests also demonstrated a strong connection between personal health and work from an individual outcome perspective. A person's health situation must be accommodated within the work environment. Supports that facilitate success in the workplace for people with disabilities are designed from an understanding of the person's physical abilities and physical and mental health needs. Work situations that do not match the person's desire for physical and mental challenge may not result in positive outcomes. Work tasks and supports may need to be modified as the person's health status changes. At a minimum, an awareness of and concern for health status supports positive employment outcomes.

In addition, personal beliefs and values influence the choice of employment and work training. The four field tests with the employment outcomes demonstrated that individual expectations about work and employment supports were often grounded in personal beliefs and values. An understanding of beliefs and values is as valuable as information about skills and physical attributes. Those individuals whose personal values and beliefs are compatible with an organization's work culture 'fit in' to the work environment. Those whose personal values conflict with the organizational culture are likely to have difficulty. For example, a person who prioritizes respect and deference to authority will perform better in a highly structured and controlled work environment than a person who values autonomy and individual learning opportunity.

Although work programmes have provided some supports in areas indirectly related to work such as social relationships, health and individual values, the framework for most work services is determined by a programmatic assessment of individual skills and disability-related needs in relation to work tasks and required work behaviour. The person-centered issues that reflect typical variables related to work success are considered only as a secondary issue. The use of outcomes elevates these concerns to primary position.

The outcomes which are most directly relevant to a person's work are determined individually. Different people attach different emphasis to the outcomes they derive from work. Some people may value money more than accomplishing personal goals. Others will emphasize free time more than economic security. Using the outcomes to design services and supports enables the organization to be responsive to individual needs. Priority outcomes expected from work are identified for each person and then supports and services are selected or created to promote priority outcomes for each person effectively.

The field-test experience revealed no strong correlations between the presence of specific outcomes, specific types of individualized organizational process, and the type of employment or work service. Outcomes originally considered indirectly linked to employment (e.g. natural supports, intimate relationships, health care) were identified as important by almost all persons interviewed during the field tests. Although the interview conversations did not always relate to employment, they did provide information that was important for problem solving and supporting the person at work.

The holistic picture of the person provided through the use of outcomes contributes to effective employment supports. This larger perspective assists staff to use limited time and resources to create maximum individual benefit. For example, information about the person's social connections outside the workplace may help employment staff to determine the importance of social connections at work. Individualized organizational processes to promote social connections are not necessary when this is not a priority for the individual. However, for people who are dissatisfied with their personal social outcomes and who may need support, information about the person's desires becomes critical. The information can assist staff to tailor employment activities to individual needs.

Using outcomes to design work and employment options for the individual

Outcome measurement has the potential for keeping the focus of employment on people and the individual dynamics that impact on success for people in the workplace. Individual outcome data enables staff to identify clearly the issues that need to be addressed through supports and services. The supports and services are then viewed as processes that enable people to achieve their prioritized outcomes. As such, organizational systems, policies and procedures become frameworks for enabling people to achieve outcomes.

Outcomes are useful for identifying individual priorities to guide the design of supports and services because they reflect the things that people typically expect in life. The individual outcome identification process requires that an active dialogue be established with each person served at the initiation of service. This information exchange and learning process continues throughout the service relationship. In individual interviews, people are asked to describe and explain the priorities in their life so that support staff can understand the unique aspects of each person's situation. This information is then used to guide additional assessment and information gathering. Although the person is always the primary source of information, discussions with other people who know the person receiving service may be needed. These individuals are asked to supplement the information provided by the person by sharing what they have learned about the person through interactions and shared experience. Other individuals may also provide insight into the person's personal history and prior experience that can influence decisions about specific service strategies. The person directs this process by providing the initial information and identifying the other people (e.g. family members, other service providers) who may provide staff with information critical to understanding the person's needs and desires.

Spending time with the person in different natural and service environments is another critical information gathering strategy. Interactions with the person and observations of the person's interactions with others provides a rich source of direct information about the person's preferences and priorities. This experiential data is used to enhance and confirm the information gathered through interviews with the person and others.

The information gathered from the person about individual outcomes is used to direct decision making about services and supports. The service planning process is an extension of the ongoing dialogue between staff and the person served. In contrast to the traditional staffing format, outcome-based service planning involves discussion of all available service options that may facilitate the person's outcomes. The service provider uses professional expertise and knowledge of the service system to assist the person to select the opportunities and services that are most compatible with his or her personal outcomes.

As service activities are implemented, individual outcome information is used to direct ongoing review and assessment of service effectiveness. Service process is judged successful when there is demonstrated progress toward the realization of desired outcomes. When no progress toward outcomes is observed, the need for a thorough review and possible redesign of service activities is warranted.

This individual, outcome-based evaluation of services plays a key role in increasing quality in the individual service process. While typical data-based measures of individual progress are effective at documenting individual gains in skill, behaviour and task completion, outcome evaluation captures the element of individual relevance. For example, traditional objective-based data may reflect how a worker is progressing with learning to complete a work task. This data may also provide information needed to make adjustments in the learning process and in aspects of the work environment to increase individual success. The specific data does not reflect whether the work task is well matched to the worker's interests and overall abilities. This kind of assessment can only be accomplished through direct interaction with the person. A combination of a traditional and outcome evaluation is necessary to provide the best overall picture of individual progress.

Outcome measurement can also be an effective tool for organizational assessment. An aggregation of individual outcome data can reveal patterns and trends in services that reflect organizational strengths and weaknesses. A pattern of outcomes and processes present for people served indicates that services are in line with individual needs. Any trends that reflect outcomes or processes not present may reflect areas where services, supports or other resources may need to be added or redesigned to be more responsive to individual needs.

The collection of individual outcome data within an organization can be an important part of an overall quality assurance and improvement system. Outcome data represents the unique perspective of the people served in a way that other programme evaluation and objective data cannot. Used in combination with other data on organizational services and accomplishments, outcome measures provide managers with a balanced assessment of performance.

The primary purpose of an employment support system is to enable people to achieve desired outcomes – such as economic resources, continuity and security, insurance, friends, participation in the life of the community and the realization of personal goals and satisfaction – through the organizational process of providing employment supports. In practice, staff sometimes become overly concerned with the implementation of services and supports. Organizational activities that seek to ensure the accurate and consistent implementation of services may inadvertently shift attention from the person to service process. Outcome-directed service activities make it more likely that service activities will remain focused on people and facilitate the attainment of outcomes.

Conclusion

Application of outcome measures in employment settings has shown that the outcomes to assist people to find, secure and sustain a meaningful employment do not differ significantly from those used to measure success in other life areas. Since outcomes function by providing a framework for understanding the person, addressing the full range of issues that may be important to people is essential to ensuring that work supports compliment other activities in the person's life. Although supports provided by the employment organization may be limited to the work setting, the knowledge of the person in all areas enables staff to ensure that the person's work situation is compatible with other activities and priorities for the person.

Ensuring the person is successfully integrated into the work environment is the primary objective of employment support, but the performance of activities at work that contribute to task and productivity is only one part of the work experience. The application of generic outcome measures to work emphasizes the view that work is a means to an end. People work to achieve individual outcomes. Work is not an end in itself. Traditional work preparation and work opportunities for people with disabilities have often treated work itself as the outcome. When work is viewed as the outcome, active engagement in any work activity can be judged as adequate. However, when providers of service look beyond work tasks to the direct and indirect outcomes that people expect from work, success and quality in employment service is defined by responsiveness to individual need.

Defining quality in terms of outcomes for people requires a change in organizational design and service practices. From an outcome perspective, quality is a design variable that shapes supports and services from the point of service initiation. Using an outcome-based approach requires organizations to address each person's priority outcomes through supports and services that facilitate individual achievement of those outcomes.

The focus on outcomes challenges the employment service organization to look beyond professional practice and programme guidelines. Whereas, in the past, employment programmes were designed according to professional criteria, an outcome approach dictates that professional expertise be used to facilitate the attainment of individual outcomes. Programme design focused on models developed by professionals – work hardening, work activity, sheltered workshops, on-the-job training – reflects generalizations about the needs of people who would use them. People sought entry into the programme that best approximated their needs. Programmes accepted people into available 'slots' instead of designing services around the needs of each person served.

In contrast, an outcome- or person-centered approach replaces the programme approach with one that is based on the discovery of specific outcomes that people expect from work and employment services. Rather than placing people in available openings or slots, organizations design supports and services that meet expectations of people seeking services. General resources such as assessment, therapies, and group learning and support activities are accessed as needed by the person served instead of routinely required as a part of programme participation. More important, organizations recognize that the measure of quality is not the delivery of a service or support, but the results that service or supports produce for each person.

Multiple choice questions

1 The term outcome measure refers to:
  (a) Units of service produced by the service organization.
  (b) Efficiency and effectiveness of services rendered.
  (c) Goals established by the interdisciplinary team.
  (d) Results of services and supports for the person.

2 The measurement of outcomes is made possible by which two of the following conditions:
  (a) Consensus on what to measure.
  (b) A 60 per cent sampling level is achieved.
  (c) Measurement is reliable and valid.
  (d) Interviews are confidential.

3 The two roles of the professional in outcome measurement are:
  (a) Identify and measure the outcome.

(b) Assist in the identification of outcomes and then facilitate the outcome.
(c) Conduct assessment and set outcome goals.
(d) Perform screenings and participate in the interdisciplinary team process.

4 The Accreditation Council developed outcome measures for people with disabilities through:
(a) Professional consensus.
(b) Individual and focus groups of people with disabilities.
(c) Regression analysis of field test and accreditation reviews.
(d) Revision of previous Accreditation Council Standards.

5 The *Outcome Based Performance Measures* are first used to:
(a) Learn about people with disabilities.
(b) Set performance expectations for people receiving services and supports.
(c) Set performance expectations for staff.
(d) Measure organizational performance.

For answers to multiple choice questions see p. 309.

Case study

Ms Henderson is a 54-year-old widow living in her own home with the support of a drop-in counsellor. She has a psychiatric diagnosis of bipolar disorder and has been hospitalized off and on for the last ten years. Her last stay was just over one year ago when she was hospitalized for four months following the death of a neighbour and close friend.

Ms Henderson is a pleasant person who speaks slowly. She is being supported at home through a community mental-health organization and attends a psychosocial programme four days a week at a second organization. She is seen monthly by a psychiatrist to monitor her medication and is receiving therapy from a counsellor at her day programme. The three medications she is prescribed – one for the bipolar disorder, one for depression and anxiety, and one to control hand tremors – are effective for control of her psychiatric difficulties but also cause her to be lethargic. Staff do not accompany her to the psychiatrist.

Ms Henderson does not indicate a strong desire to work. Her work training assignment is food service where she is responsible for cleaning tables and general clean-up in the cafeteria after meals. She reports that she enjoys the interaction with others on the days she visits the programme centre. Her limited interest in work is reflected in her attention and work performance. She has no work experience except what she has obtained through her participation at the programme centre. She was a homemaker prior to her first hospitalization and her husband provided economic support prior to his death. She can offer no suggestions when asked about other occupations she might like to try.

Two months ago, the Monroe County Department of Social Services initiated a service coordination programme. Ms Long, a service coordinator, visited Ms Henderson and began to discuss the outcomes that she expected from her services and supports.

Ms Henderson was surprised by the discussion. She had previously participated in planning meetings where professionals and service providers discussed supports and services for her. Ms Henderson realized that the community mental health organization, the psychosocial programme, and the psychiatrist provided a loosely coordinated set of services and supports that prevented rehospitalization. The community mental health centre and the psychosocial programme had recommended her for placement when there was an opening in their programmes, but the services and supports were neither individualized nor coordinated.

The psychiatrist takes care of her medications. The psychosocial programme provides job training in food service and social programmes to encourage interaction with others. The counsellor at the psychosocial programme provides therapy once a week that is focused on coping with depression and anxiety. The community mental health organization provides drop-in assistance and help in monitoring her health and medications. Each programme performs its function and discharges its responsibilities.

If you were Ms Long, how would you use outcome measures to assess services and make recommendations in this situation? What are the specific steps that you would take?

1 Interview Ms Henderson to determine what outcomes are most important in her life and what role the supports and services she receives have in facilitating these outcomes.
2 Determine whether Ms Henderson has had any exposure to or experience with other employment or work training opportunities.
3 Interview others who know Ms Henderson. Invite the psychiatrist, the counsellor, and other professionals to join you and Ms Henderson as she discusses her priorities.
4 Assist Ms Henderson in identifying the prioritized outcomes. For example, is making money more important than achievement? Is social interaction more important than both? Does Ms Henderson want full or part-time work? For her, what is the relationship between work and physical health? Will medications inhibit work? Has anyone taken the place of her neighbour and close friend who died over a year ago?
5 Once the outcomes have been identified, Ms Long will establish what methods or organizational processes the psychiatrist, the community mental health centre, the psychosocial programme, and the counsellor will use to facilitate the outcomes. For example, suppose that Ms Henderson identified the following priorities:
(a) to maintain optimum health
(b) to choose where to work on a part-time basis
(c) to have economic resources
(d) to experience continuity and security
(e) to have friends
(f) to interact with other members of the community.

Ms Long would attempt to find employment for Ms Henderson that contributed to these six outcomes. The work would be such that she could take her medications, and visit her psychiatrist and counsellor. It might be part-time work.

The work setting would promote interaction with other employees and possibly members of the community. The opportunity to make friends, and perhaps find a new close friend, would make the work setting attractive to Ms Henderson. Finally, Ms Henderson should be presented with a number of different options for work that are consistent with her desired outcomes. Opportunity for her to visit the different settings and experience the work for trial periods would be arranged. Ms Long would assist Ms Henderson to evaluate her experience in the different work settings and identify her work preferences.
6 Ms Long would communicate what she had learned about Ms Henderson's prioritized outcomes to other organizations and professionals providing services and supports to Ms Henderson. She would facilitate discussion about how services and supports were contributing to the outcomes and being responsive to Ms Henderson.

References

The Accreditation Council on Services for People with Disabilities (1993). *Outcome Based Performance Measures.* Landover, MD: The Accreditation Council.

The Accreditation Council on Services for People with Disabilities (1995). *A Guide to Using Outcome Measures in Employment Services.* Towson, MD: The Accreditation Council.

Albin, J. M. (1992). *Quality Improvement in Employment and Other Human Services: Managing for Quality through Change.* Paul H. Brookes.

Albrecht, K. (1992). *The only thing that matters: Bring the power of the customer into the center of your business.* New York: Harper Business.

Berkowitz, E. (1987). *Disabled Policy: America's Programs for the Handicapped.* Cambridge University Press.

Bell, D. (1976). *The Coming of the Post-Industrial Society: A Venture in Social Forecasting.* New York: Basic Books.

Bradley, V. J. (1994). Evolution of a New Service Paradigm. In *Creating Individual Supports for People with Developmental Disabilities* (V. J. Bradley, J. W. Ashbaugh and B. C. Blaney, eds) pp. 11–32, Paul H. Brookes.

Donabedian, A. (1980). The definition of quality and approaches to its assessment. Health Administration Press, Ann Arber, Michigan.

Kuhn, T. (1970). The structure of Scientific Revolutions, University of Chicago Press, Chicago.

Matson, J. L. and Rusch, F. R. (1986). Quality of life: does competitive employment Make a difference? In *Competitive Employment Issues and Strategies* (F. R. Rusch, ed.) pp. 331–337, Paul H. Brookes.

McLoughlin, C. S., Garner, J. B. and Callahan, M. (1987). *Getting Employed, Staying Employed*. Paul H. Brookes.

Merchant, K. (1982). The control function of management. *Sloan Management Review*, Summer 43–55.

Patton, M. Q. (1978). *Utilization-Focused Evaluation*. Sage Publications.

Peppers, D. and Rogers, M. (1993). *The one to one future: Building relationships one customer at a time*. New York: Doubleday.

Posavac, E. J. and Carey, R. G. (1980). *Program Evaluation: Methods and Case Studies*. Prentice Hall.

Ray, M. (1993). Introduction: what is the new paradigm in business? In *The New Paradigm in Business: Emerging Strategies For Leadership and Organizational Change* (M. Ray and A. Rinzer, eds) New York: Jeremy P. Tarcher/ Parigee pp. 1–10.

Rutman, L. (1977). Formative research and program evaluation. In *Evaluation Research Methods: A Basic Guide* (L. Rutman, ed.) pp. 59–71, Sage Publications.

Sakaiya, T. (1992). *The Knowledge Value Revolution: Or a History of the Future*. Kodansha International.

Sashkin, M. and Kiser, K. J. (1993). *Putting total Quality Management to Work*. Berrett-Koehler Publishers.

Schalock, R. L. (1988). Critical performance evaluation indicators in supported employment. In *Vocational Rehabilitation and Supported Employment* (P. Wehman and S. Moon, eds) pp. 163–174, Paul H. Brookes.

Schalock, R. L. and Hill, M. L. (1986). Evaluating employment services. In *Pathways to Employment for Adults with Developmental Disabilities* (J. A. Stark and W. E. Kiernan, eds) pp. 285–302, Paul H. Brookes.

Schalock, R. L. (1983). *Services for Developmentally Disabled Adults: Development, Implementation, and Evaluation*. University Park Press.

Stake, R. E. (1972). The countenance of educational evaluation. In *Evaluating Action Programs: Readings in Social Action and Education* (C. H. Weiss, ed.) pp. 31–51. Allyn and Bacon, Inc.

Suchman, E. A. (1967). Action for what? A critique of evaluative research. In *Evaluating Action Programs: Readings in Social Action and Education* (C. H. Weiss, ed.) pp. 240–56, Allyn and Bacon, Inc.

Toffler, A. (1980). *The third wave*. New York: William Morrow.

Waldrop, M. M. (1992). *Complexity: The Emerging Science at the Edge of Order and Chaos*. Simon & Schuster.

Walls, R. T. and Tseng, M. S. (1987). Measurement of client outcomes in rehabilitation. In *Handbook of Measurement and Evaluation in Rehabilitation* (B. Bolton, ed.) pp. 183–202.

Weiss, C. H. (1972). Evaluating educational and social action programs: A 'treeful of owls.' In *Evaluating Action Programs: Readings in Social Action and Education* (C. H. Weiss, ed.) pp. 1–27, Allyn and Bacon, Inc.

Wheatley, M. J. (1994). *Leadership and the new science: Learning about organizations from an orderly universe*. San Francisco: Berrett-Koehler.

Wheelen, T. L. and Hunger, J. D. (1989). *Strategic Management and Business Policy*, 3rd edn. Addison-Wesley Publishing Company.

Zuboff, S. (1988). *In the age of the smart machine: The future of work and power*. New York: Basic Books.

11

Marketing Strategies

Karen Jacobs

Learning objectives

By the end of this chapter the reader should be able to:

1 Describe the application of a SWOT analysis to work practice
2 Define basic marketing concepts and the dimension they can add to the delivery of occupational therapy services.

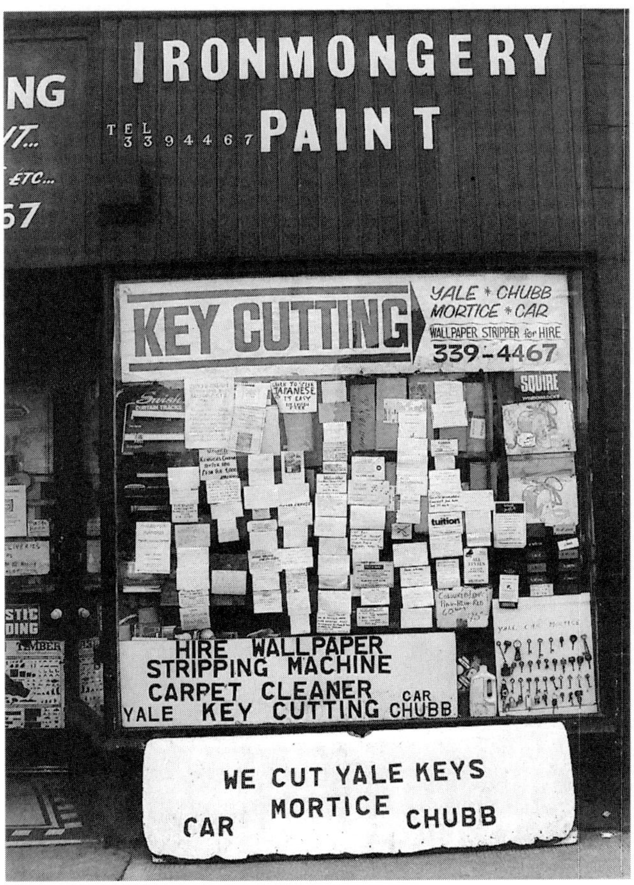

Marketing

Health care involves the exchange of a service or product for money. Although it may not be customary to perceive health care as a 'product', this is a well-recognized concept in the United States since the advent of managed care. The seller is the health-care provider and the buyer is the customer. Marketing is an attempt by either seller or buyer to influence the decision of the other party involved in the exchange (Nosse and Friberg, 1992: 177). Marketing has been a misunderstood term, most often used synonymously with public relations, selling, fund-raising, strategic planning or development. According to Kotler:

> Marketing is the analysis, planning, implementation and control of carefully formulated programs designed to bring about voluntary exchanges of values with target markets for the purpose of achieving organizational objectives. It relies heavily on designing the organization's offering in terms of the target market's needs and desires, and on using effective pricing, communication, and distribution to inform, motivate and service the markets. (1975: 5)

Paramount in this definition are needs and desires. Something that is perceived as lacking by the market (an individual or group of individuals) reflects a need; a desire is a want or personal preference. Through market research, the market is analysed as to whether it reflects an absence of a good or service or whether it prefers something in a different shape, form, time or location. According to Kiernan, Carter and Bronstein:

> Once the need or want is established, the potential buyer must view the good or service being offered as satisfying a need or want better than any other available good or service. It is the packaging and support of a good or service that assure an ongoing relationship with the customer both for purposes of repurchase and for influencing initial purchases by other potential buyers. (1989: 50)

Marketing should be viewed as a dynamic activity that includes the successful analysis of a need, the design of a good or service to meet the need, the uniting of that good or service to a potential user, and the use of a good or service by the customer. Ideally, a marketing approach is used before the development of a product. However, this is not always the case in many programmes. In particular, many work programmes have been started from a selling perspective and are now faced with the risks of having developed a product for which there is no need at that time, in that place, or at that cost (Jacobs, 1991; Jacobs and Logigian, 1994).

There are four components to a marketing approach:

1 Analysing market opportunities.
2 Researching and selecting target markets and market segments.
3 Developing marketing strategies.
4 Executing and evaluating the marketing plan.

Each of the four components of a marketing approach will now be described.

Analysing market opportunities

The first step in a marketing approach is the analysis of various elements in the marketplace. The market itself needs to be defined and may be selected simply on the basis of geographic territory. The market is all actual or potential buyers of a product, service or idea. For example, some markets for ergonomic consultation are: physicians or medical directors, occupational health or rehabilitation nurses, insurance companies, attorneys, injured workers, health-care professionals and industry, such as human resource directors, occupational health nurses or safety officers. Identifying attractive target markets includes the analysis of marketing opportunities. This analysis consists of:

1 self-audit
2 consumer analysis
3 an analysis of other providers of similar services
4 an environmental assessment.
(Jacobs, 1989; Jacobs and Logigian, 1994)

Self-audit

A self-audit assesses the strengths, weaknesses, opportunities and threats, e.g. SWOT analysis, of the individual health-care provider, specific work programme or organization.

This self-audit assists in understanding how well or poorly prepared an individual or organization is to meet the marketplace

SWOT analysis

Strengths:
1 Good reputation.
2 Clinical expertise, e.g. the therapist's qualifications, such as a master's degree; specialized training, e.g. ergonomics or human factors and biomechanics; board certification as a professional ergonomist (CPE).
3 Outcome measures.
4 Research.
5 Professionalism.
6 Commitment to quality.
7 Location of the programme to public transportation and parking.
8 Available finances.

Weaknesses:
1 Poor facilities.
2 Inadequate staffing.
3 Ineffective promotion.
4 Limited finances.

Opportunities:
1 Expansion into industry-based practice.
2 Increase in occupational stress of workers in the United Kingdom.
3 Increase in cumulative trauma disorders of workers in the United States and New Zealand.

Threats:
1 Competition for scarce resources.
2 Change in funding sources, e.g. managed care.

demands. Ascertaining what an individual or organization does well and maintaining that product or service at an optimal level is a critical aspect of marketing.

Consumer analysis

The potential consumers need to be delineated in order to understand their needs and wants for this product. Some consumers who might need, for example, ergonomic consultation might include: physicians or medical directors, occupational health or rehabilitation nurses, insurance companies, architects, attorneys, injured workers, other allied health professionals and industry, such as human resource directors or safety officers (Jacobs and Logigian, 1994).

Analysis of other providers of similar services

Identifying other providers of similar services will provide a snapshot of the kinds of services being offered in a particular locale, and analysing these services will both reduce the potential for overlap and help identify areas that are not being served. Opportunities for collaboration or joint ventures may surface at this time.

Environmental assessment

An environmental assessment attempts to predict what impact present and future demographics, political and regulatory systems, cultural and economic/financial environments, psychographics, and technology may have on your services (Jacobs and Logigian, 1994).

Researching and selecting target markets

Once the marketing opportunities have been analysed, the market's needs can be determined through research, which might include observation, survey, or even experimentation to test hypotheses. After research is completed, the market is segmented. That is, divided into target markets or groups of consumers with similar needs, wants or interests. The groups are further segmented into distinct groups of consumers who might require separate products and promotions. For example, industry can be segmented into white-collar and blue-collar businesses or service industries and manufacturing industries. Alternately, a service industry can be further segmented into those organizations within a certain catchment area. Targeting a market is the act of evaluating and selecting one or more of the markets to enter.

According to Beaton, the criteria for sementation are:

Measurability Whether the service provider can collect information on service utilization and the reasons underlying the pattern of use.

Accessibility Whether the service provider can apply marketing effort to reach a selected segment of the market.

Vocational Exploration Programme

A full formal vocational exploration programme usually takes 3 to 5 days for each person, often spread out over a number of weeks.

We also offer practical courses covering interview techniques, back care programmes and stress management etc. Some people, however, may need additional training or sheltered placement before they return to work.

Evaluating the Workplace

We can carry out an objective evaluation of the workplace (Job Site Analysis). It is a standardised method of identifying and quantifying the physical demands of any job.

After this analysis we will suggest potential changes to the work routine or organisation of the work place to accommodate the employee's disability. We will give guidance to the employer to help integrate the person with the workforce.

The benefits

Helps get employees back to work by:

- Identifying critical job demands.
- Establishing specific training requirements for the job.
- Recommending modifications to the job.

Useful in preventing injury by:

- Identifying work tasks associated with frequent injuries.
- Suggesting modifications to the workplace.

Work Placement

For those who cannot return to their previous jobs, we can provide a Work Placement Service. This programme is co-ordinated by the Vocational Placement Officer, who can make full use of existing facilities in the community.

We have a database of employers offering varied work opportunities around the country.

Our Placement Officer will liaise direct with local Employment Service representatives, the clients former employer or the referrer.

We will keep you, the referrer, fully informed at all stages and when the employee and job have been carefully matched, we will liaise, where necessary, with other agencies who can give further help with functional aids and equipment.

The total assessment programme is designed to get employees back to work as quickly as possible.

Our expert counsellors assess employees functional ability, support people adjusting back into the workforce, and help them achieve the fullest and quickest restoration of their capabilities.

For further information please contact our office.

OPEN DOOR
Mercury House
195 Knightsbridge
London SW7 1RE
Tel: 0171 589 2244
Fax: 0171 589 2255

Open Door Vocational Assessment & Guidance Centre

A Guide for Insurers

OPEN DOOR

The key to a working future

OPEN DOOR

Vocational Assessment & Guidance Centre

Open Door provides a comprehensive programme of evaluation for people who have been unable to work through injury or illness.

Our aim is to assist both employees and the self-employed to return to suitable work as early as possible. We establish their physical and mental capabilities, and develop a return to work plan, which may include modified or alternative work, or a graded work rehabilitation programme.

Key benefits

- Early intervention may prevent an insurance claim.
- Comprehensive and objective assessment may limit the extent and duration of any claim.
- Expert assessment consultants provide you with an invaluable, objective, yet accessible resource.
- The physical assessment programme uses measures based on statistical data, not subjective observations.
- The objective data provided is specific, accurate and consistently repeatable. It is so statistically reliable that it is legally defensible.
- The assessment provides clarification of an individual's work ability which will help determine whether they fulfil the definitions of incapacity.
- The assessment acts as a vital tool in communicating and substantiating claim decisions.

Open Door can greatly benefit the employer in getting staff back to work quickly and fitting the right people to the right job.

Getting people back to work involves matching the capabilities of the individual to the demands of the job and the suitability of the workplace environment.

Open Door offers an assessment of both the employee and the workplace.

Evaluating the Employee

The employee assessment programme may involve three different approaches comprising a physical evaluation (Functional Capacity Assessment), psychometric, tests and work samples (tasks which mimic the real life working environment). The assessment procedure is backed up by counselling, job placement and monitoring services.

Open Door Functional Capacity Assessment

This service is new to the U.K., but it has already established an excellent reputation in the United States, Canada and Australia where it is extensively used.

How does it work?

This assessment compares an individual's present functional abilities to the pre-accident job demands and gives a precise indication of their current work ability.

Our qualified therapists carry out an in depth assessment taking no longer than a day, based on a variety of specific, physical activities. Each of the tests has been designed with concern for the safety of the participant. The tests are conducted in a specific order, building a picture of total ability.

The equipment measures the individual's participation and effort using state of the art technology and reports the findings statistically.

What does it tell us?

After the assessment, we know whether the employee or self-employed person is:

- Fit to return to work to carry out regular duties.
- Fit to return to work if the work is modified in specific ways.
- Unfit to return to work temporarily.
- Fit to return to alternative work.
- Unfit to return to work permanently.

We can also:

- Identify any barriers in returning to work.
- Plan the future management of the employee and the work environment.

How objective is it?

- The specific activities are always followed in the same sequence.
- The assessment participant manages each test, not the therapist.
- The tests are measured technologically and the findings are reported in the form of statistics.
- The assessment is accurate, reliable and repeatable. The results are so valid that they have been defended in the US Supreme Court. Because of this objectivity, assessments of this standard have never been denied admissibility in any Court in the USA, Canada or Australia.

Figure 11.1

Stages in product life cycle

Introductory stage:	The service is introduced. Awareness is low so this is the optimal time for promoting the service using a variety of media.
Growth stage:	The service has become established. Its value is recognized and marketing awareness is fairly high. At this stage it may be useful to target key individuals for 'personal selling'. This could be aimed at clinical directors, purchasers or GP fundholders.
Maturity stage:	Market awareness of the service is at its peak. Personal selling will still benefit the service, but promotion should now be more detailed and remind the target audiences of the benefits of the service.
Decline stage:	The service is in decline and the reasons for this must be sought. If the service has become obsolete owing to changes, for example, in epidemiology, then additional promotion is only worthwhile if it is used to maintain activity levels while the providers work on developing other services in areas which show signs of growth.

Source: Beaton, J. (1995). *Marketing Handbook for Occupational Therapists*. London: College of Occupational Therapists, p. 15.

Substantiality Whether the selected services are large enough to merit a different mix of marketing activities (1995: 8–9).

Developing marketing strategies

The marketing approach continues by developing a marketing mix. The marketing mix is the particular blend of marketing variables used to meet the needs, wants or interests of this well-defined target market. It is what an individual or organization can do to influence the demand for its products or services. A marketing mix consists of what has been commonly termed the four Ps: product, price, place and promotion. Each of the four Ps will be described briefly.

Product

The product is a variable in the marketing mix that needs to be designed for the specific target market. For example, ergonomic consultation in a service industry such as a hospital, the products or product line might include job-site analysis, an audit for compliance with Title II and III of the Americans With Disabilities Act (ADA), recommending intervention for the individual worker, e.g. splinting or changes to the environment to prevent injury, e.g. adjusting the height of a table or chair, and implementing preventive programming, e.g. work-site health promotion such as stress management or physical exercise.

Each product has a life cycle. These are distinct stages in the life of product or service (Beaton, 1995: 15). An understanding of the stages in a life cycle can provide assistance in developing an appropriate marketing mix.

Place

Where the product or service is provided is the place aspect of the marketing mix. Once again, for the example of ergonomic consultation, this type of consultation is usually provided at the work site. However, on occasions, therapists will provide consultation in their own office environment or provide expert witness testimony in a court of law.

Price

The price or fee schedule for services should be based on cost, competitive factors, geographic area, and what the consumer is willing to pay. There are four major methods for establishing a fee schedule: unit value system, cost-plus or overhead, local survey or usual and customary and state code. Whatever method is selected, it is important for the price to be commensurate with perceived value.

Promotion

Promotion is the vehicle for communicating information to the consumer about the product's merits, place and price. In fact, Folts, Jeremko and Houk suggest that, 'Work programs do not sell services; rather, they sell the benefits of those services. Clients do not want therapeutic modalities, exercises, or purposeful activities. Instead, clients desire the benefits treatment provides, such as pain reduction and the ability to return to work' (1993: 13).

Instruments of promotion are:

- advertising
- sales promotion
- publicity
- personal selling.

The methods of promotion are only limited by imagination and financial resources. Jinks writes, 'First and foremost, in order to be successful in marketing OT, be creative, enthusiastic, outgoing, and most of all, have perseverance' (1995: 21).

Advertising

Advertising involves the use of a paid message presented in a recognized medium and by an identified sponsor with the purpose of informing, persuading and reminding. For example, a work programme might use some of the following advertising vehicles: brochures, direct mail, catalogues, directories, radio and television, magazine and newspaper space, and novelties, i.e. calendars. Figure 11.1 is an example of a brochure designed to advertise the services of Open Door to insurers.

Sales promotion

Sales promotion is the use of a wide variety of short-term incentives to encourage earlier and/or stronger target market response to the purchase of the product. (Kotler and Clarke, 1987). This approach is optimized when used in conjunction with advertising. Some examples of consumer sales promotion tools include: samples, coupons, gifts, contests and demonstrations.

Marketing checklist

- Introduce yourself to buyers
- Call buyer by name
- Have company prescription pads printed and send to buyers
- Speak at buyer staff meetings
- Hold inservice about work programme
- Send thank-you notes to referring physicians
- Sponsor in-house continuing education workshops
- Publish an in-house newsletter
- Be active in local government activities
- Place articles in local newspapers
- Speak on local radio and television
- Encourage satisfied customers to tell their friends
- Send birthday and special occasion cards to associates and referral sources
- Speak at support groups
- Become a student fieldwork facility
- Network with other programme professionals
- Attend symposiums on topics related to work rehabilitation/prevention

Adapted from: Jinks, P. (1995). Marketing occupational therapy in rural areas. *OT Forum*, **X**(11), June 9, p. 21.

Publicity

Publicity is often described as a marketing stepchild because it is relatively underused in relation to the real contribution it can make (Kotler, 1983). Publicity is free promotion, however despite this positive feature, one has little control over the placement of it and thus it becomes difficult to focus the message on specific target markets. For example, various radio spots on topics such as 'Preventing cumulative trauma injuries' or 'Stress management in the workplace' would be considered publicity.

Personal selling

Personal selling is the most effective form of promotion. It is face-to-face communication between the therapist and the consumer. Some examples of personal selling methods are: making presentations at meetings, providing continuing education workshops or

Marketing audit guide

The market and market segments

- How large is the territory covered by your market?
- How have you determined this?
- How is your market grouped?
  - is it scattered?
  - how many important segments are there?
  - how are these segments determined (demographics, service usage, attitudinally)?
- Is the market entirely urban, or is a fair proportion of it rural?
- What percentage of your market uses third-party payment?
  - what are the attitudes and operations of third parties?
  - are they all equally profitable?
- What are the effects of the following factors on your market?
  - age; income; occupation; increasing population; demographic shifting; decreasing birth-rate?
- What proportion of potential customers are familiar with your organization or programmes?
  - what is your image in the marketplace?
  - what are the important components of your image?

The organization

- Short history of your organization:
  when and how was it organized? what has been the nature of its growth? how fast and far have its markets expanded? where do your clients come from geographically? what is the basic policy of the organization–is its focus on 'health-care' profit? what has been the financial history of the organization? how has it been capitalized? have there been any account receivable problems? what is inventory investment? what has been the organization's success with the various services promoted?
- How does your organization compare with the health-care industry and the relevant subset of the health care industry?
  - Is the total volume (gross revenue, utilization) and/or profitability increasing, decreasing?
  - have there been any fluctuations in revenue? If so, what were they due to?
- What are the objectives and goals of the organization? How can they be expressed beyond the provision of 'good health care'?
- What are the organization's present strengths and weaknesses in:
  - medical facilities; management capabilities; medical staff; technical facilities; reputation; financial capabilities; image; interorganizational linkages?
- What is the labour environment for your organization?
  - for medical staff (nurses, physicians etc)?
  - for support personnel?
- How dependent is your organization upon the conditions of other industries? Upon other health-care delivery systems?
- Are weaknesses being compensated for and strengths being used? How? How are the following areas of your marketing function, organized?
  - structure?
  - manpower
  - reporting relationships?
  - decision-making power?
- What kind of external controls affect your organization?
  - local?
  - state?
  - federal?
  - self-regulatory?
- What are the trends in recent regulatory rulings?

Competitors

- How many competitors are in you industry?
  - how do you define your competitors?
  - has this number increased or decreased in the last four years?
  - are satellite facilities being used?
- What factors are considered in location decisions? When did you last evaluate present location?
- What distributors do you deal with (e.g. medical supply houses, etc.)?
- How large an inventory must you carry?

Source: Berkowitz, E. N. and Flexner, W. A. (1978). The marketing audit: A tool for health service organizations. *Health Care Management Review*, (Fall), 55–6.

lecturing to professional organizations. In addition, word-to-mouth recommendations by past consumers of ergonomic consultation are a powerful sales pitch. See the marketing checklist on p. 273.

Executing and evaluating the marketing plan

Once the target market has been selected and the marketing mix developed, the marketing plan is implemented. Since marketing is a dynamic activity, the plan will require periodic, ongoing re-examination to evaluate its effectiveness. A specific time frame, such as a twelve-month period, should be delineated to measure whether objectives and goals are being met. The use of marketing audit will provide assistance in this endeavour. According to Kotler and Clarke, a marketing audit is a comprehensive, systematic, independent and periodic examination of an organization's or, within an organization a, specific service's marketing environment, objectives, strategies and activities with a view to determining problem areas and opportunities and recommending a plan of action to improve the organization's marketing performance (1987: 203). The Market audit guide provides an example of some of the questions the marketing auditor might use (Jacobs and Logigian, 1994).

Conclusion

The use of a marketing approach will allow practitioners to approach the health-care environment proactively and be ready to meet the changing needs and wants of the marketplace. Limited, if any exposure to marketing is provided in the academic curricula of occupational and physical therapists, therefore it is highly recommended that therapists acquire this marketing knowledge by attending workshops, taking continuing education courses, or acquiring degrees in business. In general, practitioners need to acquire more business savvy (Jacobs and Logigian, 1994).

Practical learning activities

1 The Department of Employment has recently issued a call for tenders for a contract to provide assessment and training programmes for people with visual impairments. Prepare a draft for a poster as part of a presentation/display you will give on behalf of your OT department to try and win this contract.
2 A local mental health charity group has recently released funds for the creation of a post of Employment Adviser to assist people recovering from mental health problems to return to or find employment. Prepare a SWOT analysis you could use to demonstrate your suitability for this position when you are interviewed.
3 The Health and Safety Executive has appointed you as a private practitioner to advise local small offices on healthy workplace practices. Prepare a rough draft of a leaflet you could produce to increase awareness of any aspect of injury prevention of your choice.

4 Occupational stress is increasing nationally and many employers are undertaking initiatives to reduce this as it naturally affects employee performance. Prepare a bullet list of potential occupational therapy services which could broaden the range offered by the Employee Assistance Programme which has recently been set up in a local management consultancy firm.

References

Beaton, J. (1995). *Marketing Handbook for Occupational Therapists*. London: College of Occupational Therapists.

Clifton, D. (April/May, 1995). Diversifying for success in the '90s. *Rehab Management*, 52–3, 55, 57, 59–60.

Folts, D., Jeremko, J., Houk, D. (1993). Marketing's role in work programs. *Work* **3**(2), 13–18.

Jacobs, K. (1989). Work hardening in the health care system. In *Work Hardening: State of the Art* (L. Ogden-Niemeyer and K. Jacobs, eds), pp. 111–26, Thorofare: SLACK, Inc.

Jacobs K. (1991). A marketing approach to work practice. *Work Programs Special Interest Section Newsletter*, **5**(2), 3–4, Rockville: AOTA.

Jacobs, K. and Logigian, M. (1994) *Functions of a Manager in Occupational Therapy*. Thorofare NS: SLACK, Inc.

Jinks, P. (1995). Marketing occupational therapy in rurual areas. *Occupational Therapy Forum*, 20–1.

Kiernan, W., Carter, A., Bronstein, E. (1989). Marketing and marketing management in rehabilitation. In *Economics, Industry, and Disability*, (W. Kiernan and R. Schalock, eds), pp. 49–56, Baltimore: Brookes.

Kotler, P. (1975). *Marketing for Non Profit Organizations*. Englewood Cliffs: Prentice-Hall, Inc.

Kotler, P. (1983). *Principles of Marketing: Instructor's Manual with Cases*. Englewood Cliffs: Prentice-Hall, Inc.

Nosse, L. and Friberg, D. (1992). *Management Principles for Physical Therapists*. Baltimore: Williams & Wilkins.

Pheasant, S. (1991). *Ergonomics*. Rockville: Aspen

12

Future Considerations

Karen Jacobs, Joanne Pratt and Maree Dyson

Learning objectives

By the end of this chapter the reader should be able to:

1 Discuss common issues in work practice provided by Australian, UK and US perspectives.
2 Identify current strengths, constraints and opportunities in the environment(s) where work practice is set.
3 Identify personal learning objectives related to work practice.

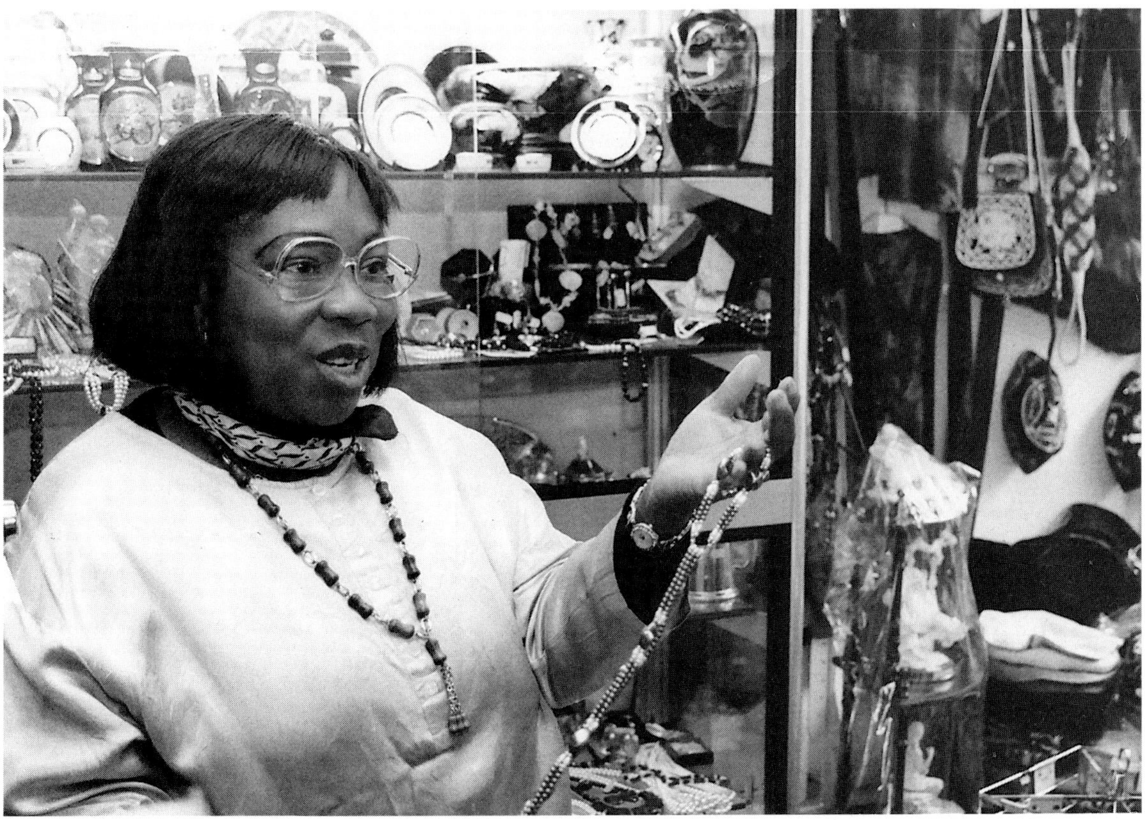

An Australian perspective

Autonomy, independence, potential for practice growth and the challenge of unpredictable and rapid change appears to be what the future holds for Australian occupational therapists in work practice. Why such opportunities and challenges? To explore the future of Australian occupational therapy work practice, it is important first to understand the base from which the current practice grew and to appreciate the political, social and economic forces which have forged and are driving practice. Against this background practice potential and future can be examined.

Work practice before the 1980s

Rather than 'work practice' Australian therapists spoke of vocational rehabilitation and, more recently, of occupational health practice. Vocational rehabilitation, predicated on such interventions as work conditioning, work hardening and work preparation, had been practised in the industrial workshops of the large psychiatric institutions since the 1950s and, subsequently, in large vocational rehabilitation centres servicing adults with physical disabilities. Such centres were traditionally funded by state and federal governments. It was from these significant bases, staffed by many of our early and prominent pioneers, that vocational rehabilitation as we now know it sprang. In the late 1970s social and political forces began to alter the perceptions of workplace safety and injury and pave the way for occupational therapists to move into industry, community-based and outreach vocational rehabilitation.

Social forces and legislation

Until the late 1970s unsafe work conditions were largely accepted as a natural part of work, for which workers were compensated by means of 'dirt pay', that is additional payments negotiated for working in unsafe and/or unpleasant conditions. Such payments were negotiated by unions under a centralized award-based system. In the late 1970s, the unions significantly shifted ground and began to demand safe workplaces and practices for their members. The concept of 'dirt pay' was no longer acceptable and unions focused on the creation of safe work places and the prevention of injury. At the same time, there was a growing view from the unions and the community that compensation alone, for injury, was inadequate, that efforts needed to be made to rehabilitate and return injured workers to work.

In the early 1980s, small private companies, locally established or internationally based, began to offer rehabilitation services to injured workers and negotiate with insurers payments for such services. A small but significant change had occurred and a few occupational therapists moved from the more traditional vocational rehabilitation centres to these new, community-based or outreach-focused services.

With the unions' connections to the Australian Labor Party, these new emphases were reflected in changes to the workers' compensation legislation as Labor governments were elected through the early 1980s (see for example, Accident Compensation Act, 1985). Varying in the specifics across state and federal jurisdictions, these pieces of legislation commonly addressed the themes of injury prevention, compensation and rehabilitation.

The demand for occupational therapists in these jurisdictions grew rapidly as therapists' skills in task analysis, workplace assessment and management of return to work were recognized. Social forces empowered through legislation created this growth and laid the groundwork for the future.

Practice drivers in the 1990s and beyond

Legislation has remained a key driver for current vocational rehabilitation practice. In states where the legislation has not changed to reflect an emphasis on rehabilitation, the practice growth has been small. The driver of politics and legislation has meant that the field is subject to rapid change. Job vacancies for therapists have grown enormously virtually overnight, and disappeared in equally short time frames as governments of different political persuasions have come and gone. Governments have exercised increasing control in vocational rehabilitation, directing service philosophies and thereby practice, controlling payments and setting standards. This interest is likely to remain and, therefore, the volatility of the field is likely to be a continuing feature of practice for occupational therapists into the twenty-first century.

Although the initial developments in this field may be traced to social and political influences, the economic impact of time lost through injuries, injury rate and cost-based insurance premiums, and the risk of unfunded liabilities, have driven the more recent developments. Given the economic importance of workers' compensation to industry, a continuing strong interaction between political and economic influences in driving practice is probable. This interaction is the most frequently cited driver of practice identified by therapists working in the field.

Worker's compensation authorities and larger organizations have come to appreciate the cost benefits associated with prevention of injury. Although work practice is still strongly based in rehabilitation, therapists identify services in injury prevention and early intervention as a steadily growing field of practice. Therapists routinely describe involvement in the development and presentation of programmes aimed at injury prevention. Prominent practitioners, consulted for their views, have noted that, to develop this market further, therapists need to become more effective in demonstrating the economic benefits through well-researched cost–benefit analyses.

The social influences operating are not as easily identified by practitioners as the political and economic influences. Nevertheless, their impact is profound and likely to impact on practice through the following:

1 The expectations of equal opportunity for people with disabilities.
2 The way in which work is changing.
3 The impact of work changes on the industrial relations system, including industrial awards.
4 The new technologies.
5 The development of accreditation programmes.
6 Graduate and specialist training.

Each of these will be considered in turn.

Equal opportunity for people with disabilities

In 1993, the Burdekin Report: Human Rights drew attention to the disadvantages experienced by people with psychiatric disabilities. Of interest in the discussion of work practice is the problems identified by Burdekin (1993) in employment opportunities and vocational rehabilitation. He identified a lack of targeted services and an inability, on the part of generic services, to meet the specific vocational needs of people with a psychiatric disability. As specialist services are developing and are likely to increase towards the end of the century, to address long-standing imbalances, there is scope for growth in this field of work practice for occupational therapists. Similarly, there is opportunity for field-based research by therapists. Sherwin (1993) notes there is a lack of research into employment and return to work for people with psychiatric disabilities.

In keeping with various pieces of anti-discrimination legislation, employers are increasingly expected to undertake reasonable accommodations to make employment accessible to people with disabilities (see, for example, Disability Discrimination Act, 1992). A small growth in identifying necessary accommodations and negotiating with employers, together with people with disabilities, is discernible. As the impact of this legislation is felt more widely and comes directly and subtly to influence behaviour, increased practice in this field may be expected. Recent changes to the award system (that is, the national central system under which minimum salaries and employment conditions are set) to recognize productivity-based payments to people with disabilities are similarly likely to provide growth opportunities for therapists in work practice (Hannan, 1994).

The changing nature of work

Handy describes the way in which work is changing through his description of the 'Shamrock organization'. In *The Age of Unreason* (1990) he postulated the growth of the shamrock organization. Symbolically, the three leaves of the shamrock represent the core workers (of whom there will be fewer working longer hours), the contractual fringe (taking in specialist and technical services), and the flexible labour force. In Australia in the 1990s we are seeing organizations restructuring as described by Handy; and it is this restructuring that is opening opportunities for occupational therapists in work practice.

Small therapist-based private practices and large multidisciplinary practices are successfully contracting with organizations to provide services. Typically, such services include: case management for injured workers, general and work capacity assessments, return-to-work management and the earlier mentioned preventative and early intervention programmes. Models of payment for such services vary from hourly rates to an outcome-linked or based fee. Many of these models were suggested by Handy in his view of payments to the 'contractual fringe' as being 'for results not time, in fees not wages'. Although Handy wrote of organizations 'putting boring work out on contract' this does not seem to be the case for work practice contracts offered to occupational therapists (Handy, 1990: 77–8). More typically, organizations would seem to be using contacting as a means of gaining access to specialists, who become familiar with the work and its demands, without needing to have such people on staff. As one therapist described it, working as a contractor is 'like being a member of the extended family'. Contracts are usually long term and initially negotiated on some sort of competitive tendering basis, renegotiation seems to be strongly based on past results.

As the 'core' works harder (Handy, 1990, 1994; Farnworth, 1995), the increasing workload and stress is leading to health problems (Powell, 1995). It is in this area that opportunities in work practice have opened and continue to grow for occupational therapists. The development and implementation of stress management, positive health and health promotion programmes are described as being an expanding field of practice.

Industrial relations

As the nature of work is changing, so too are aspects of the industrial relations system. In 1994, Australia introduced its first telecommuting award. The development of home-based offices, mobile services and telecommuting may well raise unexpected issues of occupational health and safety and again provide challenges to therapists in the field of work practice.

As Australia moves from a centrally-based award system to a system of enterprise bargaining, it is important to note that occupational health and safety is included in a substantial number of newly created agreements. Such inclusion indicates an ongoing need for services related to work practice and therefore for occupational therapy services.

Unions have undoubtedly played a central role in the recent developments in occupational health and safety and, thereby, in the development of occupational therapy work practice. The impact of declining unionism (Deery and Plowman, 1991; Jost, 1994) on practice is not yet discernible. It may be that therapists have established a sufficient workplace role and occupational health a sufficiently high political and economic profile for there to be little impact.

The new technologies

Lansbury and Davis (1984) write of the new information technologies as having the capacity to democratize information or increase control by a small powerful elite. In the light of such a comment, it is interesting to note the work being undertaken by therapists in the development of interactive training programmes, video-based training and virtual reality safety training. A few leading practitioners are applying the new technologies to the democratization of information in work practice and it is to be hoped that such developments continue.

Accreditation and graduate qualifications

An increasing focus on quality, accreditation, accountability and service is impacting on how work is regulated and organized and how practitioners provide services and differentiate themselves in the marketplace.

Some compensation systems require therapists to apply for recognition from a central instrumentality, such as a state or federal government department, before being able to practise in the field of vocational rehabilitation. In some instances, such recognition is extended into a specification of fields in which various disciplines are qualified to practise. At an individual level documented, service plans must generally be approved and audits may be conducted to review practice standards. Although mechanisms vary across Australia, there is a discernible move to formal accreditation processes of disciplines, practitioners, practices and plans.

Therapists in the field generally comment that this is not a field for new graduates, unless the employing organization is large and has a strong mentor and peer review programme. Even so, few new graduates seem to venture directly into the field of work practice. The emphasis placed on formal graduate qualifications seems to vary on their availability in particular regions. Certainly there is a strong emphasis on ongoing graduate training and a preference for graduate qualifications, where practical. Formal graduate qualifications are cited by private practitioners as a useful tool in market differentiation.

Impact on practice

McLaren and Keaney (1992) wrote of occupational therapy intervention in occupational health as occurring at four levels: assessment; treatment; facilitation of the work re-entry process; and follow up and closure. While these areas continue to provide the core of practice, there are clear shifts in emphasis within this core and beyond.

There is an escalating emphasis on assessment, specifically in the area of functional or work capacity assessments as industry, government and therapists seek a more structured approach to the determination of suitable duties and ability to work. Broad-based individual treatments, such as relaxation training, have tended to decline as the legislation increasingly emphasizes vocational rather than general rehabilitation. The legislation details the philosophy of work practice and thereby the actual practice. The strong emphasis on workplace re-entry and follow up remain cornerstones of vocational practice.

Beyond the core, practice is growing in the areas of early intervention services, the design, development and implementation of injury prevention programmes and, slowly, health promotion and positive health programmes. It is this author's view that these areas will continue to grow and be joined by growth in workplace services to people with psychiatric disabilities, employee assistance programmes and equal opportunity programmes.

Experience to date would indicate a growth of small-scale private practices offering specialist contractual services. The area of work practice currently contributes the greatest number of private practitioners to the Victorian Association of Occupational Therapists Private Practice Register (1994). Private practitioners in work practice are increasingly operating on a contractual basis both in the work they gain and in the staff they engage.

Large government-based rehabilitation services are similarly developing the contractual market and training their staff to operate in this arena. Competitive forces on these organizations will ensure continued growth in this area.

Beyond the private practice and large organization rehabilitation base referred to earlier, occupational therapists skilled in work practice are currently working in diverse management positions in large companies. For example, as the prevention programmes manager with a large insurer, as the national manager of occupational health and safety for a large retail chain, as the national manager of occupational health and safety for a large service company, as a regional manager for a national safety organization and as a senior government adviser. With graduate qualifications and experience in work practice, it seems more opportunities are opening for therapists in management through their work practice experience.

Practitioners consistently cite the autonomy this field of work offers for their continuing interest in work practice. The autonomy seems to be linked to the flexibility of working arrangements, the control over workload and cases and the independence afforded by contracting services rather than being employed. Also frequently described were the challenges provided by the changing nature of the work, social and government influences, the high professional profile afforded in work practice and the breadth of skills demanded.

Work practice has, in the last decade, grown from an institutional base into a community-based or outreach-focused service. It has afforded, and continues to afford, therapists the opportunity to provide core vocational rehabilitation services.

The future is likely to offer increasing opportunities in the development of injury prevention, early intervention, health promotion and positive health programmes, together with opportunities to provide services linked to equal opportunity for people with psychiatric and physical disabilities. Increasingly, therapists will find themselves contracting for services and working for multiple organizations, service-based industries, mobile services and the telecommuters of the future. Therapists will continue to enjoy the autonomy and flexibility inherent in such work and cope with the frequent changes arising in an area in which government takes such an interest. Many therapists will use their skills and experience in service provision to move into management-related fields.

The future holds enormous opportunities, however work practice is unlikely, in the foreseeable future, to be a field of practice for those seeking stability or predictability.

Acknowledgement

The therapists who gave of their valuable time to participate in interviews to construct much of this material are gratefully acknowledged.

References

Accident Compensation Act, reprint no 5 (1985). Incorporating amendments to Act No 62/1994. Melbourne: Printing and Publishing Services Victoria.

Burdekin, B. (1993). *Burdekin Report: Human rights*. Canberra: Australian Government Publishing Service.

Deery, S. and Plowman, D. (1991). *Australian Industrial Relations*, 3rd edn., Sydney: McGraw Hill.

Disability Discrimination Act, No 135/1992 (1992). Canberra: Australian Government Publishing Service.

Farnworth, L. (1995). An exploration of skill as an issue in unemployment and employment. *Journal of Occupational Science: Australia*, **2**(1), 22–9.

Handy, C. (1990). *The Age of Unreason*. London: Arrow Books.

Handy, C. (1994). *The Empty Raincoat: Making Sense of the Future*. London: Random House.

Hannan, E. (1994). Job pact gives disabled a chance. *The Australian*, 21 July, 5.

Jost, J. (1994). Time for the unions to pay their dues. *Australian Business Monthly*, March, 25–8.

Lansbury, R. and Davis, E. (1984). *Technology, Work and Industrial relations*. Melbourne: Longman Cheshire.

McLaren, S. and Keaney, A. (1992). Occupational therapist role in worker rehabilitation. In *Victorian Association of Occupational Therapists: Convention*. Melbourne: Victorian Association of Occupational Therapists.

Register of private practitioners (1994). Melbourne: Victorian Association Occupational Therapists (Inc).

Powell, S. (1995, April 8&9). The age of overwork. *The Weekend Australian*, Review, 8–9 April, 1–2.

Sherwin, J. L. (1993). Paid integrated open employment for people who have a psychiatric disability. Brisbane: Community Resource Unit.

A United Kingdom perspective

The UK approaches the new century in a state of major transition in the realms of health care, social care and employment practices. Coupled with this, the nature of education programmes for occupational therapy students has also experienced significant paradigm shifts throughout the 1980s and 1990s. All these factors deserve consideration as each will naturally have an impact on work practice in occupational therapy. The profession's own adaptation to these changes, by integrating occupational therapy philosophy within this environment, is a major challenge to be faced.

Employment practices

The nature of work in Britain is experiencing significant change as we leave the twentieth century. An informal survey of media reports over the past six months reveals that these changes are chronicled almost weekly. Timmins (1996) describes the current period as an educational and work revolution which is tending to shorten working lives while the population ages. The industry bywords in Britain in the 1990s include 'downsizing' and 'delayering'. Tough managerial initiatives of the past decade have found many company structures adopting a modular shape, whereby only the essential cores of staff are employed. Workforces have therefore shrunk so that businesses are in a position to expand through contracting of services when opportunities arise. This is part of the new culture of management consultancy with the managerial/professional group now forming a third of the workforce. Advances in telecommunications ensure information can be transferred at unprecedented rates. In addition, Britain continues to debate its commitment to and position within the European Union which brings with it extensive industry regulations.

The psychosocial consequences of the current business climate for the individual include: the disappearance of 'jobs for life', redundancy, increased workloads, decreased career advancement and fear of job loss (Clement, 1995a). Occupational stress is considered the industrial disease of the 1990s in Britain. It is estimated that this stress costs industry £5.3 billion annually due to absenteeism and reduced work performance. The ratio of lost work days between stress-related illnesses and strikes now approaches 130:1 (Health and Safety Executive, 1995). Toynbee (1995) reports that Britons:

> work longer hours than in any other EC country, on average 44 hours per week. Sixty per cent of men work more than 40 hours, whereas in the rest of Europe fewer than half work that long, a third of British women work more than 40 hours, while only 14 per cent of the women in the rest of Europe work so long. The EC is trying to bring in a 48-hour maximum working week for all. The Government is resisting it fiercely.

She concludes that such legislation might help break the upward spiral seen in this employment practice which is desirable as, somewhere in the past twenty years, the balance between the getting of time and the spending of money has been lost.

In contrast, and according to the most recent British Social Attitudes Survey, 74 per cent of people said they would still work at a paid job even if they had enough money without employment. Only 36 per cent said a job was just a way of earning a living with 64 per cent saying it meant more to them than that (Blanchflower and Oswald, 1986). There has, however, been a perceptible shift in what is considered preferred work by school leavers and new graduates. Health and social-care professions have replaced the more traditional ones of law, medicine and accounting as the most desired. As the time spent in education lengthens, however, working life, especially for men, is shortening (Timmins, 1996). Only 51 per cent of men aged 60 to 64 years now work, this proportion is expected to fall below a half by the year 2000. This contrasts with the situation twenty-five years ago when four out of five men in this age bracket was in gainful employment. While work is shrinking for men, the reverse is true for women. Factors which account for this are the rise in part-time work, women having fewer children, delaying having them and/or being more likely to return to work after having a child (Timmins, 1996).

Debate continues on the call for the introduction of a minimum wage in Britain (Clement, 1995b). While some workers earn as little as £1.50 an hour there is no consensus on whether a minimum wage should be set. Those opposed argue that job losses would be the real cost of the £4.15 minimum desired by supporters.

There is also a change in the perceived role of unions:

> Seven years ago, in 1989, 28 per cent of those questioned listed improving pay as the most important thing they thought trade unions should do. By 1994, that had changed dramatically. More than twice as many (37 per cent) wanted unions to concentrate on protecting jobs. (Timmins, 1996)

Health and social care

Two pieces of legislation provided, until the late 1980s, the cornerstones of rehabilitation and employment services for people with disabilities. These were the National Health Service Act (1948) and the Employment of Disabled Persons Act (1944). The first led to the establishment of a range of health and social services to meet the needs of the country's citizens from the 'cradle to the grave'. Such services were funded through taxation and administered nationally by the government's Department of Health and Social Services. These two departments have acted as the traditional and largest employers of occupational therapists to the present day. Pay scales and career structure were set at this national level in line with that of other paramedical professions. The second piece of legislation was enacted in response to the needs of disabled veterans returning from the war effort. The resources required to assist them to return to paid work, undertake rehabilitation or training, be assessed for benefits or allowances continued to be administered and funded through the Department of Employment. Disability employment advisor posts and placement, assessment, counselling teams were created by this department through the 1980s and 1990s to continue to address the needs of people with disabilities.

In 1990 the government introduced the most significant policy shift since the creation of the National Health Service in 1948 which was embodied in two White Papers, Working for Patients and Care in the Community. These have served since that time to propel the culture of health and social-care services towards one of consumerism. With the focus on service structures driven by client needs the government is attempting to create an internal market of service providers and service purchasers. Hospitals have been required to achieve self-governing trust status in order to act as service providers. Government local authorities and general practitioners have also become fundholders in order to act as service purchasers. This culture of consumerism has been imported from industry into health care with its attendant foundations of standards, policy and procedure delineations, quality assurance mechanisms and outcome measurement systems. At the present time, it could be argued that the intended benefits of increased accountability, efficiency and cost-effectiveness are offset by the constraints of insensitive quality-of-care indicators and a perceived lack of ownership by staff in the new culture. Clients and patients can only be considered vulnerable consumers in this environment where they are dependent on the negotiating skills of their GPs practice. By contrast, however, this policy shift has also created opportunities for the development of independent service providers, private health coverage schemes as well as a potential new group of service purchasers. All are finding their growing place in the new environment. Occupational therapists and their multidisciplinary colleagues are increasingly seeking and obtaining employment in this new sector.

In July 1995, following a government cabinet reshuffle, it was announced that the discrete and autonomous Department of Employment would cease to exist and instead would be absorbed by the Department of Education and the Department of Trade and Industry. The implications of this, while unknown at this time, are likely to be far-reaching for work practice in the UK. Present government policy is based on a training-for-work model for people with disabilities. Projects which are developed to undertake this training can be funded as service providers by Local Enterprise Companies (LECs) in Scotland and Training Enterprise Companies (TECs) in England. Occupational therapists have been working successfully in the 1990s as project managers, training officers, and development officers in these services. Innovative and creative partnerships have been forged with many local colleges to provide clients with training packages to meet their levels of ability. It is to be hoped that these relationships will be strengthened and not pressed to realign as competitors with this policy change.

Additionally, there is increasing recognition that school leavers with disabilities are not currently well served when making the transition into employment. Tisdall (1994) has argued that three negative statuses are typically attributed to young people during this transition stage: of being crisis-riddent adolescents; of being needy clients; and of being marginalized members of society. A possible cause for this in the past has been government-funding mechanisms which, owing to their mainly linear structures, have led to criticisms of fragmentation in the delivery of services. The needs of service users are also changing, with the rise in the number of HIV+ children representing a small but distinct case in point.

Disability advocates have in the main been frustrated in their attempts to introduce legislation which would establish and protect the rights of members of the disability community. Critics say the Disability Discrimination Act (1995) falls far short of a Disabled Rights Bill, which could have taken us a long way towards a citizenship model for the members of our society with disabilities. Instead, we are left with a piece of legislation which has made a convoluted and complex response to the need to translate medical theory into social reality (Light, 1996). Richard Light has also described the DDA as providing us with a skeletal frame, upon which Regulations and a Code of Practice, once published, will act as the flesh. It is hoped that the responsibilities introduced by the Act will become far clearer.

Occupational therapy education

Occupational therapy education programmes have been delivered in Britain for more than sixty years. Originally they were funded and administered by government health boards, frequently in small autonomous schools and headed by a principal. Until 1981 and in keeping with government policy, all three-year training programmes led to a diploma award. During the 1980s and 1990s: there has been a threefold increase in the number of educational programmes available, rising from ten to more than thirty. Many programmes are now delivered in the higher education sphere and all these undergraduate qualifications are at degree level. The focus has moved from a basis in the training of technical expertise towards one which supports the development of research-based practice.

Given the changing health and social care environment described earlier, it behoves educators to prepare students to recognize changing patterns in employment opportunities. The new culture of consumerism means that not only will graduates require a strong sense of professional identity, they will also require the ability to market themselves and their profession. Largely due to the care in the community policy, the new graduate is more likely to find employment in community-based multidisciplinary teams as the sole occupational therapist. Supervision may or may not be provided by a senior occupational therapist. This contrasts with traditional hospital-based employment, where occupational therapy services, however small, were usually based in autonomous departments. Professional support was in-built in this environment. Many aspects of work practice will be delivered through a range of services like training projects, vocational rehabilitation programmes, occupational health departments in industry, and employer services. This again marks a departure from traditional occupational therapy practice in Britain, where work performance is largely considered as part of general rehabilitation. The changing environment requires practitioners to design, market, provide and evaluate services based on specific client needs. Holistic approaches to patient care have been a particularly valued part of practice philosophy in this country and have to be reconciled with the new culture of consumerism.

Practitioners have already begun to identify and develop roles in many aspects of work practice. Following the European Union's directive on moving and handling, several therapists are contracting independently as trainers to industry. Industry is undertaking initiatives which maintain or improve employee's work performance through injury prevention programmes, job-site analysis and adaptation, employee assistance programmes, health promotion campaigns and wellness forums. A small number of dynamic practitioners around the country are successfully accessing these employment opportunities which until now have been considered non-traditional areas of practice.

Conclusion

The end of the 1990s sees many aspects of the British employment and health environments in a period of transition and, occasionally, turbulence. Such periods in history can drive or propel change if managed successfully. Occupational therapists in Britain are facing this challenge with a greater awareness of their professional skills and abilities, due in part to the development of their knowledge base through initial research activity in this country as well that provided by colleagues where this is better established. The rest of their success is being built on their tenacity and strong professional values.

References

Blanchflower, D. G., Oswald, A. J. (1989). International patterns of work. In *British Social Attitudes Survey: Special International Report*, 6th Report (R. Jowell, S. Witherspoon and L. Brook, eds), Gower, England.

Clement, B. (1995a). Clash of ideologies in minimum wage battle. *Independent*, 14 September.

Clement, B. (1995b). Employees reluctant to give up the idea of a job for life. *Independent*, 27 October.

Cusick, J., (1995). Union seeks staff cuts 'to reduce stress'. *Independent*, 13 September.

Firth-Cozens, J. (1995). *Employees' Health and Organisational Practice*. London: Institute of Business Ethics.

Fowler, R. (1995). Modest millionaires who work work work. *Independent*, 18 November.

Light, R. (1995). Non-discrimination in Employment: responsibilities and duties imposed by the DDA 1995, Vol. 40, winter.

Northern Ireland Committee of College of Occupational Therapists (1992). *Employment Assessment and Preparation in Occupational Therapy*. College of Occupational Therapists.

Social Trends (1996). London: HMSO.

Tisdal, E. K. M. (1994). Why not consider citizenship? A critique of post-school transitional models for young disabled people, *Disability and Society*, **9**, 3–17.

Timmins, N. (1995). Rediscovering the missing underclass. *Independent*, 7 July.

Timmins, N. (1996). Education takes more time as work shrinks. *Independent*, 25 January.

Toynbee, P. (1995). Whatever happened to nine to five? *Independent Magazine*, 10 June.

A United States perspective

A United States perspective of this chapter is based on three previously written articles/chapters by Karen Jacobs. They are: Jacobs, K. (1992). A 21st century survival kit. *Rehab. Management*, Oct/Nov, 121–122; Niemeyer, L. and Jacobs, K. (1992). Trends in work practice for the twenty-first century. *Orthopaedic Physical Therapy Clinics*, 1(1), 149–154; Jacobs, K. (1995). Preparing for return to work. In *Occupational Therapy for Physical Dysfunction* (C. Trombly, ed.), Baltimore: Williams and Wilkins, pp 329–349.

The future: work practice in the United States

The world of health care in the United States is changing. Practitioners are affected by its vulnerabilities as well as its strengths (Baum, 1985: 4). This chapter will describe the changing US health-care system, then focus more specifically on the changes in work practice, and finally offer some ways to manage through these changes.

The US health-care system

The US health-care system is currently changing from a provider to a payer-driven system which will eventually change to a consumer-driven system (De Jong and Sutton, 1994). Managed-care contracting, insurance reform, and capitation payment systems are currently at the forefront of this changing health-care environment. Practitioners must have a clear understanding of these issues and concepts if they are to position their services appropriately and be prepared for the future (Baum, 1985).

Change as a *constant* is something you can depend on! Preparing for the future requires us to pay attention to the 'winds of change'. These 'winds of change' are: managed care, size and role of the government, globalization, demographics, crises facing humankind, and shifts in societal values.

Managed care

Health maintenance organizations (HMOs), point-of-service plans and preferred provider organizations are all examples of managed-care systems with a focus on managed competition. The assumption in managed care is that economic incentives will determine how consumers use and providers deliver health care. Over half of all insured employees in the US are participants in managed-care programmes of some type. It is predicted that, within ten years, the major rehabilitation organizations will either be linked contractually to the insurance industry or replaced by facilities managed directly by the insurer. Because of rising costs, and the growing emphasis on accountability and outcomes, the health-care industry has become an object of scrutiny by the government as well as the public (Jacobs, 1996). Outcomes are simply the result of care. There are three types of outcome: cost; patient satisfaction; and technical. The first two are self-explanatory, but I'd like to elaborate more on the third, technical outcomes. Technical outcomes affect cost and satisfaction, and are the clinical results of care that reflect a model of health and disease. An example might make this more clear. The World Health Organization (WHO) has six technical outcomes. They are: prevention; cure; symptom control; elimination of impairment; elimination of disability; elimination of the resulting disadvantage (Jacobs, 1996).

Practitioners are all competing for a shrinking health-care dollar. Improving function, which has long been the mission of occupational therapy, is now being used in documentation by other professionals as a means to receive third-party payment. Now more than ever it is important for practitioners to *know* and be able to articulate *how* our profession is unique (Jacobs, 1996).

Size and role of the government

The dramatic change in the makeup of the US Congress, with a Republican majority in both the House and Senate for the first time in 40 years, is having a profound impact on the size and role of government. It is anticipated that power will shift to the states; and more public and private partnerships will emerge (Jacobs, 1996).

Globalization

Movement of products, information, capital and technology information, and ideas around the world will continue at a record pace and global competition will intensify. Distance learning will be commonplace and will facilitate global collaboration in academic training, clinical practice and research. Fair and accurate empirical research to support our intervention strategies will occur through this sharing of information (Jacobs, 1992; 1996).

Demographics

Another wind of change is that baby boomers will dominate the workplace. Baby boomers are those individuals born between the end of the Second World War and the early 1960s. We are finding that our society is becoming increasingly diverse and that entry-level workers are becoming less educated. Diversity and an ageing population will increase. As the current population ages, practitioners will continue to provide programmes to increase independence and maintain function of the elderly, thus hopefully decreasing long-term management health costs. One third of the current United States population will be senior citizens by the year 2030. These individuals will remain in the workforce longer then previous cohorts (Niemeyer and Jacobs, 1994: 153). As a result of the normal ageing process, however, we may encounter an increased incidence of injuries in older workers that require special considerations, such as job rescheduling, rotation, sharing or restructuring.

Crises facing humankind

Violence in the workplace, AIDS as an epidemic, and poverty are anticipated to increase. One in five infants and children in the US are at risk due to poverty. As in New Zealand, head trauma is a social problem. Breakdowns in morality, education and literacy are expected to continue. Unfortunately, terrorism has now become a real threat in the US (Jacobs, 1996).

Shifts in societal values

A quality revolution, consumer protection, and emphasis on grass-roots will all intensify. However, life can be confusing and values will be tested. One area of concern is ethics. Ethical dilemmas are part of the fabric of our activities of daily living, not only for us as practitioners, but as members of society. Just pick up a newspaper or professional newsletter or listen to the news to confirm this reality! (Jacobs, 1996.)

Managed care has precipitated the dilemma of limited or fewer resources to carry out what we want to do as professionals. Some common ethical issues seen in the practice of occupational and physical therapy include: the types of services provided by non-licensed or non-professional staff; large staff-to-supervisor ratios or one supervisor with many supervisees located geographically in multi-facilities and in multiple states; and the fraud or misappropriation of funds through false or improper billing practices. In challenging times ethics become even more important (Jacobs, 1996).

Work practice: present and future

If work practice were compared to any art form, it would be analogous to a tapestry. There is complexity of patterns, but there are unifying threads as well. The field of practice has been adapted to a wide variety of settings and clientele. Some unifying characteristics and future predictions of work practice in the United States will now be shared.

Unidisciplinary to transdisciplinary

We have seen a movement from unidisciplinary to multidisciplinary, where there is shared information, to interdisciplinary, where there are shared goals, to transdisciplinary involvement, the sharing of expertise. Originally, work programmes were run solely by occupational or physical therapists or vocational evaluators; however, many have expanded their staffing to include other disciplines. Teams have become a unifying thread in work programmes. In today's fast-paced health-care market, the demand for some disciplines is declining, for others it is expanding. This has created competition among team members, as well as role blurring in which boundaries among disciplines become unclear as staff try to fill roles traditional to other disciplines (Niemeyer and Jacobs, 1992).

Uniform terminology

Another unifying thread is the continued movement toward more uniform terminology and programming. With terminology, I shall first begin with the definition of work. Work refers to skill and performance in participating in socially purposeful and productive activities. (AOTA, 1994).

Two important elements constitute the concept of work: work behaviours and work skills, aptitudes and physical capacities. Work behaviours, also referred to as prevocational readiness, are those behaviours that are necessary for successful participation in a job or independent living. They include but are not limited to cooperative behaviour, attention span, motivation and productivity. Work behaviours are the antecedents to specific work skill development (Jacobs, 1991).

Work skills, aptitudes and physical capacities, frequently referred to as vocational skills, are required to perform the tasks of the actual job. More specifically, work skills are capabilities that the worker has learned or has the potential to learn, such as typing or sewing. Work aptitudes are abilities that are, to one degree or another, possessed by nearly all workers. They include coordination, dexterity and intelligence (Jacobs, 1991).

Physical capacities or demands are factors defined by the United States Department of Labor. Seven physical demands: standing, walking, sitting, lifting, carrying, pushing and pulling, are expressed in terms of five levels of strength. These are sedentary, light work, medium work, heavy work and very heavy work. Other physical demands include climbing, balancing, stooping, kneeling, crouching, crawling, reaching, handling, fingering, feeling, talking, hearing, acuity, depth perception, visual accommodation, colour vision and field of vision (Jacobs, 1991; 1995).

The terms previously described are considered performance components and, as such, have formed the basis for the majority of work assessments. However, this reductionist view is presently under question. A better approach would be to assess occupational performance, that is activities of daily living, work and leisure, and the individual's role performance, such as a worker, volunteer, student or homemaker. This may be conceptualized as occupational functioning. A unifying thread is the need to develop better instrumentation to measure role performance and occupational functioning (Jacobs, 1995).

Continuing with uniform terminology, when we begin to look at intervention strategies, the terms work hardening, work conditioning and transition work come to the forefront.

Work hardening

Work hardening is a work-oriented treatment programme, the outcome of which is measured in terms of improvement in the client's productivity (Matheson *et al.*, 1985; Ogden-Niemeyer and Jacobs, 1989). The ultimate goal is to help the person achieve a level of productivity that is acceptable in the competitive labour market. It is a comprehensive interdisciplinary (e.g. occupational therapist, physical therapist, psychologist, and vocational specialist) approach that uses graded work simulation to address the biomedical and psychosocial problems of the injured worker.

The clients who benefit from this type of programming are those who are seriously deconditioned after an impairment caused by an injury or disease and those people who have major discrepancies between their symptoms and objective findings (Matheson, 1985). Improvement in productivity is achieved through graded activity designed to increase work tolerances, improve work rate, master pain, improve work habits, increase confidence and proficiency with work adaptations or assistive devices. It involves the client in highly structured, simulated work tasks in an environment where expectations for basic worker behaviours (timeliness, attendance and dress) are in keeping with workplace standards. Programme duration varies from two to twelve weeks average with daily participation ranging from two to eight hours (Bettencourt, 1991; Jacobs, 1995).

Work conditioning

When a client has an uncomplicated injury but physical limitations preclude return to work, work conditioning may be an appropriate intervention (Darphin, Smith and Green, 1992). Work conditioning is typically provided as a unidisciplinary or bidisciplinary (occupational and/or physical therapy) half-day programme which uses exercise, aerobic conditioning, education and limited work tasks to restore an individual's systemic and neuromusculoskeletal function (strength, endurance, movement, flexibility and motor control) so that the client can return to work or become physically reconditioned so vocational services can commence (Darphin *et al.*, 1992; Jacobs, 1995).

Transition work

Transition work is any job or combination of tasks and functions that may be performed safely and with remuneration by an employee whose physical capacity to perform functional job demands has been compromised. Clinical expertise is brought to the work site to upgrade progressively the level of real-work activities to eventual full duty

Outcome

A call for functional outcome data has been a unifying thread. In the twenty-first century, all programmes will be receiving the same payment and it will be quality that is the deciding variable. Research on the effectiveness of work hardening programmes has been systematically gathered since the mid-1980s. Return-to-work statistics obtained from individual programmes range from 50–60 per cent to 85–88 per cent (Ogden-Niemeyer and Jacobs, 1989). By far the strongest variable related to return to work in clients entering work hardening programmes was length of disability, whether measured as time since date of injury or last date worked (Niemeyer *et al.*, 1994).

The future

Unparalleled opportunities in work practice await us in the twenty-first century. Changing demographics, technological advances, and limited financial resources will all play a role in shaping the profile of work practice. *Cost control*, however, will be of primary importance. At present, work-related injury in the United States has reached epidemic proportions, and the increase in the cost of workers' compensation, our major insurance avenue for injured workers, is already overloading the system in many states (Niemeyer and Jacobs, 1992: 149).

According to the National Institute on Occupational Safety and Health (NIOSH), by the twenty-first century, half of the US workforce will suffer some type of occupational disorder. Unfortunately some of the most powerful strategies for reducing costs in the long term will require more financial commitment initially (Jacobs, 1992: 71). These strategies include:

1 Widespread adoption of the biopsychosocial model of practice.
2 Injury prevention and health and wellness promotion programmes.
3 Ergonomic design in the workplace.
4 More intensive case management.
5 Implementation of the Americans with Disabilities Act (ADA), a major American Civil Rights Law for persons with disabilities.
6 Increasing business savvy (Niemeyer and Jacobs, 1992: 149).

To be successful in work practice, practitioners will need to become familiar with these cost control strategies and the windows of opportunity that they represent. Each of these areas will be discussed in turn.

Adoption of biopsychosocial model of practice

A current and alarming development in job-related injury has been the increasing incidence of cumulative trauma disorders and other chronic disorders. There is growing evidence that evaluation and treatment of chronic disorders is best guided by a biopsychosocial model using an interdisciplinary perspective, rather than by the more traditional and much narrower medical model (Feverstein, 1991). When a health professional approaches assessment and remediation of disorder using this framework, he or she looks at the whole person within a context consisting of psychologic, social and behavioural variables that influence the development and maintenance of pain and disability. For example, factors such as fear of reinjury, sick-role familiarity, depression, or anxiety regarding discrimination or dismissal on returning to work can contribute to what has been called delayed recovery or disability exaggeration. Hazard *et al.* found that disability exaggeration did not predict poor outcomes for patients with chronic low back pain when multidisciplinary care was used. On the contrary, the authors suggest disability exaggeration will predict poor outcomes of treatments such as surgery, manipulation and exercise that neglect psychological components. If, by the twenty-first century, the present US workers' compensation system persists with the narrow biomedical focus, it will be contributing to the very problems it is trying to remedy. In the twenty-first century, practitioners who maintain a holistic perspective can be primary lobbyists for the revamping of the workers' compensation model of practice (Niemeyer and Jacobs, 1992: 150).

Injury prevention and health and wellness promotion programmes

In the twenty-first century, injury prevention and health and wellness promotion services will become a more viable alternative to injury management. Health and wellness promotion will no longer be something that 'only fringe companies install'. In fact, there is strong evidence that supports the cost-saving benefits of employee health programmes. In-house prevention and health and wellness promotion programmes in industry that have been developed and successfully marketed by therapists will be more commonplace in the twenty-first century. However, there will be obstacles to overcome. Practitioners will need to gain an understanding of the industrial environments and learn to develop marketing approaches and sales techniques that address industry's priorities, and communicate with industry effectively (Niemeyer and Jacobs, 1992: 151; Melnik, 1991).

Changes in the nature of the supervisor–employee relationship will help support the development of injury prevention programmes. There will be more communication between upper management and the worker, more supervisory personnel will have safety identified as an essential function of their job and more accountability for personal safety and participation in safety programmes will be at the level of the individual worker (Niemeyer and Jacobs, 1992: 151; M. Melnik, personal communication, 1991).

Ergonomic design in the workplace

The efficacy of ergonomic design in prevention of cumulative trauma disorders and maximizing of productivity has already been recognized. In the twenty-first century, more specific ergonomic guidelines, as well as stronger sanctions against ergonomically poor work environments that place the worker at risk, will be established. Practitioners who have acquired additional expertise in ergonomics will find job opportunities. Many will elect to obtain advanced degrees or certification in human factors or ergonomics. Dual certification in human factors/ergonomics and occupational or physical therapy may become available, just as we are witnessing the introduction of course work in this area into undergraduate and graduate programmes. Academic programmes may evolve into providing specialization in ergonomics for musculoskeletal disorders. A strength in this specialization will be the therapist's knowledge of normal and abnormal development and the musculoskeletal system, the impact of disability and task analysis (Niemeyer and Jacobs, 1992: 151).

More intensive case management

Better coordination of services for injured workers, particularly those with chronic disorders, will control costs. Intensive case management in a managed-care environment will attempt to insure timely and appropriate provision of services and prevent service gaps that can lead to delayed recovery. The case manager 'coordinates service, analyses fiscal benefits, advocates for essential services, advises the client, family, or caregiver, and monitors the use of resources.' In addition, case managers can help promote prevention and early diagnosis and treatment as well as quality care. This approach to injured-worker care will be more widely accepted in the twenty-first century, although we see the beginnings now. More practitioners will find their way into case management positions traditionally held by rehabilitation nurses and vocational counsellors because of their skills in functional assessment, task analysis and intervention planning, and their ability to integrate the biomechanical and psychosocial aspects of an injured worker's case (Niemeyer and Jacobs, 1992: 151–152).

Implementation of the Americans with Disabilities Act (ADA)

By the twenty-first century, the Americans with Disabilities Act (ADA) will have been implemented for eight years. Once again, this is landmark civil rights legislation for Americans with disabilities in the areas of: employment, public accommodations, transportation, telecommunication and state and local government. During the time since its implementation, practitioners will have rallied to position themselves as the primary players in the dissemination of information to the business sector. Many will have added consultation on the ADA to their product line and will be working collaboratively with professionals such as architects, human services personnel, and rehabilitation engineers. Ergonomic principles will be incorporated into the selection of reasonable accommodations for individuals with disabilities. After many court cases, the ADA's impact on the workplace will have been established. Therapists will have played key roles as expert witnesses for the Equal Employment Opportunity Commission (EEOC) (Niemeyer and Jacobs, 1992: 152).

Strategies for managing through change

Managing through change will require us to answer the question, 'What do you want to have happen in the future?' As it is stated in the Koran, 'If you don't know where you are going, any road will take you there.' What road do you want to take? Heeding the call of the wild, I spent some time on a wilderness adventure in the US West. As I unpacked from this trip, I was struck by how closely the contents of my backpack resemble those items practitioners will need to manage through change as we enter into the twenty-first century. Each item seemed metaphorically to suggest a particular skill that is crucial. Instead of a tent, sleeping bag, compass or wind- and water-proof matches, we will require greater tools in order to survive in a more technologically complex, chaotic, demanding and accountable environment. Preparing for the twenty-first century is like a first-aid kit, but without labels on the contents to show what they are used for and without certainty that all the necessary items are included. My survival backpack would include specialized knowledge and skills in areas such as technology, marketing, ergonomics, gerontics and the government and legal systems (Jacobs, 1992b: 121).

Paramount to managing through change will be an understanding of creativity, leadership, *communication* and *negotiation skills*. Creativity would be the wind- and water-proof matches in my backpack. A prerequisite to managing through change is the ability to be creative. Robert Cooper, author of *The Performance Edge*, provides suggestions for developing a creative attitude. These are establishing and maintaining an open mind and spirit of enquiry; removing hidden obstacles to creative thinking; laughing more, looking for anomalies and rejecting old explanations; asking creative questions; listening and paying attention; continually expanding and developing your expertise both in work and play; to be willing to be uncertain, to gather data and to be goal directed, *yet* not goal-governed (Jacobs, 1992b: 121).

Like tents used in camping, leadership in the twenty-first century will take many different forms. However, the commonality for all leaders will be for them to be visionary and a lover of change. Successful leaders will need to follow the suggestions of Tom Peters, author of *Thriving on Chaos*. Peters writes that to survive in this chaotic world everything should be piloted, innovation should be *fostered*, involve everybody in everything so you have a collective responsibility, *listen*, *celebrate* and recognize achievement, develop self-managing teams, recruit well, train and retrain, provide everyone with incentive pay, guarantee employment, delegate, evaluate everyone based on their love of change and measure what's important. These strategies will facilitate growth-oriented, collegial environments which are critical ingredients to managing through change (Jacobs, 1992b: 121).

Advancements in technology will become the gateway to sophisticated communication services. Video, audio and data transmission will increasingly be integrated into a single fiberoptic telephone system. The potential benefits to be gained from technology in the twenty-first century almost defy the imagination. Technologic advances in biomechanical engineering will facilitate developments in workplace design that will more effectively match the capacities of the human worker. Their use will have a significant impact on reducing worker injury (Niemeyer and Jacobs, 1992b: 152–153).

Technology may completely dominate those work activities that are 'routine, uninteresting, and perhaps hazardous to physical and mental health' (Christianson, 1987). Most importantly, technology will help provide the means whereby individuals with severe disabilities can function as productive workers. Technology will continue to have an impact on diagnosis and treatment of work injuries. Computer-guided machines are now available that provide accurate back evaluation and that generate a wide variety of simulated physical demands of work while providing objective and reliable data on work output. These machines will in the twenty-first century become a valuable part of many programmes geared toward evaluation and treatment of injured workers. We must keep in mind, however, that the research on these devices regarding normative data and clinical use and benefits is still in its early stages. Not all data generated by high-technology equipment is infallible, valid or useful; nor do we at present understand all the issues involved in interpreting that data. We must also not lose sight, in the twenty-first century, of the importance of the human element in practice. As Susan Isernhagen, renowned physical therapist has stated: 'While we strive to become more scientific and research oriented, we must never forget that it is the ability of the therapist to combine science/client parameters and professional skills into a healing art. Therefore, high technology equipment which is scientific in nature should be integrated into our art, rather than substituted for it.' (S. J. Isernhagen, personal communication, 1991; Niemeyer and Jacobs, 1992: 152–153.)

A compass is imperative for survival in the wilderness and provides the backpacker with the ability to negotiate the terrain. A key to managing through change will be the ability to negotiate. Principles negotiation, as described by Roger Fisher and William Ury, authors of *Getting to Yes*, is one successful technique. In principles negotiation the participants are problem solvers, problems are separated from people, there is always a willingness to explore options with the focus on interest, not positions, and results are reached based on objective criteria. By itself, each item in the backpack will not *guarantee* survival, but the combination of items might be a barometer for success (Jacobs, 1992b: 122).

Conclusion

In all times of change, there is a chance for great opportunity. Change starts with self-examination. You will need to examine your creative talents and energy. Managing through change will require a strong sense of self. A relatively new book, entitled *How to be your own Best Friend*, suggests that you learn to give yourself boundless encouragement, kindly patience, and unqualified support. Forgive yourself when you make mistakes and reward yourself when you do well. Managing through change will require that you take an active role within your professional organizations. To survive this changing health-care climate, practitioners will need to take a better look at how they position themselves in the health-care environment. They will need to develop business savvy.

Product development that takes place in response to the public's changing needs and wants is part of a marketing approach. In the last decade, marketing has become more commonplace in health-care organizations and in fact has become a necessary component in order to stay competitive in the American health-care system. Traditionally, practitioners and health-care organizations developed their products based on what they thought the customer wanted relative to their own plans. Marketing reverses this process. Marketing is an important aspect of the delivery of services in today's changing health-care environment, and it is critical that all practitioners have an understanding of it. Practitioners need to learn tools and techniques of marketing just as they needed to go to school to learn the tools and techniques of their profession (Jacobs, 1993).

The twenty-first century is a very significant time for work practice. We must respond with confidence that the people we serve are being given the opportunity to gain meaningful lives. We need to continue to assume a responsible role in lending support and direction to health care, insurance and legislative changes.

References

American Occupational Therapy Association. (1994). Uniform terminology for occupational therapy 3rd edn. *American Journal of Occupational Therapy,* **48,** 1047–1059.

Baum, C. (1985). The Evolution of the U.S. Health Care System. In *The Occupational Therapy Manager.* pp. 3–25. Rockville: AOTA.

Bettecnourt, C. (1991). Chronic back pain, disability, and rehabilitation of the injured worker. In *Occupational Therapy: Work Related Programs and Assessments* (K. Jacobs, ed.) pp. 257–273. Boston: Little, Brown & Co.

Christensen, J. (1987). The human factors profession. In *Handbook of Human Factors* (G. Salvendy, ed.) New York: John Wiley & Sons.

Darphin, L., Smith, R. and Green, E. (1992). Work conditioning and work hardening. *Orthopaedic Physical Therapy Clinic,* **1**, 105–124.

DeJong, G. and Sutton, J. (1994, November 23), REHAB 2000: The evolution of medical rehabilitation in American health care. Paper presented at the National Rehabilitation Hospital Research Center, Washington, DC.

Feuerstein, M. (1991). A multidisciplinary approach to the prevention, evaluation, and management of work disability. *Journal of Occupational Rehabilitation*, **1**(1) 5–12.

Jacobs, K. (1991). *Occupational Therapy: Work-Related Programs & Assessments*, 2nd edn. Boston: Little, Brown & Co.

Jacobs, K. (1995). Preparing for Return to Work. In *Occupational Therapy for Physical Dysfunction* 4th edn. (C. Trombly, ed.) pp. 329–349. Baltimore: Williams & Wilkins.

Jacobs, K. (1996). The Evolution of the Occupational Therapy Delivery System. In *The Occupational Therapy Manager* 2nd edn. pp. 3–48. Bethesda: AOTA.

Jacobs, K. (Feb/Mar, 1992a). Work Practice for the New Millennium. *Rehab Management*. pp. 71–72.

Jacobs, K. (Oct/Nov, 1992b). A 21st Century Survival Kit. *Rehab Management*. pp. 121–122.

Jacobs, K. (Oct/Nov, 1993), Getting the Word Out. *Rehab Management*. pp. 128–129.

Jacobs, K. (May 4, 1996b). *Managing Through Change*. Keynote Address. Georgia Occupational Therapy Association. Calloway Gardens, GA.

Matheson, L., Ogden, L., Violette, K. and Schultz, K. (1985). Work hardening: Occupational therapy in industrial rehabilitation. *American Journal of Occupational Therapy*, **39**, 314–321.

Melnik, M. (1991). Marketing injury prevention services to industry. Work Programs Special Interest Section Newsletter, **5**(4), 1–3.

Niemeyer, L. and Jacobs, K. (1992). Trends in work practice for the twenty-first century. *Orthopaedic Physical therapy Clinics*, **1**(1), 149–154.

Niemeyer, L., Jacobs, K., Reynolds-Lynch, K., Bettencourt, C., Lang, S. (1994). Work hardening: Past present and future. The national work hardening outcome study. *American Journal of Occupational Therapy*, **48**(4), 327–336.

Ogden-Niemeyer, L. and Jacobs, K. (1989), *Work Hardening: State of the Art*. Thorofare: SLACK, Inc.

Appendices

A: Team Members

Maree Dyson and Dorothy Ferguson

B: Resources

Joanne Pratt

Learning objectives

At the end of this section the reader should be able to:

1 State which professionals may contribute to the work practice team.
2 Define the role of each member of the team.
3 Discuss the complimentary roles of the team members.
4 Relate knowledge of the work practice team to client care.
5 Describe equipment which can be used to support interventions.

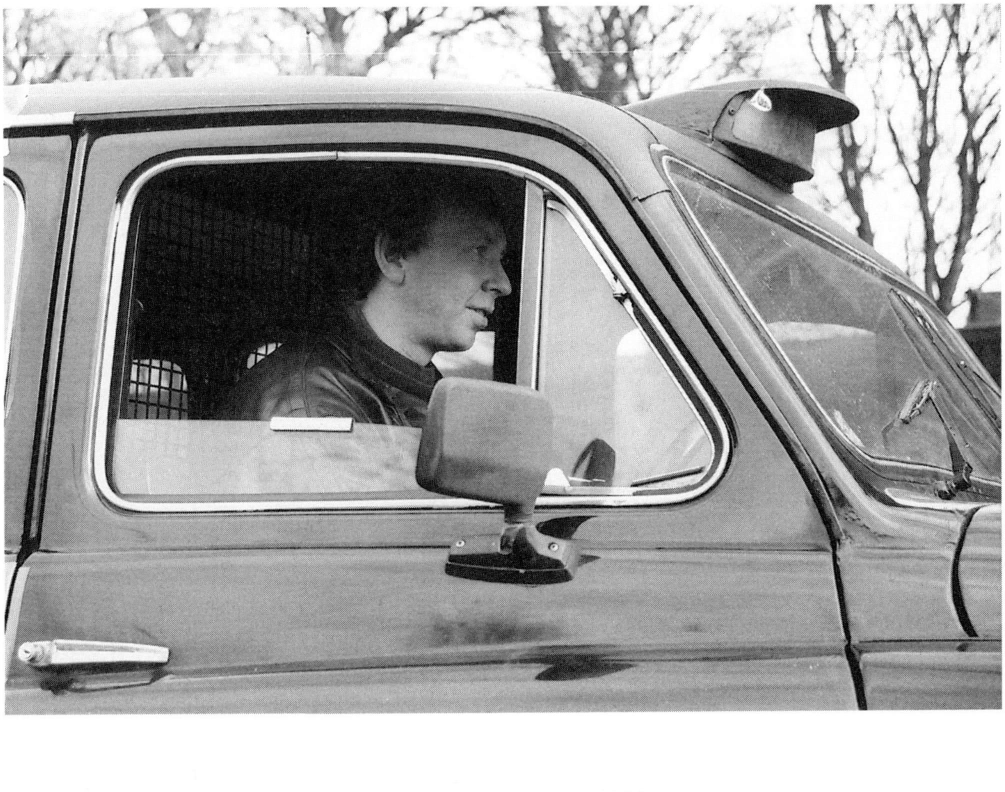

Appendix A

Team Members

An Australian perspective

Ergonomists

Ergonomists typically come from a background in engineering or health sciences and usually hold graduate qualifications in this discipline. Those with an engineering background are usually the practitioners whose advice is sought in risk assessment and design or major redesign of work systems. Although engineering ergonomists work in a range of fields in workplace design there is a strong emphasis on the health-and-safety-based approaches. Ergonomists with a health worker background would usually bring their health and ergonomics skills to bear in the workplace adjustments aimed at assisting a particular worker, for example a worker returning to work after an injury, a worker seen to be at risk of injury, or a worker with disabilities. While the above refers to general practice it is noted that some practitioners have successfully expanded their skills and bases from their traditional areas. For all discipline backgrounds training, again based around health and safety, is an aspect of services.

Occupational health nurses

Occupational health nursing 'is the application of specialised nursing knowledge and skills for the purpose of conserving, promoting and restoring the health of persons at their place of work' (ACHON, 1988: 2). Occupational health nursing is recognized as an area of advanced nursing and practice standards are supported by the Australian College of Occupational Health Nursing.

Frequently the occupational health nurse is the sole occupational health and safety professional on site. As such, the occupational health nurse plays a key role in overall service planning, service provision, coordination of specialist external services and programme evaluation. Where a worker has been injured the occupational health nurse may be involved in assessment, engagement of specialist services, case management and monitoring return to work programmes.

Occupational physicians

Occupational medicine is recognized as an area of specialization under the Australasian Faculty of Occupational Medicine. Occupational physicians provide services as salaried employees in industry or government, as consultants to industry or government, in academic posts and/or in private occupational medicine practice. Although occupational physicians play a key role in diagnosing and managing work or environmentally related injuries or illnesses, their work extends beyond the realm of any given workers' compensation system.

Occupational physicians are involved in management and development of occupational health programmes, workplace health surveillance (including identification of those at increased risk, early detection of disease and evaluation of the effectiveness of control measures), health promotion in industry, management of alcohol and other drug-related problems, and health assessments for work, with an emphasis on individual capabilities and individual tasks to optimize worker and task match.

Occupational therapists

Occupational therapy intervention focuses on assessment, treatment, facilitation of the work re-entry process, and follow-up and closure. There is an escalating emphasis on functional or work capacity assessments as industry, government and therapists seek a more structured approach to the determination of suitable duties and ability to work. Practice is growing in the areas of early intervention services and the design, development and implementation of injury prevention programs.

Typically, therapists work as consultants to an employer or as a member of an employee's rehabilitation team. The completion of graduate studies in rehabilitation, ergonomics, occupational health practice, etc. is not uncommon among occupational therapists working in this field.

Psychologists

Although some psychologists are involved in work place training and health promotion their services are most frequently accessed as part of an overall rehabilitation program for an individual worker. Interventions from a psychologist may include post-traumatic stress and pain management, grief counselling, occupational rehabilitation and guidance, vocational counselling, neuropsychological assessment and treatment, treatment of anxiety, mood and other accident related psychological disorders, associated social and family readjustment counselling.

Physiotherapists

Trained as they are in human movement physiotherapists help employees reach the fitness levels that enable them to work effectively and minimise the occurrence of injury. Physiotherapists provide services in employee pre-placement assessments, work task and work place evaluation, remedial and preventative training, functional assessments, work conditioning and vocational rehabilitation services. As employees or consultants industrial physiotherapists may work with individual employees or groups of employees.

Physiotherapists practising in the field of occupational health have often completed graduate studies in such fields as rehabilitation, ergonomics, occupational health practice, etc.

Rehabilitation counsellors

Rehabilitation counselling would usually be provided in the context of an overall externally based rehabilitation programme and focus on capabilities and opportunities.

Rehabilitation counselling may address case management, vocational assessment and guidance, job development and placement, vocational counselling, vocational education and training, vocational monitoring, lifestyle and work adjustment counselling and avocational counselling and placement.

Acknowledgment

The assistance of the various organizations who contributed to the above section is gratefully acknowledged.

References

Australian College of Occupational Health Nurses (1988). Information sheet: definitions. Rozelle, New South Wales.

Australian Physiotherapy Association (1992). Looking after your industrial athlete. Melbourne: Ergonomic and Occupational Health Group (Victorian Chapter).

The Australasian Faculty of Occupational Medicine (1993). The training of occupational physicians. Sydney.

The Australasian Faculty of Occupational Medicine (1995). The occupational physician relative value study of medical benefit items. Sydney.

A United Kingdom perspective

Abstract

Occupational health teams within the United Kingdom vary in size and in composition. Within this section the variety of professional expertise which may contribute to such teams is explored. The contribution of the differing members is examined and their specific role explained.

Although many health-care services in the UK are funded by government and provided with some degree of uniformity, occupational health (OH) does not form part of that National Health Service provision. Many organizations have long-established OH services, some have recently developed facilities, while yet others offer no provision for the health of the employee at work. The recent increase in legislation relating to health and safety at work (see Chapter 5) has encouraged some employers to address this issue and it is to be hoped that others will soon follow this example. In those organizations where occupational health services do exist, the nature of the provision will vary with the size, nature and financing of the occupational setting.

In this chapter the contribution of a variety of professionals to occupational health will be explored. Having briefly stated the types of services which may exist, the staff which may be employed will be described and their particular expertise identified. The impact on client care will then be assessed.

Types of services

Occupational health services may be based within one organization (an 'in-house' service) or may take the form of an independent service which offers care to several separate industries (a 'group' service). There may be a team approach to the care, or the care may be offered by an occupational health nurse working alone. These are not exclusive categories but will exist in a variety of combinations.

'In-house' services

There are, within the UK, many examples of in-house services, both large and small. In some smaller companies the OH provision exists on the one site which the company owns, whereas several large organizations have occupational health services organized nationally but operating at the various local work locations. Royal Mail, for example, has an occupational health service which is administered centrally with devolved responsibilities at the local level. The team members have both local and national duties and regularly attend both local and national team meetings and conferences. The 'team' composition may vary from one region to another, but will consist of at least an occupational health physician, one or more occupational health nurses and secretarial support. In some regions a physiotherapist is also employed. At a national level such teams may be expanded by the membership of an ergonomist, an industrial hygienist or a clinical psychologist who will be available to advise staff locally and nationally.

Smaller organizations may offer an in-house service which is based entirely within that organization and contained at one location. The service may involve any combination of the range of professionals discussed below as a team service, or may be a nurse-led service where the care is delivered and the service is managed by an occupational health nurse. As Johnson and Christie (1995) emphasize, 'if the nurse is trained and competent in this field, then the service can well be one of excellence.' Unfortunately, many services are still being provided by personnel who have not undertaken specialist training in occupational health.

Group services

Smaller industries or organizations for whom it would not be cost effective to provide an occupational health service may employ a 'group service' to provide care for their workforce. The 'group' would consist of occupational health professionals who have established their own organization and contracted out their services to those purchasers of care. The service offered would be negotiated between the management and the group and would relate to such aspects as the size and nature of the company, the hazards dealt with in the work process and the demography of the working population.

Potential OH team members

As with any health-care setting, there is potential within occupational health for contributions to care from a wide range of professionals. Some of these professions have specialist training available within the field of occupational health, while others bring their existing expertise and apply it within this novel setting. In some settings teams exist, in others the occupational health nurse works alone and so the role of the occupational health nurse is the first to be examined here.

Occupational health nurse

The Health and Safety Commission (1990) define a qualified occupational health nurse as one who is a registered general nurse and who holds a recognized occupational health nursing qualification. The United Kingdom Central Council for Nursing, Midwifery and Health Visiting (the body which governs nursing in the UK) includes occupational health nursing within the sphere of 'specialist community nursing practice' (UKCC, 1994). To undertake specialist training in this field, the nurse must first be a registered general nurse and have undertaken a period of professional practice. Specialist occupational health nurse training is then undertaken on a course approved by the National Board of Nursing, Midwifery and Health Visiting for the appropriate country.

Chard suggests that occupational health nursing 'takes a holistic view of the work process unifying job requirements to applicant ability with the aim of creating a match that eliminates the risk of sickness or injury as much as possible' (1993: 122). The Royal College of Nursing (1991) emphasizes that the role of the occupational health nurse is not a static one confined by lists of tasks or duties but will vary with the occupational setting in which that nurse is working. Rogers (1994) suggests that occupational health nursing is grounded in public health practice, focusing on prevention, health teaching and the elimination of health hazards within the workplace.

The specific nature of the nurse's job will vary with the employment situation. There may be provision for pre-employment screening (such as that recommended by the Allitt Inquiry (1991) for nurses when they obtain their first post after qualifying). Among the other health screening procedures which may be undertaken are audiometric screening, fitness to drive, respiratory function, visual acuity and general fitness. Specific screening tests may be required under the Control of Substances Hazardous to Health Regulations (COSHH) 1988.

Most occupational health nurses are involved in health promotion in a variety of ways. Counselling is a feature of most occupational health nurses' duties, although as Goldman (1993) suggests, it may also be necessary to refer the employee for services outside the occupational setting. Newton-Livens and Brown (1994) describe the implementation of a workplace exercise programme in which the occupational health nurse made use of a variety of health promotion strategies. Ramsarran and Wilson (1993) suggest that appropriate immunization procedures further help in promoting wellness. The immunization offered will vary with the nature of the work process and the structure of the workforce. Health-care workers, for example, should now be immunized against Hepatitis B whereas this would be inappropriate in a workforce where exposure to the virus does not exist.

Risk assessment is a feature of recent legislation and is to be undertaken in relation to such varied aspects of care as manual handling and lifting, exposure to blood products, working with visual display units or any other health-and-safety issue. Meusz (1995) extends this aspect of practice to the disabled at work, demonstrating the contribution of the occupational health nurse to the employment of those with disability.

Occupational health nurses are involved in advising management and individual workers on aspects of illness and injury at work. This may include supervision or provision of first aid services, the monitoring of accident reports, and aspects of sickness absence, including return to work and rehabilitation. Davies (1993) proposes improvements in the return-to-work process and emphasizes the role of occupational health in encouraging early rehabilitation. Some occupational health nurses offer a treatment service, although this has become a less important feature of modern services which emphasize preventive and health promoting aspects of care. Environmental monitoring forms part of the preventive function, ensuring that the temperature, atmosphere and general surroundings are suitable for healthy functioning.

Although many occupational health nurses work alone, most will have a medical officer on whom they can call or to whom they can refer as necessary. If no medical officer is retained by the organization the nurse will refer to the client's general practitioner.

The occupational health physician

Medical service provision within occupational health demonstrates a similar variety of qualifications to that described above in relation to nurses. Harrington and Gill (1992) point out that to practise occupational medicine in the UK only a registerable medical qualification is required, although the establishment of the Faculty of Occupational Medicine (FOM) in 1978 has resulted in ongoing improvements in the education and standards of practice for doctors within occupational health.

Some doctors will have undertaken postgraduate training and have qualified as members of the Faculty of Occupational Medicine. Others may have undertaken a short introductory course in occupational medicine. Others will be general practitioners with no specialist knowledge of this particular area of medicine. Those employed as occupational health consultants within the National Health Service, will have followed an approved course as laid down by the Faculty of Occupational Medicine (BMA, 1982). The availability of the physician also varies from service to service. Some of the larger national services may employ full-time occupational health physicians while others employ the doctor on a sessional basis. Others may have a full-time occupational health physician based in their head office but employ local doctors to undertake the delivery of medical care at the local level.

Within the current legislation some tasks are specified to be undertaken by the medical officer, e.g. medical assessment of drivers of heavy goods vehicles or forklift trucks (Harrington and Gill, 1992). Many of the tasks within occupational health are shared by the nurse and the doctor, the specific delivery of care altering with the setting, the skills of the available personnel, the times they are available, etc. Both the nurse and the doctor, for example, will contribute to screening, to health surveillance, to counselling and so on. In most services, there is co-operation and negotiation to ensure the best provision for the care of the worker.

The occupational hygienist

The occupational hygienist is a member of the occupational health team, focusing on the identification and control of hazards in the workplace. Some larger occupational health services may employ a hygienist on a full-time basis while smaller services may only access such specialist advice as required.

The World Health Organization describes the occupational hygienist as 'a person with a university degree in engineering, physics, or chemistry or an equivalent science degree . . . with specialist training in the recognition, evaluation and control of hazards that arise in and out of the workplace' (1981: 28). Vincent suggests that 'the science and art of occupational hygiene is about the interaction between man and his working environment' (1980: 1). The main role then of the hygienist is related to the control of hazards. The hazards may be physical, chemical, biological, ergonomic or psychological in origin. (For a useful summary see Harrington and Gill, 1992.)

Cook (1989) describes the hygienist's activities in measuring exposure through sampling and interpretation of results. Measures taken may include general preventative actions, such as good housekeeping or dust suppression, or specific with the introduction of filters. In companies where no occupational hygienist is available, the role of the occupational health nurse in hazard identification and monitoring is crucial (Rogers, 1994).

The ergonomist

Dixon and Price define ergonomics as 'the study of the relationship between man and his working environment and the equipment he uses' (1984: 247). Harrington and Gill suggest that 'ergonomics is the study and design of the working situation in order to benefit the worker-user' (1992: 9). Ergonomists then attempt to ensure that the machinery used by the worker does not prove to be hazardous to his or her health. The ergonomist seeks to ensure that the environment in which the worker functions does not cause undue physical or mental strain. This may involve advice on the design or position of machinery or of furniture, or ensuring that the best fit for the specific worker is available. In seeking to fit men and women to machines within the working environment, the ergonomist aims to reduce incidence of such problems as repetitive strain injury (Brodie, 1994).

The physiotherapist

Many occupational health services now employ a physiotherapist on either a full-time or sessional basis. The physiotherapist may utilize ergonomic principles when advising the worker or management on work-related issues. Bullock (1990) and Eastlake (1994) demonstrate that the physiotherapist's contribution to occupational health is not restricted to treatment but may include prevention of injury and relevant research as well. Boyling (1994) highlights the role of the physiotherapist in industry in the identification of those situations at work which put workers at risk of musculoskeletal problems within the context of the recent campaign by the Health and Safety Executive to 'lighten the load'. He further discusses the benefits of the on-site treatment and rehabilitation services of a physiotherapist from the managerial, financial and client perspective. Physiotherapy available within the workplace should help prevent musculoskeletal problems from arising. Where injury does occur, whether within the workplace or outside working hours, the presence of the physiotherapist in the workplace allows prompt referral and treatment, speeding recovery and assisting in the rehabilitation process.

The toxicologist

Chemicals have the potential to affect the body adversely. Stacey defines occupational toxicology as 'the study of the adverse effects of agents that may be encountered by workers during the course of their employment, (1993: 3). He goes on to note the rise in the number of chemicals in use within our society and therefore the increased potential for toxic exposure.

Occupational exposure limits for toxic substances are set, summaries of which are published by the Health and Safety Executive (1993). The toxicologist will advise management and the occupational health team on the interpretation of such documents, the implementation of the relevant regulations and the monitoring of the workplace to ensure the worker is not exposed to toxic levels. In those areas where a toxicologist is not employed, the other members of the occupational health team must be aware of the basic principles of toxicology and employ their skills in this aspect of care, which forms part of the education of both occupational health nurses and physicians. (A useful summary of the basic principles is contained in Harrington and Gill, 1992).

Other potential members of the occupational health team

Maintaining the health of the individual at work is a complex activity and can involve many members of the caring professions, the unions and the management of the organization, as well as many consultants both external and internal.

It may be that legal advice is required, either about an aspect of medical or nursing practice (such as an aspect of record keeping), or concerning an issue related to the workplace (for example equal opportunities), or related to a worker (for example compensation for injury) (Kloss, 1994). In such situations the advice and counsel of a lawyer is imperative. While large organizations may employ a lawyer, smaller businesses may relay on consultation with an external law firm. In work-related issues the advice of a lawyer specializing in occupational health law is to be advised.

Health physicists, microbiologists, epidemiologists, safety engineers, audiologists, chiropodists and fitness advisers may all contribute to the health of the worker. WHO (1981) expands this list to include administrators, architects, designers, chemists, engineers, social workers and psychologists. There may be such professionals employed on a full- or part-time basis or available for consultation as required. As yet, few occupational health services in the UK employ an occupational therapist. It is to be hoped that this will alter in the near future, thus expanding the expertise available and improving the care of the worker.

Impact on client care

It should not be assumed that the occupational health service which employs the largest number of a variety of professionals will offer the best occupational health care. In small industries a qualified occupational health nurse caring for a specific workforce with hazards clearly identified and controlled, and health actively promoted, may provide a service of excellence. The focus may vary from that provided in a large organization employing all available occupational health expertise to the nurse working alone, who undertakes a more varied role fulfilling a wider variety of functions.

In smaller settings the nurse will have the advantage of knowing all the workers and being more readily available to them for consultation or advice. In larger settings the professional may rely on the client's or manager's making appropriate referrals. However, the provision on site of services such as physiotherapy or chiropody minimizes the time spent away from work to keep appointments, thus appealing to management, and speeds up the referral time, thus pleasing the workers.

Rehabilitation should begin as soon as possible and employ the skills of all the professionals. The knowledge of the work process and the workplace which the occupational health professional has should be utilized early in the process to ensure the speediest and most effective rehabilitation for the worker. This can only be achieved when professionals work together for the clients benefit. This is another sphere in which the role of the occupational therapist has much to contribute and it is hoped that books such as this will enhance the development of the role of the occupational therapist within the occupational health team.

References

The Allitt Inquiry. (1991). HMSO.

Boyling, J. (1994). Lightening the load: physiotherapy in industry. *Occupational Health*, **46**(10), 342–6.

British Medical Association (1982). *The Occupational Physician*, 2nd edn, British Medical Association.

Brodie, D. (1994). *Health Matters at Work.* Tudor Business Publishing.

Bullock, M. I. (ed.) (1990). *Ergonomics: The Physiotherapist in the Workplace.* Churchill Livingstone.

Chard, C. (1993). *Health and Safety for Nurses.* Chapman & Hall.

Cook, P. (1989). *Trevick's Occupational Health Hazards: A Practical Guide.* Heinemann Medical.

Davies, B. (1993). Restoration of occupational capacity in post-cardiac patients. *Occupational Health*, **45**(10), 330–4.

Dixon, W. M. and Price, S. M. G. (1984). *Aspects of Occupational Health.* Faber & Faber.

Eastlake, A. (1994). Role of the physiotherapist in industry. In *Physiotherapy in Occupational Health* (B. Richardson and A. Eastlake, eds) Butterworth Heinemann.

Goldman, J. (1993). A friend in need or a counsellor? *Occupational Health*, **45**(8), 263–5.

Harrington, J. M. and Gill, F. S. (1992). Occupational Health: Pocket Consultant, 3rd edn. Blackwell Scientific.

Health and Safety Commission (1988). *Control of Substances Hazardous to Health Regulations.* HMSO.

Health and Safety Commission (1990). *First Aid at Work: Health and Safety (First Aid) Regulations 1981 and Guidance.* HMSO.

Health and Safety Executive (1993). *Occupational Exposure Limits: document summaries.* HMSO.

Johnson, G. and Christie, D. (1995) Statutory right of access to OH services. *Occupational Health*, **47**(1), 15–16.

Kloss, D. (1994). *Occupational Health Law*, 2nd edn. Blackwell Scientific.

Meusz, C. (1995). Disability and work: risk assessment. *Nursing Standard*, **9**(26), 38–41.

Newton-Livens, M. and Brown, P. (1994). Fine-tuning a health promotion to local needs. *Occupational Health*, **46**(7), 240–3.

Ramsarran, B. and Wilson, S. (1993). Promoting wellness in the OH setting. *Occupational Health*, **45**(10), 335–6.

RCN Society of Occupational Health Nursing. (1991). *A Guide to an Occupational Health Nursing Service*. Scutari Projects.

Rogers, Bonnie (1994). *Occupational Health Nursing: Concepts and Practice*. W. B. Saunders Co.

Stacey, N. (1993). *Occupational Toxicology*. Taylor & Francis.

UKCC (1994). *The Future of Professional Practice – The Council's Standards for Education and Practice following Registration*. UKCC.

Vincent, J. H. (1980). The physics of gases and aerosols. In *Occupational Hygiene: An Introductory Text* (H. A. Waldron and J. M. Harrington, eds) pp. 1–37, Blackwell Scientific.

World Health Organization (1981). Education and training in occupational health, safety and ergonomics. *WHO Technical Report Series 663*, WHO.

Appendix B

Resources

Seating

Name	*Description*	*Supplier*
Posturite Opera Range	A range of three chairs designed to avoid back pain and promote healthy posture. Adjustment possible for chair height, back and seat. Armrests optional, supports bodyweight up to 16 stone (224lbs/100kgs).	Posturite (UK) Ltd
Hag Credo Range	A range of chairs which tilt backward and forward, lockable in three positions. Adjustment possible to seat depth, back height, seat height and armrests.	Posturite (UK) Ltd
Karanorm Kneeling Chair	Designed to encorage correct posture and ease of movement. Has a forward sloping seat and knee support which are adjustable. Used for secretaries, students and those with backache.	Posturite (UK) Ltd
Tripp Trapp chair (for children)	Chair which adjusts to suit the growing child. Seat and footplate height and depth are moveable for positioning relative to body size.	Posturite (UK) Ltd SitSmart Ltd and Disability Care Services
Variable balans chair; Pendulum chair; Oposit balans chair; Wing balans chair; Flysit chair; Duo balans chair; Gravity balans chair; Multi balans chair; Thatsit balans chair; Ekstrem chair; Move chair	From the original Norwegian designers of the Tripp Trapp chair, this is a series designed for adult users at home or work. Designed to promote good posture and support, these chairs are innovative in design and widely used in Europe.	Stokke Fabrikker and SitSmart Ltd
Savo chair series	A range of tilting chairs designed to provide support during prolonged sitting activities. Adjusts to weight, size and shape.	SitSmart Ltd, Savo Kontorstoler

Work surfaces and work station accessories

Name	*Description*	*Supplier*
Ropox group table; Ropox minitable; Ropox column table; Bed and wheelchair table; Carpenter's bench; Nursing table; Adjustable work center; Ironing board	A series of Danish designed adjustable height tables and workplaces which vary in height for better postural fit.	Scanflex Ltd and Ropox ApS
PC Printer Desk; Spacemaster workstation; CAD workcenter; Footrests; Copyholders	Office equipment which complies with the minimum EC (European Community) due in place by December, 1996.	INMAC (UK) Ltd

Keyboards and accessories

Name	*Description*	*Supplier*
Mountbatten Brailler	A brailler designed to meet the needs of a wide variety of visually impaired users.	RNC Ent. Ltd and QT Pty Ltd
Communication aids; Computer keyboards; Keyboard emulators; Input devices	A wide range of devices used to enhance computer technology for people with physical, cognitive or sensory performance deficits.	QED Ltd
Ergonomic keyboards	A range of ergonomically designed keyboards designed to reduce strain and workload. Compatible with most computers.	PCD Maltron Ltd
Copyholders; Adjustable wrist rest; Incline mouse pad; Monitor stands; Anti-glare filters; Monitor arms	Computer accessories designed to comply with EC (European Community) requirements, due in place by December, 1996.	INMAC (UK) Ltd

Suppliers addresses

Disability Care Services Ltd
3 Radley Road Industrial Estate
Abingdon
Oxfordshire OX14 3RY
England
Tel: 01235 523353/554527
Fax: 01235 531019

INMAC (UK) Ltd
Executive Office
Westerly Point
Bracknell
Berkshire RG12 1EW
England
Tel: 01344 424333
Fax: 01344 483709

PCD Maltron Ltd
15 Orchard Lane
East Molesey
Surrey KT8 OBN
England
Tel: 0181 398 3265

Posturite (UK) Ltd
PO Box 468
Hailsham
East Sussex BN27 4LZ
England
Tel: 01323 833353

Quantum Technology Pty Ltd
5 South Street
Rydalmere 2116
South Australia
Tel: 02 684 2077
Fax: 02 684 4717

Quest Enabling Designs Ltd
Ability House
242 Gosport Rd
Fareham
Hampshire PO16 OSS
England
Tel: 01329 828444
Fax: 01329 828800

RNC Enterprises Ltd
College Rd
Hereford HR1 1EB
England
Tel: 01432 265725
Fax: 01432 353478

Savo Kontorstoler AS
Fyrstikkbakken 7
PO Box 161
Bryn
N-0611 Oslo
Norway
Tel: 47 22 64 70 20
Fax: 47 22 63 12 09

Scanflex Ltd
2 Thursby Rd
Croft Business Park
Bromborough
Wirral L62 3PW
England
Tel: 0151 343 1523
Fax: 0151 343 1514

SitSmart Ltd
2 Oak Mead
Godalming
Surrey GU7 3RL
England
Tel: 0483 419990

Stokke Fabrikker AS
N-6260 Skodje
Norway
Tel: (47) 70 27 59 00
Fax: (47) 70 27 58 01

The BackShop Clinic Ltd
24 New Cavendish Street
London W1M 7LH
England
Tel: 0171 935 9120
Fax: 0171 224 1903

Reference

Barret, J. and Herriotts, P. (1994). *Employment and the Workplace*. Oxford: Disability Information Trust.

Answers to Multiple Choice Questions

Chapter 2

1 b, 2 c, 3 a, 4 b, 5 c

Chapter 3

1 c, 2 d, 3 e, 4 a

Chapter 4

1 a, b and c, 2 c, 3 all correct, 4 d, 5 d

Chapter 9

1 d, 2 a, 3 c, 4 b, 5 d

Chapter 10

1 d, 2 a and c, 3 b, 4 b, 5 b

Index